50% OFF Online CEN Prep Course!

Dear Customer,

We consider it an honor and a privilege that you chose our CEN Study Guide. As a way of showing our appreciation and to help us better serve you, we have partnered with Mometrix Test Preparation to offer **50% off their online CEN Prep Course**. Many CEN courses are needlessly expensive and don't deliver enough value. With their course, you get access to the best CEN prep material, and you only pay half price.

Mometrix has structured their online course to perfectly complement your printed study guide. The CEN Prep Course contains **in-depth lessons** that cover all the most important topics, **video reviews** that explain difficult concepts, **over 700 practice questions** to ensure you feel prepared, and **over 450 digital flashcards**, so you can study while you're on the go.

Online CEN Prep Course

Topics Include:	*Course Features:*
• Cardiovascular Emergencies	• CEN Study Guide
• Respiratory Emergencies	○ Get content that complements our best-selling study guide.
• Neurological Emergencies	• 5 Full-Length Practice Tests
• Gastrointestinal, Genitourinary, Gynecology and Obstetrical Emergencies	○ With over 700 practice questions, you can test yourself again and again.
• Psychosocial and Medical Emergencies	• Mobile Friendly
• Maxillofacial, Ocular, Orthopedic and Wound Emergencies	○ If you need to study on the go, the course is easily accessible from your mobile device.
• Environment and Toxicology Emergencies, and Communicable Diseases	• CEN Flashcards
• Professional Issues	○ Their course includes a flashcard mode consisting of over 450 content cards to help you study.

To receive this discount, visit their website: mometrix.com/university/cen and add the course to your cart. At the checkout page, enter the discount code: **TPBCEN50**

If you have any questions or concerns, please don't hesitate to contact them at universityhelp@mometrix.com.

Sincerely,

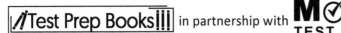 in partnership with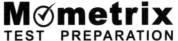

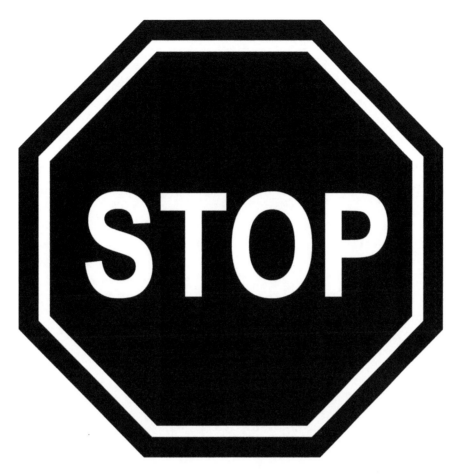

FREE Test Taking Tips DVD Offer

To help us better serve you, we have developed a Test Taking Tips DVD that we would like to give you for FREE. **This DVD covers world-class test taking tips that you can use to be even more successful when you are taking your test.**

All that we ask is that you email us your feedback about your study guide. Please let us know what you thought about it – whether that is good, bad or indifferent.

To get your **FREE Test Taking Tips DVD**, email freedvd@studyguideteam.com with "FREE DVD" in the subject line and the following information in the body of the email:

> a. The title of your study guide.
>
> b. Your product rating on a scale of 1-5, with 5 being the highest rating.
>
> c. Your feedback about the study guide. What did you think of it?
>
> d. Your full name and shipping address to send your free DVD.

If you have any questions or concerns, please don't hesitate to contact us at freedvd@studyguideteam.com.

Thanks again!

CEN Review Book

CEN Study Guide and Practice Test Questions for the Certified Emergency Nurse Exam [3rd Edition Prep]

TPB Publishing

Interested in buying more than 10 copies of our product? Contact us about bulk discounts:
bulkorders@studyguideteam.com

ISBN 13: 9781628459050
ISBN 10: 1628459050

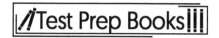

Table of Contents

Quick Overview

As you draw closer to taking your exam, effective preparation becomes more and more important. Thankfully, you have this study guide to help you get ready. Use this guide to help keep your studying on track and refer to it often.

This study guide contains several key sections that will help you be successful on your exam. The guide contains tips for what you should do the night before and the day of the test. Also included are test-taking tips. Knowing the right information is not always enough. Many well-prepared test takers struggle with exams. These tips will help equip you to accurately read, assess, and answer test questions.

A large part of the guide is devoted to showing you what content to expect on the exam and to helping you better understand that content. In this guide are practice test questions so that you can see how well you have grasped the content. Then, answer explanations are provided so that you can understand why you missed certain questions.

Don't try to cram the night before you take your exam. This is not a wise strategy for a few reasons. First, your retention of the information will be low. Your time would be better used by reviewing information you already know rather than trying to learn a lot of new information. Second, you will likely become stressed as you try to gain a large amount of knowledge in a short amount of time. Third, you will be depriving yourself of sleep. So be sure to go to bed at a reasonable time the night before. Being well-rested helps you focus and remain calm.

Be sure to eat a substantial breakfast the morning of the exam. If you are taking the exam in the afternoon, be sure to have a good lunch as well. Being hungry is distracting and can make it difficult to focus. You have hopefully spent lots of time preparing for the exam. Don't let an empty stomach get in the way of success!

When travelling to the testing center, leave earlier than needed. That way, you have a buffer in case you experience any delays. This will help you remain calm and will keep you from missing your appointment time at the testing center.

Be sure to pace yourself during the exam. Don't try to rush through the exam. There is no need to risk performing poorly on the exam just so you can leave the testing center early. Allow yourself to use all of the allotted time if needed.

Remain positive while taking the exam even if you feel like you are performing poorly. Thinking about the content you should have mastered will not help you perform better on the exam.

Once the exam is complete, take some time to relax. Even if you feel that you need to take the exam again, you will be well served by some down time before you begin studying again. It's often easier to convince yourself to study if you know that it will come with a reward!

Test-Taking Strategies

1. Predicting the Answer

When you feel confident in your preparation for a multiple-choice test, try predicting the answer before reading the answer choices. This is especially useful on questions that test objective factual knowledge. By predicting the answer before reading the available choices, you eliminate the possibility that you will be distracted or led astray by an incorrect answer choice. You will feel more confident in your selection if you read the question, predict the answer, and then find your prediction among the answer choices. After using this strategy, be sure to still read all of the answer choices carefully and completely. If you feel unprepared, you should not attempt to predict the answers. This would be a waste of time and an opportunity for your mind to wander in the wrong direction.

2. Reading the Whole Question

Too often, test takers scan a multiple-choice question, recognize a few familiar words, and immediately jump to the answer choices. Test authors are aware of this common impatience, and they will sometimes prey upon it. For instance, a test author might subtly turn the question into a negative, or he or she might redirect the focus of the question right at the end. The only way to avoid falling into these traps is to read the entirety of the question carefully before reading the answer choices.

3. Looking for Wrong Answers

Long and complicated multiple-choice questions can be intimidating. One way to simplify a difficult multiple-choice question is to eliminate all of the answer choices that are clearly wrong. In most sets of answers, there will be at least one selection that can be dismissed right away. If the test is administered on paper, the test taker could draw a line through it to indicate that it may be ignored; otherwise, the test taker will have to perform this operation mentally or on scratch paper. In either case, once the obviously incorrect answers have been eliminated, the remaining choices may be considered. Sometimes identifying the clearly wrong answers will give the test taker some information about the correct answer. For instance, if one of the remaining answer choices is a direct opposite of one of the eliminated answer choices, it may well be the correct answer. The opposite of obviously wrong is obviously right! Of course, this is not always the case. Some answers are obviously incorrect simply because they are irrelevant to the question being asked. Still, identifying and eliminating some incorrect answer choices is a good way to simplify a multiple-choice question.

4. Don't Overanalyze

Anxious test takers often overanalyze questions. When you are nervous, your brain will often run wild, causing you to make associations and discover clues that don't actually exist. If you feel that this may be a problem for you, do whatever you can to slow down during the test. Try taking a deep breath or counting to ten. As you read and consider the question, restrict yourself to the particular words used by the author. Avoid thought tangents about what the author *really* meant, or what he or she was *trying* to say. The only things that matter on a multiple-choice test are the words that are actually in the question. You must avoid reading too much into a multiple-choice question, or supposing that the writer meant something other than what he or she wrote.

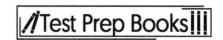

5. No Need for Panic

It is wise to learn as many strategies as possible before taking a multiple-choice test, but it is likely that you will come across a few questions for which you simply don't know the answer. In this situation, avoid panicking. Because most multiple-choice tests include dozens of questions, the relative value of a single wrong answer is small. As much as possible, you should compartmentalize each question on a multiple-choice test. In other words, you should not allow your feelings about one question to affect your success on the others. When you find a question that you either don't understand or don't know how to answer, just take a deep breath and do your best. Read the entire question slowly and carefully. Try rephrasing the question a couple of different ways. Then, read all of the answer choices carefully. After eliminating obviously wrong answers, make a selection and move on to the next question.

6. Confusing Answer Choices

When working on a difficult multiple-choice question, there may be a tendency to focus on the answer choices that are the easiest to understand. Many people, whether consciously or not, gravitate to the answer choices that require the least concentration, knowledge, and memory. This is a mistake. When you come across an answer choice that is confusing, you should give it extra attention. A question might be confusing because you do not know the subject matter to which it refers. If this is the case, don't eliminate the answer before you have affirmatively settled on another. When you come across an answer choice of this type, set it aside as you look at the remaining choices. If you can confidently assert that one of the other choices is correct, you can leave the confusing answer aside. Otherwise, you will need to take a moment to try to better understand the confusing answer choice. Rephrasing is one way to tease out the sense of a confusing answer choice.

7. Your First Instinct

Many people struggle with multiple-choice tests because they overthink the questions. If you have studied sufficiently for the test, you should be prepared to trust your first instinct once you have carefully and completely read the question and all of the answer choices. There is a great deal of research suggesting that the mind can come to the correct conclusion very quickly once it has obtained all of the relevant information. At times, it may seem to you as if your intuition is working faster even than your reasoning mind. This may in fact be true. The knowledge you obtain while studying may be retrieved from your subconscious before you have a chance to work out the associations that support it. Verify your instinct by working out the reasons that it should be trusted.

8. Key Words

Many test takers struggle with multiple-choice questions because they have poor reading comprehension skills. Quickly reading and understanding a multiple-choice question requires a mixture of skill and experience. To help with this, try jotting down a few key words and phrases on a piece of scrap paper. Doing this concentrates the process of reading and forces the mind to weigh the relative importance of the question's parts. In selecting words and phrases to write down, the test taker thinks about the question more deeply and carefully. This is especially true for multiple-choice questions that are preceded by a long prompt.

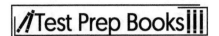

9. Subtle Negatives

One of the oldest tricks in the multiple-choice test writer's book is to subtly reverse the meaning of a question with a word like *not* or *except*. If you are not paying attention to each word in the question, you can easily be led astray by this trick. For instance, a common question format is, "Which of the following is…?" Obviously, if the question instead is, "Which of the following is not…?," then the answer will be quite different. Even worse, the test makers are aware of the potential for this mistake and will include one answer choice that would be correct if the question were not negated or reversed. A test taker who misses the reversal will find what he or she believes to be a correct answer and will be so confident that he or she will fail to reread the question and discover the original error. The only way to avoid this is to practice a wide variety of multiple-choice questions and to pay close attention to each and every word.

10. Reading Every Answer Choice

It may seem obvious, but you should always read every one of the answer choices! Too many test takers fall into the habit of scanning the question and assuming that they understand the question because they recognize a few key words. From there, they pick the first answer choice that answers the question they believe they have read. Test takers who read all of the answer choices might discover that one of the latter answer choices is actually *more* correct. Moreover, reading all of the answer choices can remind you of facts related to the question that can help you arrive at the correct answer. Sometimes, a misstatement or incorrect detail in one of the latter answer choices will trigger your memory of the subject and will enable you to find the right answer. Failing to read all of the answer choices is like not reading all of the items on a restaurant menu: you might miss out on the perfect choice.

11. Spot the Hedges

One of the keys to success on multiple-choice tests is paying close attention to every word. This is never truer than with words like almost, most, some, and sometimes. These words are called "hedges" because they indicate that a statement is not totally true or not true in every place and time. An absolute statement will contain no hedges, but in many subjects, the answers are not always straightforward or absolute. There are always exceptions to the rules in these subjects. For this reason, you should favor those multiple-choice questions that contain hedging language. The presence of qualifying words indicates that the author is taking special care with his or her words, which is certainly important when composing the right answer. After all, there are many ways to be wrong, but there is only one way to be right! For this reason, it is wise to avoid answers that are absolute when taking a multiple-choice test. An absolute answer is one that says things are either all one way or all another. They often include words like *every*, *always*, *best*, and *never*. If you are taking a multiple-choice test in a subject that doesn't lend itself to absolute answers, be on your guard if you see any of these words.

12. Long Answers

In many subject areas, the answers are not simple. As already mentioned, the right answer often requires hedges. Another common feature of the answers to a complex or subjective question are qualifying clauses, which are groups of words that subtly modify the meaning of the sentence. If the question or answer choice describes a rule to which there are exceptions or the subject matter is complicated, ambiguous, or confusing, the correct answer will require many words in order to be expressed clearly and accurately. In essence, you should not be deterred by answer choices that seem excessively long. Oftentimes, the author of the text will not be able to write the correct answer without

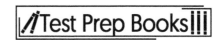

offering some qualifications and modifications. Your job is to read the answer choices thoroughly and completely and to select the one that most accurately and precisely answers the question.

13. Restating to Understand

Sometimes, a question on a multiple-choice test is difficult not because of what it asks but because of how it is written. If this is the case, restate the question or answer choice in different words. This process serves a couple of important purposes. First, it forces you to concentrate on the core of the question. In order to rephrase the question accurately, you have to understand it well. Rephrasing the question will concentrate your mind on the key words and ideas. Second, it will present the information to your mind in a fresh way. This process may trigger your memory and render some useful scrap of information picked up while studying.

14. True Statements

Sometimes an answer choice will be true in itself, but it does not answer the question. This is one of the main reasons why it is essential to read the question carefully and completely before proceeding to the answer choices. Too often, test takers skip ahead to the answer choices and look for true statements. Having found one of these, they are content to select it without reference to the question above. Obviously, this provides an easy way for test makers to play tricks. The savvy test taker will always read the entire question before turning to the answer choices. Then, having settled on a correct answer choice, he or she will refer to the original question and ensure that the selected answer is relevant. The mistake of choosing a correct-but-irrelevant answer choice is especially common on questions related to specific pieces of objective knowledge. A prepared test taker will have a wealth of factual knowledge at his or her disposal, and should not be careless in its application.

15. No Patterns

One of the more dangerous ideas that circulates about multiple-choice tests is that the correct answers tend to fall into patterns. These erroneous ideas range from a belief that B and C are the most common right answers, to the idea that an unprepared test-taker should answer "A-B-A-C-A-D-A-B-A." It cannot be emphasized enough that pattern-seeking of this type is exactly the WRONG way to approach a multiple-choice test. To begin with, it is highly unlikely that the test maker will plot the correct answers according to some predetermined pattern. The questions are scrambled and delivered in a random order. Furthermore, even if the test maker was following a pattern in the assignation of correct answers, there is no reason why the test taker would know which pattern he or she was using. Any attempt to discern a pattern in the answer choices is a waste of time and a distraction from the real work of taking the test. A test taker would be much better served by extra preparation before the test than by reliance on a pattern in the answers.

FREE DVD OFFER

Don't forget that doing well on your exam includes both understanding the test content and understanding how to use what you know to do well on the test. We offer a completely FREE Test Taking Tips DVD that covers world class test taking tips that you can use to be even more successful when you are taking your test.

All that we ask is that you email us your feedback about your study guide. To get your **FREE Test Taking Tips DVD**, email freedvd@studyguideteam.com with "FREE DVD" in the subject line and the following information in the body of the email:

- The title of your study guide.
- Your product rating on a scale of 1-5, with 5 being the highest rating.
- Your feedback about the study guide. What did you think of it?
- Your full name and shipping address to send your free DVD.

Introduction to the CEN

Function of the Test

The Certified Emergency Nurse (CEN) exam is designed to assess the knowledge that nurses have obtained in the specialty area of emergency medicine and who are interested in pursuing a certification in this field. A nonprofit corporation, known as the Board of Certification for Emergency Nursing (BCEN), grants this certification to individuals who successfully pass the exam and who have a current RN (registered nurse) license or a nursing certificate equivalent in good standing in the United States or its Territories. Although not required, it is recommended that test takers have two years of work experience in the emergency department.

It is possible for individuals who are retired from the nursing profession to sit for this exam and earn a CEN (Ret) credential. In order to be eligible for such a designation, individuals must have a current RN (registered nurse) license in good standing in the United States or its Territories, have held a CEN certification for a full certification term (four years) before applying, and be retired from nursing (and teaching) or are planning to retire.

The current pass rate for the CEN exam is around 61 percent.

Test Administration

The CEN test is only offered as a computer-based (online) exam. It is administered at numerous Pearson VUE test centers throughout the world. Before scheduling an appointment at a test center, a test taker must first complete an online application through his or her Board of Certification for Emergency Nursing (BCEN) account or register by calling Pearson VUE.

There is no limit to the number of times that an individual can retake the CEN test. However, test takers must wait 90 days between attempts, and they can only take the exam a maximum of two times during any six-month period. Once the exam is successfully passed, the CEN certification is good for four years.

All of the Pearson VUE test centers are wheelchair-accessible. Individuals taking an exam are also allowed to take breaks in order to address any type of medical need. It is important to note that no additional time is granted for breaks during the test. The time is deducted from the available test-taking time. Any additional accommodations that may be needed by test takers can be requested by completing a Testing Accommodation Form available on the BCEN website (http://www.bcencertifications.org) and emailing the completed form to bcen@bcencertifications.org.

Test Format

The CEN exam takes three hours to complete and consists of 175 multiple-choice questions, 25 of which are unscored and used to gather data for future versions of the exam. The test questions are broken

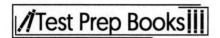

down into eight subject areas (and several subtopics within each of those subject areas) as outlined in the table below.

Sections of the CEN Test	
Subject Area	*# of Questions*
Psychosocial & Medical Emergencies	25
Gastrointestinal, Genitourinary, Gynecology & Obstetrical Emergencies	21
Maxillofacial, Ocular, Orthopedic & Wound Emergencies	21
Cardiovascular Emergencies	20
Neurological Emergencies	16
Professional Issues	16
Respiratory Emergencies	16
Environment & Toxicology Emergencies and Communicable Diseases	15
Total Questions – 150	Time: 3 hours

Scoring

Individuals are not penalized for guessing. A passing score is achieved when a little more than 70 percent of the scored questions are answered correctly. Scores are displayed on the computer immediately upon completion of the exam.

Study Prep Plan for the CEN Exam

1 **Schedule** - Use one of our study schedules below or come up with one of your own.

2 **Relax** - Test anxiety can hurt even the best students. There are many ways to reduce stress. Find the one that works best for you.

3 **Excecute** - Once you have a good plan in place, be sure to stick to it

Sample Study Plans

One Week Study Schedule

Day 1	Care Delivery and Reimbursement Methods
Day 2	Psychosocial Concepts and Support Systems
Day 3	Quality Outcomes Evaluations and Measurements
Day 4	Rehabilitation Concepts and Strategies
Day 5	Ethical, Legal, and Practice Standards
Day 6	Review Answer Explanations
Day 7	**Take Your Exam!**

Two Week Study Schedule

Day 1	Adherence to Care Regimen	Day 8	Functional Capacity Evaluation
Day 2	Case-Management Process and Tools	Day 9	Affordable Care Act
Day 3	Behavioral Change Theories And Stages	Day 10	Risk Management
Day 4	Client Self-Care Management	Day 11	Practice Questions
Day 5	Accreditation Standards and Requirements	Day 12	Review Answers
Day 6	Healthcare Analytics	Day 13	Review Explanations
Day 7	Assistive Devices	Day 14	**Take Your Exam!**

One Month Study Schedule					
Day 1	Adherence to Care Regimen	Day 11	Support Programs	Day 21	Affordable Care Act
Day 2	Case-Management Process and Tools	Day 12	Accreditation Standards and Requirements	Day 22	Case Recording
Day 3	Managed Care Concepts	Day 13	Cost-Benefit Analysis	Day 23	Ethics Related to Care Delivery
Day 4	Private Benefit Programs	Day 14	Data Interpretation and Reporting	Day 24	Risk Management
Day 5	Abuse and Neglect	Day 15	Healthcare Analytics	Day 25	Standards of Practice
Day 6	Behavioral Health Concepts	Day 16	Program Evaluation and Research Methods	Day 26	Practice Questions
Day 7	Conflict Resolution Strategies	Day 17	Types of Quality Indicators	Day 27	Practice Questions
Day 8	End-of-Life Issues	Day 18	Assistive Devices	Day 28	Review Answers
Day 9	Interpersonal Communication	Day 19	Functional Capacity Evaluation	Day 29	Review Explanations
Day 10	Interview Techniques	Day 20	Vocational and Rehabilitation Service Delivery System	Day 30	**Take Your Exam!**

Cardiovascular Emergencies

Cardiovascular emergencies are life-threatening conditions. Any condition that impedes circulation has the potential to damage the myocardium, or heart muscle. A damaged myocardium may be unable to meet the oxygen demands of the body. It is important to quickly identify any patient exhibiting symptoms indicative of such emergencies so that they can receive prompt treatment to prevent further cardiovascular injury or death. Every patient presenting to the emergency department with possible cardiovascular symptoms should immediately be given a focused assessment followed by a history and physical. Simultaneously, an intravenous (IV) line should be established and an electrocardiogram (ECG) and laboratory and radiographic studies should be performed. The triage, assessment, diagnostics, and treatment of such patients must be prioritized to preserve cardiac function and, ultimately, life.

Acute Coronary Syndrome

Acute coronary syndrome (ACS) is the term used to describe the clinical symptoms caused by the sudden reduction in blood flow to the heart, but it is also known as **acute myocardial ischemia**. The causes of the ischemia include stable and unstable angina (UA), non-ST elevation myocardial infarction (NSTEMI), and ST elevation myocardial infarction (STEMI), which is shown in the figure below.

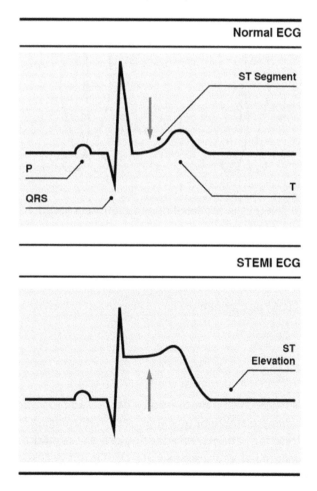

Common symptoms of a patient presenting with ACS include:

- Chest pain or discomfort in the upper body that radiates to the arms, back, neck, jaw, or stomach, as shown in the image below

Typical Pain Radiation Patterns of Acute Coronary Syndrome

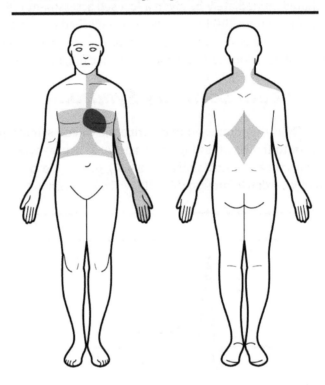

- Dizziness, syncope, or changes in the level of consciousness (LOC)

- Nausea or vomiting

- Palpitations or tachycardia

- Shortness of breath (SOB) or dyspnea

- Unusual fatigue

Angina

Angina is the term used to describe chest pain caused by decreased blood flow to the myocardium. The two primary categories of angina are stable or unstable, with stable angina being more common. It presents in a predictable pattern for patients, responds quickly to cessation or exertion or medication, and while it increases the likelihood of a future heart attack, it is not necessarily indicative of such an event occurring imminently. Unstable angina is often more frequent and severe. It may occur without physical exertion and be unresponsive to medication or activity cessation. It should be treated as an emergency and can signal an imminent heart attack.

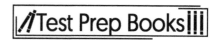

Treatment for angina depends on the severity of the symptoms and can range from lifestyle modifications to surgical intervention. Pharmacological treatments for angina include beta-blockers, calcium channel blockers (CCBs), angiotensin-converting enzyme (ACE) inhibitors, statins, and antiplatelet and anticoagulant medications. These medications treat the symptoms related to angina by lowering blood pressure (BP), slowing heart rate (HR), relaxing blood vessels, reducing strain on the heart, lowering cholesterol levels, and preventing blood clot formation. Generally, the risk factors for the development of angina include:

- Diabetes
- Dietary deficiency (fruits and vegetables)
- Excessive alcohol consumption
- Family history of early coronary heart disease
- Hypertension (HTN)
- High LDL (low-density lipoprotein)
- Low HDL (high-density lipoprotein)
- Males
- Obesity
- Old age
- Sedentary lifestyle
- Smoking

Stable Angina

Atherosclerotic buildup generally occurs slowly over time. Because the buildup is gradual, the heart can usually continue to meet the body's oxygen demands despite the narrowing lumen of the vessel. However, in situations with increased oxygen demand, such as exercise or stress, the myocardium may not be able to meet the increased demands, thereby causing angina. The angina subsides with rest. Stable angina is predictable; it occurs in association with stress or certain activities. It does not increase in intensity or worsen over time. Nitroglycerine is effective in the treatment of stable angina because it dilates the blood vessels, reducing the resistance to blood flow, which decreases the demand on the myocardium. Lifestyle modifications such as smoking cessation and a regular exercise program are needed to slow atherosclerotic buildup.

Unstable Angina

Unstable angina (UA) is a more severe form of heart disease than stable angina. The angina associated with UA is generally related to small pieces of atherosclerotic plaque that break off and cause occlusions. The occlusions suddenly decrease blood flow to the myocardium, resulting in angina, without causing an actual MI. The pain symptomatic of UA occurs suddenly without a direct cause, worsens over a short period of time, and may last 15 to 20 minutes. Dyspnea (shortness of breath) and decreased blood pressure are also common. Because the angina is related to an acute decrease in blood flow, rest does not alleviate symptoms. Generally, UA does not respond to the vasodilatory effect of nitroglycerine. Laboratory values are typically negative for cardiac enzymes related to cardiac damage, but they can be slightly elevated. Therefore, a comprehensive history and physical exam that properly identify pertinent risk factors are critical for early diagnosis and treatment.

Depending on the severity of symptom presentation, pharmacological treatment for UA will include one or more antiplatelet medications and a cholesterol medication. In addition, medications to treat

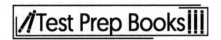

hypertension, arrhythmias, and anxiety may be necessary. The recommended intervention is angioplasty with coronary artery stenting. A coronary artery bypass grafting (CABG) surgery may be necessary in the case of extensive occlusion of one or more of the coronary arteries.

NSTEMI

The NSTEMI does not produce changes in the ST segment of the EKG cycle. However, troponin levels are positive. Patients with a confirmed NSTEMI are hospitalized. Morphine, oxygen, nitroglycerin, and aspirin (MONA protocol) is administered. Additional pharmacological agents for treatment are beta-blockers, ACE inhibitors, statins, and antiplatelet medications. Coronary angiography and revascularization may be necessary.

The primary difference between UA and a NSTEMI is whether the ischemia is severe enough to damage the myocardium to the extent that cardiac markers indicative of injury are released and detectable through laboratory analysis. A patient is diagnosed with a NSTEMI when the ischemia is severe enough to cause myocardial damage and the release of a myocardial necrosis biomarker into the circulation (usually cardiac-specific troponins T or I). In contrast, a patient is diagnosed with UA if such a biomarker is undetectable in his or her bloodstream hours after the ischemic chest pain's initial onset.

STEMI

The STEMI is the most serious form of MI. It occurs when a coronary artery is completely blocked and unable to receive blood flow. Emergent revascularization is needed either through angioplasty or a thrombolytic medication.

Unstable angina and NSTEMIs generally indicate a partial-thickness injury to the myocardium, but a STEMI indicates injury across the full thickness of the myocardium, as shown in the image below. The etiology behind ischemia is partial or full occlusion of coronary arteries.

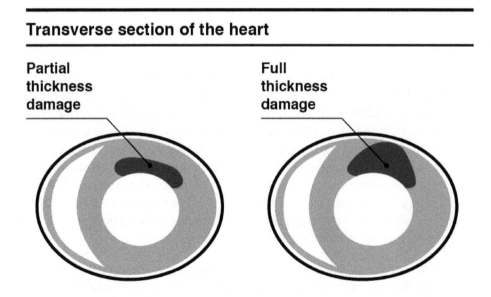

Differentiation Between Non-ST and ST MIs

Transverse section of the heart

Partial thickness damage

Full thickness damage

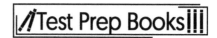

Treatment and Risk Scoring

Treatment for UA and NSTEMI is planned according to a risk score using the Thrombolysis in Myocardial Infarction (TIMI) tool. In the presence of UA or a NSTEMI, seven categories are scored: age, risk factors, a prior coronary artery stenosis, ST deviation on ECG, prior aspirin intake, presence and number of angina episodes, and elevated creatinine kinase (CK-MB) or troponins. In the presence of a STEMI, the TIMI tool scores eleven categories: age, angina history, hypertension, diabetes, systolic BP, heart rate, Killip class, weight, anterior MI in an ECG, left bundle branch block (LBBB) in an ECG, and a treatment delay after an attack. The Global Registry of Acute Coronary Events (GRACE), or ACS risk calculator, is a common tool used to predict death during admission and six months, as well as three years after a diagnosis of Acute Coronary Syndrome (ACS).

ACS can be life threatening. Treatment and survival are time-dependent. Quick recognition by the nurse followed by a thorough focused assessment that includes evaluation of pain type, location, characteristic, and onset is essential. The MONA protocol is implemented immediately. The nurse should obtain a family, social, and lifestyle assessment to identify high-risk patients. An evaluation of recent medical history is imperative, since most ACS patients experience prodromal symptoms a month or more prior to the acute event. Establishing IV access is paramount for rapid administration of medications. Obtaining and reviewing an ECG and drawing and reviewing labs including troponins, CK-MB, complete blood count (CBC), C-reactive protein (CRP), electrolytes, and renal function will provide critical diagnostic data. A chest x-ray and echocardiogram will also add to the differential diagnosis. Immediate and long-term complications of ACS are cardiac dysrhythmia, heart failure (HF), and cardiogenic shock. Education should be provided to each patient about the diagnosis, risk factors, lifestyle modifications, and medications once the acute event has stabilized.

Aneurysm/Dissection

An aneurysm is an abnormal bulge or ballooning that can form within an artery, as seen in the image below. Depending on the location, the rupture of an aneurysm can result in hemorrhage, stroke, or death. The most common places for the formation of an aneurysm are the left ventricle (LV) of the heart, the aorta, the brain, and the spleen.

Blood Vessel with an Aneurysm and Rupture

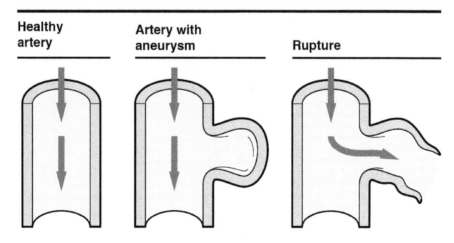

15

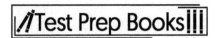

Anatomical Review

Generally, arteries carry oxygenated blood away from the heart to the organs and tissues of the body. The largest artery is the aorta, which receives blood directly from the LV of the heart. Oxygen-carrying blood continues to travel down the arterial system through successively smaller arteries that supply organs, ending with the arterioles that empty into the capillary bed.

Pulmonary and Systemic Circulation

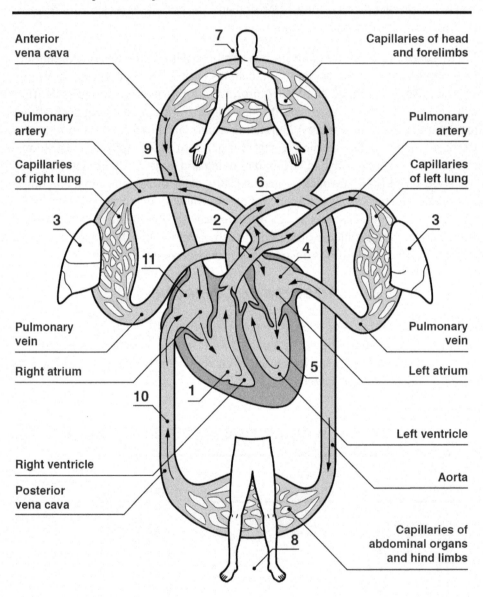

The capillary beds are drained on their opposite side by the venules, which return the now-deoxygenated blood back to the right atrium through progressively larger veins, ending in the great veins of the heart, known as the superior and inferior vena cava. The deoxygenated blood from the great veins moves into the right atrium, then the right ventricle, which pumps the blood to the lungs via

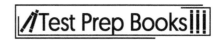

the pulmonary artery to become oxygenated once again. The oxygenated blood flows from the pulmonary vein into the left atrium, then the LV, and into the aorta to repeat the cycle.

Arteries and Veins

There are three tissue layers in the structure of arteries and veins. The endothelium, or tunica intima, forms the inner layer. The middle layer, the tunica media, contains elastin and smooth muscle fibers, and connective tissue forms the outside coating called the tunica externa.

Arteries have a thicker elastin middle layer that enables them to withstand the fluctuations in pressure, which result from the high-pressure contractions of the LV. Arterioles regulate blood flow into the capillary bed through constriction and dilation, so they are the primary control structures for blood pressure regulation. Meanwhile, the venous side of circulation operates under very low pressures, so veins have no elastin in their structure; instead, they use valves to prevent backflow in those vessels working against gravity, as shown in the image below.

Structure of an Artery and Vein

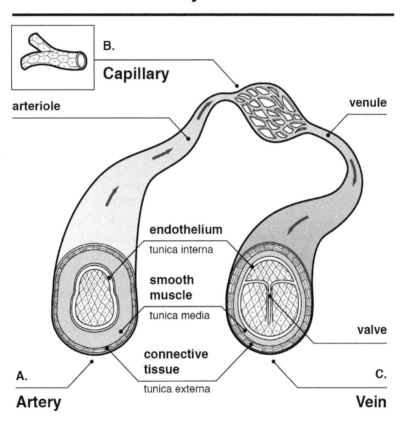

Left Ventricular Aneurysm

A left ventricular aneurysm (LVA) is a bulge or ballooning of a weakened area of the LV, generally caused by an MI. There are no symptoms of an LVA, which should be diagnosed with an echocardiogram and angiogram. Small LVAs usually do not require treatment. Clot formation is a common occurrence with LVAs. In the body's attempt to repair the aneurysm, the inflammatory process and the clotting cascade

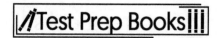

are initiated, both of which increase the propensity for clot formation. Patients are most likely prescribed anticoagulants. Rapid treatment for an MI reduces the incidence of LVA formation.

Aorta

The aorta stretches from the LV through the diaphragm into the abdomen and pelvis. In the groin, the aorta separates into two main arteries that supply blood to the lower trunk and the legs. An aneurysm can occur anywhere along the aorta; an abdominal aortic aneurysm (AAA) is the most common. Atherosclerosis, hypertension, diabetes, infection, inflammation, and injury such as from a fall or auto accident are frequent causes. The most common presenting symptoms with an AAA are chest pain and back pain. The clinician may be able to palpate a pulsating bulge in the abdomen. Nausea and vomiting may be present. Other symptoms include lightheadedness, confusion, dyspnea, rapid heartbeat, sweating, numbness, and tingling. When an AAA develops slowly over a period of years, it is less likely to rupture, in which case the patient should be regularly monitored with ultrasound imaging. Aneurysms greater than 2 inches (5.5 centimeters) will generally require surgical repair.

A thoracic aortic aneurysm occurs in the stretch of the aorta that lies within the chest cavity. The critical size for surgical intervention of a thoracic aortic aneurysm is 2.3 inches (6 centimeters). As with all surgeries in such close proximity to the heart, the risk-to-benefit ratio must be carefully weighed.

Treatment Options

If the AAA is small and slow-growing, a watch-and-wait approach is often taken. An abdominal ultrasound, computed tomography (CT), and MRI will aid in the determination of the most appropriate treatment. Surgical repair involves removing the damaged portion of the aorta and replacing it with a graft. Another minimally-invasive technique involves reinforcing the weakened area with metal mesh.

Brain

Bulging or ballooning in a blood vessel within the brain is the second most common site for an aneurysm. Another common site for aneurysms is where the internal carotid artery (ICA) enters the cranium; it branches into a system of arteries that provide blood flow to the brain, known as the **circle of Willis**. Most small brain aneurysms do not rupture and are found during various tests. An aneurysm may press on brain tissue and present with ocular pain or symptoms. However, a rupture is a medical emergency that can lead to stroke or hemorrhage. The most common symptom described by patients is "the *worst* headache of my life." A sudden, severe headache, stiff neck, blurred or double vision, photophobia, seizure, loss of consciousness, and confusion may also be reported.

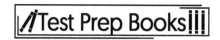

Here's a graphic of the circle of Willis, which are interconnecting arteries at the base of the brain:

Circle of Willis

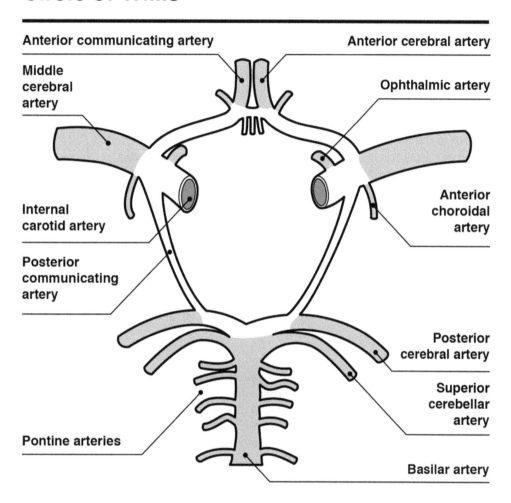

Risk Factors

A family history of aneurysm and certain other aneurysm risk factors are genetic. Other predisposing factors are an arteriovenous malformation (AVM) at the circle of Willis, polycystic kidney disease (PKD), and Marfan syndrome. Poor lifestyle choices, such as smoking and cocaine use, greatly increase the risk for aneurysm formation. There is a higher risk for individuals over the age of forty, women, patients who have experienced a traumatic head injury, and patients with hypertension.

Treatment Options

Depending on a brain aneurysm's cause, size, and symptoms, and the patient's general health, there are several treatment options. The most common surgical treatment is clipping. The bulge is clipped at the base to prevent blood from entering. The clip remains in place for life. Eventually, the bulge will shrink.

If the artery has been damaged by the aneurysm, an occlusion and bypass surgical procedure may be performed. The affected artery is closed off, and a new route that allows circulation to bypass the damage is created. The artificial development of an embolism, known as **endovascular embolization**, is another treatment option. A variety of substances such as plastic particles, glue, metal, foam, or balloons are coiled and inserted into the aneurysm to block blood flow.

A liquid embolic surgical glue is a new option to the standard coiling procedure: Onyx HD 500 is a vinyl alcohol copolymer that solidifies on contact with the blood in the aneurysm, sealing it. In the case of smaller aneurysms, a watch-and-wait approach may be taken. Bleeding, vasospasm, seizures, and hydrocephalus are the main complications related to a brain aneurysm.

Spleen

The spleen plays an important role in the regulation of red blood cells. The filtration action of the spleen removes worn-out or damaged red blood cells and microbes. It is also an important organ in the immune system, producing the white blood cells that fight infection and synthesize antibodies.

Although very rare, the spleen is the third most common site of an aneurysm. The exact cause of a splenic arterial aneurysm is unknown. However, the aneurysm represents a damaged splenic artery. Portal hypertension and multiple pregnancies produce an increase in intra-abdominal pressure that is thought to damage the splenic artery, leading to the formation of an aneurysm. Trauma and autoimmune disease are also known causes.

A splenic aneurysm is generally asymptomatic and found incidentally on diagnostic studies. An aneurysm of the splenic artery is treated by clipping.

Dissection

Dissection is a condition in which the layers of the arterial wall become separated and blood leaks in between the layers of the vessel. A dissection represents damage through more than one layer of an artery. It is a more serious form of aneurysm because all the layers are compromised.

A dissection is different from a rupture. With a dissection, blood leaks in and through the layers of an artery, but the artery remains structurally intact, albeit weakened. Blood is still contained within the vessel. When a rupture occurs, it is similar to the popping of a balloon. The integrity of the artery is disrupted, and blood leaks out of the artery. Dissections increase the risk of rupture. Medical management with beta-blockers is the treatment of choice for stable aortic dissections.

Summary

Symptoms of an aneurysm/dissection may be absent, vague, or difficult to identify. The consequences of a rupture are life-threatening. The expert clinician will ascertain a thorough patient and family history, including social factors and lifestyle choices. Autoimmune disorders, age, gender, a sedentary lifestyle, smoking, and drug or alcohol abuse are contributing factors to the development of an aneurysm. Rapid assessment, diagnosis, and treatment are essential. Vital signs, neurological status, and loss of consciousness should be closely monitored.

Cardiopulmonary Arrest

Cardiopulmonary arrest is a life-threatening emergency characterized by the sudden unexpected cessation of heart function, breathing, and consciousness caused by a disturbance in the electrical conduction of the heart. Immediate basic life support (BLS) followed by current advanced cardiac life

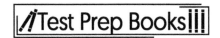

support (ACLS) protocol is the treatment. Defibrillation is the treatment choice for cardiopulmonary arrest caused by ventricular tachycardia, or fibrillation. The time between patient collapse and initiation of resuscitation efforts is the most important factor in patient survival.

The brain is the first organ impacted by loss of blood flow and oxygenation. Cardiac arrest lasting longer than 8 minutes has poor survival rates. A diagnostic work-up during and after stabilization will include an ECG, arterial blood gases (ABGs), troponins counts, CBC, electrolyte counts, and renal function labs.

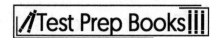

Dysrhythmias

Dysrhythmia, also known as **arrhythmia,** is abnormal electrical activity of the heart. The heartbeat may be regular or irregular, too fast, or too slow.

Normally, the electrical conduction system of the heart begins with an impulse known as the **action potential** at the pacemaker sinoatrial (SA) node. The impulse travels across the right and left atria before activating the atrioventricular (AV) node.

Cardiac Conduction Cycle

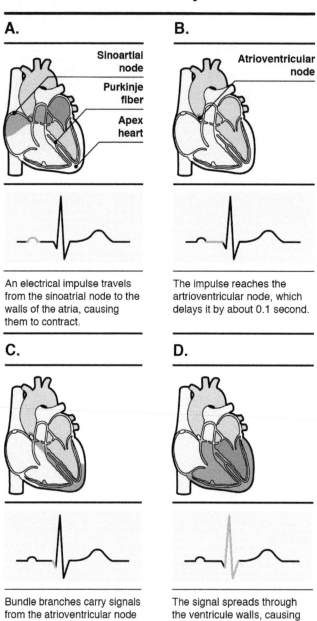

A.

Sinoartial node
Purkinje fiber
Apex heart

An electrical impulse travels from the sinoatrial node to the walls of the atria, causing them to contract.

B.

Atrioventricular node

The impulse reaches the artrioventricular node, which delays it by about 0.1 second.

C.

Bundle branches carry signals from the atrioventricular node to the heart apex.

D.

The signal spreads through the ventricule walls, causing them to contract.

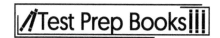

The pathway from the SA to the AV node is visualized on the ECG as the P wave. From the AV node, the impulse continues down the septum along cardiac fibers. These fibers are known as the **bundle of His**. The impulse then spreads out and across the ventricles via the Purkinje fibers. This is represented on the ECG as the QRS complex. The T wave represents the repolarization or recovery of the ventricles.

Electrical Events of the Cardiac Cycle

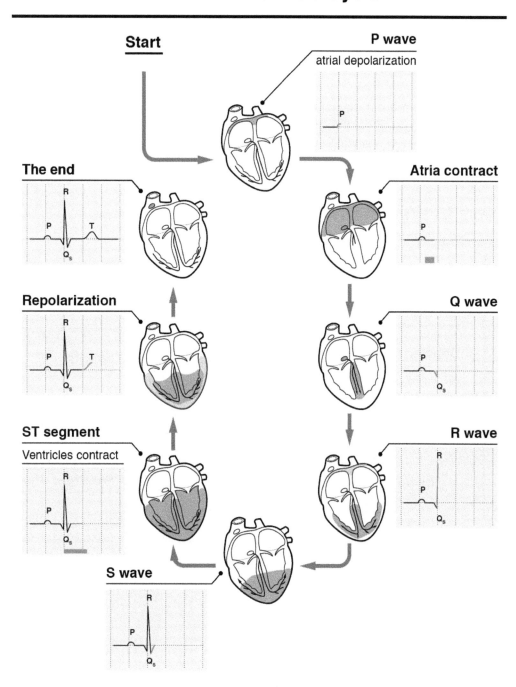

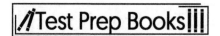

Properties of Cardiac Cells

Cardiac cells have four important properties: excitability, conductivity, contractility, and automaticity. **Excitability** allows the heart to respond to stimuli and maintain homeostasis. **Conductivity** is the ability to transfer the electrical impulse initiated at the SA node across cardiac cells. **Contractility** is the cardiac cells' ability to transform an action potential into the mechanical action of contraction and relaxation. **Automaticity** is the ability of cardiac cells to contract without direct nerve stimulation. In other words, the heart initiates its own impulse. If the SA node fails to initiate the impulse, the AV node will fire the impulse at a slower rate. If neither the SA nor the AV node fires the impulse, the cells within the bundle of His and the Purkinje fibers will fire to start the impulse at an even slower rate.

Action Potential

The action potential is a representation of the changes in voltage of a single cardiac cell. Action potentials are formed as a result of ion fluxes through cellular membrane channels, most importantly, the sodium (Na^+), potassium (K^+), and calcium (Ca^{2+}) channels. Electrical activity requires an action potential. Contraction of the cardiac muscle fibers immediately follows electrical activity.

Phases of an Action Potential

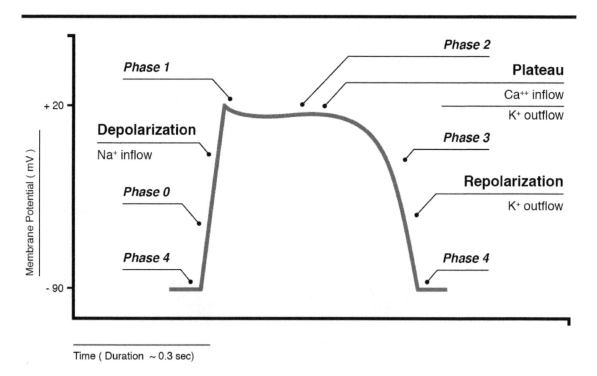

Phase 0: Depolarization

- Rapid Na^+ channels are stimulated to open.

- The cardiac cell is flooded with Na^+ ions, which change the transmembrane potential.

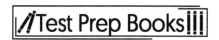

- The shift in potential is reflected by the initial spike of the action potential.

- Depolarization of one cell triggers the Na^+ channels in surrounding cells to open, which causes the depolarization wave to propagate cell by cell throughout the heart.

Phases 1–3: Repolarization phases

- During these phases, represented as the plateau, Ca^{2+} and some K^+ channels open.

- Ca^{2+} flows into the cells, and K^+ flows out.

- The cell remains polarized, and the increased Ca^{2+} within the cell trigger contraction of the cardiac muscle.

Phase 4: Completion of repolarization

- Ca^{2+} channels close.
- K^+ outflow continues.
- The cardiac cell returns to its normal state.

The cardiac cycle of **depolarization-polarization-depolarization** is represented on the ECG by the P wave, QRS complex, and T wave. A dysrhythmia can occur anywhere along the conduction system. It can be caused when an impulse from between the nodes or fibers is delayed or blocked. Arrhythmias also occur when an ectopic focus initiates an impulse, thereby disrupting the normal conduction cycle. Additional sources of damage to the conduction system include MIs, hypertension, coronary artery disease (CAD), and congenital heart defects.

Overview of Dysrhythmias

Abnormalities in the electrical conduction system of the heart may occur at the SA node, the AV node, or the His-Purkinje system of the ventricles. Careful evaluation of the ECG will aid in determining the location and subsequent cause of the dysrhythmia.

Dysrhythmias that occur above the ventricles in either the atria or the SA/AV nodes are known as **supraventricular dysrhythmias**. Common arrhythmias in this category are sinus bradycardia, sinus tachycardia, atrial fibrillation, atrial flutter, junctional rhythm, and sustained supraventricular tachycardia (SVT). **Atrioventricular (AV) blocks**, known as **heart blocks,** occur when the impulse is delayed or blocked at the AV node. The three types of **heart block** are first degree, second degree, and third degree, with first degree being the least severe and third degree being the most severe.

Ventricular dysrhythmias can be life-threatening because they severely impact the heart's ability to pump and maintain adequate cardiac output (CO). A bundle branch block (BBB), premature ventricular complexes (PVCs), sustained ventricular tachycardia (V-tach), ventricular fibrillation (V-fib), Torsades de pointes, and digoxin-induced ventricular dysrhythmias are the most common ventricular arrhythmias.

Supraventricular Dysrhythmias

Sinus Bradycardia
Sinus bradycardia occurs when the SA node creates an impulse at a slower-than-normal rate—less than 60 beats per minute (bpm). Causes include metabolic conditions, calcium channel blockers (CCB) and

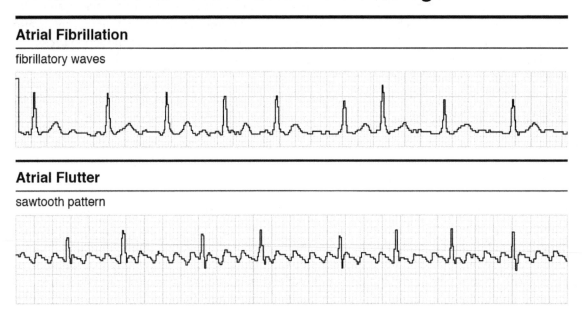
beta-blocker medications, MIs, and increased intracranial pressure. If symptomatic, treatment involves transcutaneous pacing and atropine.

Sinus Tachycardia

Sinus tachycardia occurs when the SA node creates an impulse at a faster-than-normal rate, also characterized as a rate greater than 100 bpm. Causes include physiological stress such as shock, volume loss, and heart failure, as well as medications and illicit drugs. Sinus tachycardia is typically treated by treating the underlying cause.

Atrial Fibrillation

Atrial fibrillation is the most common sustained dysrhythmia. It is caused when multiple foci in the atria fire randomly, thereby stimulating various parts of the atria simultaneously. The result is a highly irregular atrial rhythm. Ventricular rate may be rapid or normal. Fatigue, lightheadedness, chest pain, dyspnea, and hypotension may be present. Treatment goals are to improve ventricular pumping and prevent stroke. Beta-blockers and CCBs impede conduction through the AV node, thereby controlling ventricular rates, so they are the medications of choice. Cardioversion and ablation are also treatment options.

Atrial Fibrillation and Flutter ECG Tracings

Atrial Fibrillation

fibrillatory waves

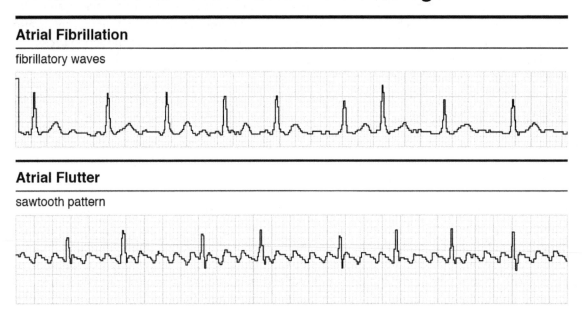

Atrial Flutter

sawtooth pattern

Atrial Flutter

Atrial flutter is caused by an ectopic atrial focus that fires between 250 and 350 times a minute. The AV node is unable to transmit impulses at that speed, so typically only one out of every two impulses reach the ventricles. Cardioversion is the treatment of choice to convert atrial flutter back to a sinus rhythm. CCBs and beta-blockers are used to manage ventricular rates.

Junctional Dysrhythmias

If either the SA node slows or its impulse is not properly conducted, the AV node will become the pacemaker. The heart rate for an impulse initiated at the AV junction will be between 40 and 60 bmp.

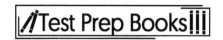

The P wave will be absent on an EKG. Suggested treatment is similar to that of sinus bradycardia: transcutaneous pacing, atropine, and epinephrine.

Supraventricular Tachycardia

Sustained supraventricular tachycardia (SVT) is usually caused by an AV nodal reentry circuit. Heart rate can increase to 150 to 250 bpm. Interventions that increase vagal tone such as the Valsalva maneuver or carotid massage may slow the heart rate. Adenosine, beta-blockers, and CCBs may be administered intravenously for immediate treatment, while beta-blockers and CCBs may be taken orally to prevent reoccurrence.

Heart Block

In first-degree heart block, the impulse from the SA node is slowed as it moves across the atria. On an ECG, the P and R waves will be longer and flatter. First-degree block is often asymptomatic.

Second-degree heart block is divided into two categories known as Mobitz type I and Mobitz type II. In Mobitz type I, the impulse from the SA node is increasingly delayed with each heartbeat until eventually a beat is skipped entirely. On an ECG, this is visible as a delay in the PR interval. The normal PR interval is 0.12–0.20. The PR interval will get longer until the QRS wave doesn't follow the P wave. Patients may experience mild symptoms with this dysrhythmia.

When some of the impulses from the SA node fail to reach the ventricles, the arrhythmia is a Mobitz type II heart block. Some impulses move across the atria and reach the ventricles normally, and others do not. On an ECG, the QRS follows the P wave at normal speed, but some QRS complexes are missing because the signal is blocked. Patients experiencing this dysrhythmia usually need a pacemaker.

A third-degree heart block is also known as complete heart block, or complete AV block. The SA node may continue to initiate the impulses between 80 and 100 bpm, but none of the impulses reach the ventricles. The automaticity of cardiac cells in the Purkinje fibers will prompt the ventricles to initiate an impulse; however, beats initiated in this area are between 20 and 40 bpm. The slower impulses initiated from the ventricles are not coordinated with the impulses from the SA node. Therefore, third-degree heart block is a medical emergency that requires a temporary to permanent pacemaker.

Bundle Branch Block

A bundle branch block (BBB) occurs when there is a delay or defect in the conduction system within the ventricles; a BBB may be designated as "left" or "right" to specify the ventricle at fault or as "complete" or "partial." The QRS complex will be widened or prolonged. Treating the underlying cause is the goal.

Premature Ventricular Complex

A premature ventricular complex (PVC) occurs when a ventricular impulse is conducted through the ventricle before the next sinus impulse. This may be caused by cardiac ischemia, heart failure, hypoxia, or hypokalemia. Treatment is to correct the cause, and long-term treatment is not indicated unless the patient is symptomatic. It should be noted that while single PVCs happen occasionally and are often harmless, frequent PVCs pose a significant risk of eventual heart failure or sudden cardiac death.

Ventricular Tachycardia

Ventricular tachycardia (V-tach) occurs from a single, rapidly firing ectopic ventricular focus that is typically at the border of an old infarct (MI). This dysrhythmia is usually associated with CAD. Ventricular rates can be 150 to 250 bpm. However, the heart cannot pump effectively at those increased rates. Immediate cardioversion is the treatment of choice. Antidysrhythmic medications such as amiodarone,

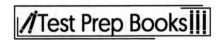

lidocaine, or procainamide may be given. An implantable cardioverter defibrillator (ICD) may be necessary.

Ventricular Tachycardia and Fibrillation ECG Tracings

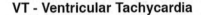

VT - Ventricular Tachycardia

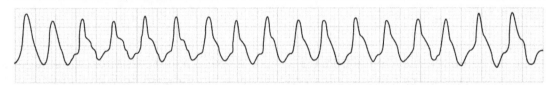

VF - Ventricular Fibrillation

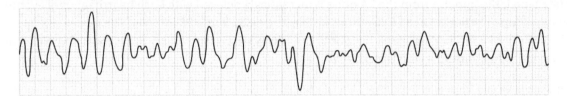

Ventricular Fibrillation

Ventricular fibrillation (V-fib) is a life-threatening emergency that requires immediate treatment. It is caused by multiple ventricular ectopic foci firing simultaneously, which forces the ventricles to contract asynchronously. Coordinated ventricular contraction is impossible in this scenario. The result is reduced cardiac output, and defibrillation is required. Lidocaine, amiodarone, and procainamide may be used.

Torsade de Pointes

Torsade de pointes is an atypical rapid undulating ventricular tachydysrhythmia. This rhythm has a prolonged QT interval. A variety of drugs cause QT-interval prolongation. The treatment is intravenous magnesium and cardioversion for sustained V-tach.

Torsade de Pointes ECG Tracing

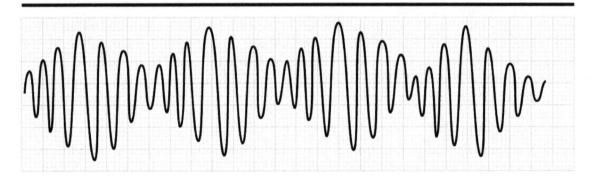

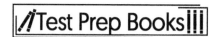

Digoxin-Induced Ventricular Dysrhythmias

Digoxin is a cardiac glycoside medication that increases the strength and regularity of the cardiac rhythm. It has a very narrow therapeutic range. Toxicity occurs when therapeutic levels are exceeded. Digoxin toxicity can mimic all types of dysrhythmias. Digoxin acts by increasing automaticity in the atria, ventricles, and the His-Purkinje system. It also decreases conduction through the AV node. Therefore, an AV block is the most common form of presenting dysrhythmia in the general population. Among the elderly, chronic toxicity is common as well, as it can be easily caused by drug-to-drug interactions and declining renal function.

Summary

Dysrhythmias range from asymptomatic to life-threatening. They can be divided into three major groups: **supraventricular dysrhythmias**, **heart block**, and **ventricular dysrhythmias**. Treatment is necessary when ventricular pumping and cardiac output are impacted. There are two phases of treatment. The first is to terminate the dysrhythmia using medications, defibrillation, or both. The second is long-term suppression with medications.

A complete medical history with an emphasis on current medications, comorbidities, and family history is paramount. Immediate nursing priorities include establishing IV access, monitoring vital signs, and administering oxygen as needed. Evaluation of the ECG, chest x-ray, and both laboratory and diagnostic values is required. Defibrillation, cardioversion, and transcutaneous pacing are other possibilities.

Endocarditis

By definition, endocarditis is the inflammation of the endocardium, or innermost lining of the heart chambers and valves. It is also called **infective endocarditis,** or **bacterial endocarditis**.

To review, there are three layers of tissue that comprise the heart. A double-layer serous membrane, known as the **pericardium**, is the outermost layer. The pericardium forms the pericardial sac that surrounds the heart. The middle and largest layer is the **myocardium**. Since an MI occurs when the heart muscle is deprived of oxygen, the myocardial layer of the heart is where the damage due to lack of oxygen occurs. The innermost layer that lines the heart chambers and also the heart valves is called the **endocardium**. Endocarditis occurs when the endocardial layer and heart valves become infected and inflamed.

The most common cause of endocarditis is a bloodstream invasion of bacteria. **Staphylococci** and **Streptococci** account for the majority of infective endocarditis occurrences. During medical or dental procedures—such as a colonoscopy, cystoscopy, or professional teeth cleaning—bacteria may enter the bloodstream and travel to the heart. Inflammatory bowel disease and sexually transmitted diseases also foster bacterial transmission to the bloodstream and, ultimately, the heart.

Risk factors for the development of endocarditis include valve and septal defects of the heart, an artificial heart valve, a history of endocarditis, an indwelling long-term dialysis catheter, parenteral nutrition or central lines in the right atrium, IV drug use, and body piercings. Patients taking steroids or immunosuppressive medications are susceptible to fungal endocarditis. Regardless of the source, the bacteria infect the inside of the heart chambers and valves. Clumps of infective bacteria, or vegetation, develop within the heart at the site of infection. The heart valves are a common infection site, which often results in incomplete closure of the valves.

The classic symptoms of endocarditis are fever, cardiac murmur, and petechial lesions of the skin, conjunctiva, and oral mucosa. However, symptoms can range in severity. Flu-like symptoms, weight loss, and back pain may be present. Dyspnea and swelling of the feet and ankles may be evident. Endocarditis caused by **Staphylococcus** has a rapid onset, whereas **Streptococcus** occurs more slowly with a prolonged course.

Layers of the Heart Wall

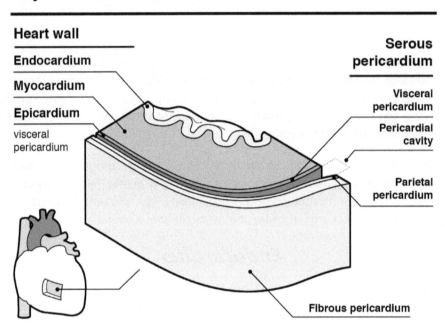

Antimicrobial treatment for four to six weeks is the standard of care. In some cases, two antimicrobials are used to treat the infection and prevent drug resistance. The objective of treatment is to eradicate the infection and treat complications. Surgery may be required for persistent recurring infections, one or more embolic occurrences, or if heart failure develops.

Left untreated, endocarditis can result in stroke or organ damage, as the vegetation breaks off and travels through the bloodstream and blocks circulation. The spread of infection and subsequent formation of abscesses throughout the body may also occur. Heart failure may develop when the infection hampers the heart's ability to pump effectively or with perforation of a valve.

A complete history and physical that includes inquiry about medications, recent surgeries, screening, and diagnostic testing may provide the crucial piece of information that identifies endocarditis in the face of otherwise vague symptom presentation. The nurse should anticipate the order for blood cultures, an erythrocyte sedimentation rate (ESR), a CBC, an ECG, a chest x-ray, and a transthoracic or transesophageal echocardiogram to identify the location of the infected area.

An in-depth patient interview and assessment by the nurse are essential. Diagnostic and laboratory results coupled with data from the patient interview will aid in early recognition and treatment of endocarditis. Because an incident of endocarditis places one at a higher risk for future infections, patient teaching should include informing all providers and dentists prior to treatment. Antibiotic prophylaxis may be indicated.

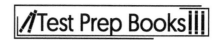

Heart Failure

Mechanism

Defined as the failure of the heart to meet the metabolic demands of the body, **heart failure** (HF) is a general term that refers to the failure of the heart as a pump. Heart failure is a syndrome with diverse clinical features and various etiologies. The syndrome is progressive and often fatal. It may involve either or both sides of the heart. Based on an ejection fraction (EF), it can be further categorized as **diastolic** or **systolic** HF.

Left-sided HF is also referred to as congestive heart failure (CHF) because the congestion occurs in the **pulmonary** capillary beds. As mentioned previously, oxygenated blood flows from the pulmonary artery into the left atrium, then the LV, and into the aorta for distribution through the systemic circulation.

Once the oxygenated blood has been delivered to end-point tissues and organs, it arrives at the capillary bed. The now-deoxygenated blood begins the return journey back to the heart by passing from the capillary beds into small veins that feed into progressively larger veins and, ultimately, into the superior and inferior vena cava. The vena cava empties into the right atrium. From the right atrium, blood flows into the right ventricle and then into the pulmonary system for oxygenation.

When the right ventricle is impaired, it cannot effectively pump blood forward into the pulmonary system. The ineffective forward movement of blood causes an increase of venous pressure. When venous pressures rises, the blood backs up and leaks into the tissues and the liver. The end result is edema in the extremities and congestion within the liver.

When the LV is impaired, it cannot effectively pump blood forward into the aorta for systemic circulation. The ineffective forward movement of blood causes an increase in the pulmonary venous blood volume, which forces fluids from the capillaries to back up and leak into the pulmonary tissues. This results in pulmonary edema and impaired oxygenation.

Ejection fraction (EF) is the percentage of blood volume pumped out by the ventricles with each contraction. The normal EF is 50 to 70 percent. An EF of 60 percent means that 60 percent of the available blood volume was pumped out of the LV during contraction. It is an important measurement for diagnosing and tracking the progression of HF. The EF also differentiates between diastolic and systolic HF.

Diastolic HF is currently referred to as HF with normal ejection fraction (HFNEF). The heart muscle contracts normally, but the ventricles do not adequately relax during ventricular filling. In systolic HF, or heart failure with reduced ejection fraction (HFrEF), the heart muscle does not contract effectively, so less blood is pumped out to the body.

Variables

There are several variables that both impact and are impacted by HF. A review of these variables will provide the backdrop for a closer look at the classification, sequelae, symptoms, and treatment of HF.

Cardiac output (CO, or Q) is the volume of blood being pumped by the heart in one minute. It is the product of heart rate multiplied by stroke volume. **Stroke volume** (SV) is the amount of blood pumped out of the ventricles per beat; $CO = HR \times SV$. Normal CO is between four and eight liters per minute. Both CO and SV are reduced in HF.

Systemic vascular resistance (SVR) is related to the diameter and elasticity of blood vessels and the viscosity of blood. For example, narrow and stiff vessels and/or thicker blood will cause an increase in SVR. An increase in SVR causes the LV to work harder to overcome the pressure at the aortic valve. Conversely, larger and more elastic vessels and/or thin blood will decrease SVR and reduce cardiac workload.

Pulmonary vascular resistance (PVR) is the vascular resistance of the pulmonary circulation. It is the difference between the mean pulmonary arterial pressure and the left atrial filling pressure. Resistance and blood viscosity impact both SVR and PVR. However, pulmonary blood flow, lung volume, and hypoxic vasoconstriction are unique to the pulmonary vasculature.

Preload is defined as the amount of ventricular stretch at the end of diastole, or when the chambers are filling. In other words, preload is the amount of pressure from the blood that is being exerted against the inside of the LV. It is also known as left ventricular end-diastolic pressure (LVEDP) and reflects the amount of stretch of cardiac muscle sarcomeres. **Afterload** is the amount of resistance the heart must overcome to open the aortic valve and push the blood volume into the systemic circulation.

Classification

HF is closely associated with chronic hypertension, CAD, and diabetes mellitus. The New York Heart Association (NYHA) classification tool is most frequently used to categorize the stages and symptom progression of HF as it relates to heart disease.

- Stage I: Cardiac disease; no symptoms during physical activity
- Stage II: Cardiac disease; slight limitations on physical activity
- Stage III: Cardiac disease; marked limitations during physical activity
- Stage IV: Cardiac disease; unable to perform physical activity; symptoms at rest

Sequelae

Heart failure may have an acute or chronic onset, but it is progressive. When CO is diminished, tissues are not adequately perfused, and organs ultimately fail. When the LV works harder because of increased preload or afterload, its muscular walls becomes thick and enlarged, resulting in ventricular hypertrophy. Ventricular hypertrophy causes ventricular remodeling (cardiac remodeling), which is a change to the heart's size, shape, structure, and physiological function.

The sympathetic nervous system responds to a diminished CO by increasing the heart rate, constricting arteries, and activating the renin-angiotensin-aldosterone system (RAAS). Elevated angiotensin levels raise BP and afterload, thereby prompting the heart to work harder. The reduced CO caused by HF can diminish blood flow to the kidneys. The kidneys respond to the decreased perfusion by secreting renin and activating the RAAS. As a result, the increase in aldosterone signals the body to retain Na^+ and water. Retained Na^+ and water leads to volume overload, pulmonary congestion, and hypertension. The body's response to reduced CO caused by HF can perpetuate a downward spiral. However, there are naturally-occurring natriuretic peptides that are secreted in response to elevated pressures within the heart. These peptides counteract fluid retention and vasoconstriction.

Atrial natriuretic peptide (ANP) is secreted by the atria. **B-type natriuretic peptide** (BNP) is secreted by the ventricles. Both ANP and BNP cause diuresis, vasodilation, and decreased aldosterone secretion, thereby balancing the effects of sympathetic nervous system response and RAAS activation. Elevated levels of BNP are a diagnostic indication of HF.

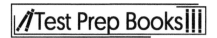

Symptoms of Heart Failure

Either an MI or a dysrhythmia can precipitate HF. The clinical presentation reflects congestion in the pulmonary and/or systemic vasculature. Treatment depends on the clinical stage of the disease. Common symptoms include:

- Dyspnea on exertion
- Fatigue
- Pulmonary congestion, which causes a cough and difficulty breathing when lying down
- Feelings of suffocation and anxiety that are worse at night
- Peripheral edema

The most common cause of HF exacerbation is fluid overload due to nonadherence to sodium and water restrictions. Patient education is extremely critical to avoiding and managing exacerbations. Congestive heart failure is a core measure, tied to patient satisfaction, patient education, subsequent readmissions in a defined period of time, and ultimately, to reimbursements.

Treatment

Therapy for HF focuses on three primary goals: reduction of preload, reduction of afterload (SVR), and inhibition of the RAAS and vasoconstrictive mechanisms of the sympathetic nervous system. Pharmacotherapy includes ACE inhibitors, angiotensin II receptor blockers (ARBs), diuretics, beta-blockers, vasodilators, and a cardiac glycoside.

The ACE inhibitors and ARBs interfere with the RAAS by preventing the body's normal mechanism to retain fluids and constrict blood vessels. Diuretics decrease fluid volume and relieve both pulmonary and systemic congestion. Beta-blockers and cardiac glycosides slow the HR and strengthen the myocardium to improve contractility. Vasodilators decrease SVR. In addition to a thorough physical exam and complete medical history, a clinical work-up will include a chest x-ray, a BNP and other laboratory values, an ECG, and perhaps an echocardiogram or multigated acquisition (MUGA) scan to measure EF.

Summary

HF is a common debilitating syndrome characterized by high mortality, frequent hospitalizations, multiple comorbidities, and poor quality of life. A partnership between providers, nurses, and patients is paramount to managing and slowing disease progression. Patient education should include a discussion of the disease process, prescribed medications, diet restrictions, and weight management. Patients should know which symptoms require immediate medical care. Self-care can be the most important aspect of HF management. The nurse as educator performs an essential role in this and all disease management.

Hypertension

Hypertension (HTN) is an abnormally high BP (140/90 mmHg or higher). The diagnosis is based on two or more accurate readings that are elevated. HTN is known as **the silent killer** because it is asymptomatic. Several variables impact BP, and understanding them is essential.

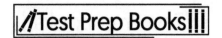

Variables

Blood pressure is the product of CO multiplied by SVR; $BP = CO \times SVR$. Cardiac output is the volume of blood being pumped by the heart in one minute. It is the product of HR multiplied by SV; $HR \times SV = CO$. Stroke volume is the amount of blood pumped out of the ventricles per beat.

SVR is related to the diameter of blood vessels and the viscosity of blood. The narrower the vessels or the thicker the blood, the higher the SVR. Conversely, larger-diameter vessels and thinner blood decrease SVR.

Mechanism

For HTN to develop, there must be a change in one or more factors affecting SVR or CO and a problem with the control system responsible for regulating BP. The body normally maintains and adjusts BP by either increasing the HR or the strength of myocardial contraction or by dilating or constricting the veins and arterioles.

When veins are dilated, less blood returns to the heart, and subsequently, less blood is pumped out of the heart. The result is a decrease in CO. Conversely, when veins are constricted, more blood is returned to the heart, and CO is increased. The arterioles also dilate or constrict. An expanded arteriole reduces resistance, and a constricted arteriole increases resistance. The veins and arterioles impact both CO and SVR. The kidneys contribute to the maintenance and adjustment of BP by controlling Na⁺, chloride, and water excretion and through the RAAS. Management of HTN will focus on one or more of the factors that regulate BP. Those regulatory factors are SVR, fluid volume, and the strength and rate of myocardial contraction.

Classification

HTN is classified as **primary** or **secondary** depending on the etiology. In primary HTN, the cause is unknown, but the primary factors include problems related to the natriuretic hormones or RAAS or electrolyte disturbances. Primary HTN is also known as **essential** or **idiopathic** HTN.

In secondary HTN, there is an identifiable cause. Associated disease states include kidney disease, adrenal gland tumors, thyroid disease, congenital blood vessel disorders, alcohol abuse, and obstructive sleep apnea. Products associated with secondary HTN are nonsteroidal anti-inflammatory drugs (NSAIDs), birth control pills, decongestants, cocaine, amphetamines, and corticosteroids.

HTN normally increases with age, and it is more prominent among African Americans. BP is classified according to treatment guidelines as normal, pre-HTN, Stage 1 HTN, and Stage 2 HTN. **Pre-HTN** is defined as systolic pressures ranging from 120 to 139 mmHg and diastolic pressures ranging from 80 to 89 mmHg. **Stage 1 HTN** ranges from 140 to 159 mmHg systolic and 90 to 99 mmHg diastolic pressures. In the more severe Stage 2 HTN, systolic pressures are 160 mmHg or higher, and diastolic pressures are 100 mmHg or higher.

Sequelae

Systolic pressure is the amount of pressure exerted on arterial walls immediately after ventricular contraction and emptying. This represents the highest level of pressure during the cardiac cycle. Diastolic pressure is the amount of pressure exerted on arterials walls when the heart is filling. This

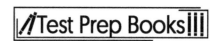

represents the lowest pressure during the cardiac cycle. In general, hypertension increases the risk of cardiovascular disease; diastolic HTN poses a greater risk.

Prolonged HTN damages the delicate endothelial layer of vessels. The damaged endothelium initiates the inflammatory response and clotting cascade. As mentioned, the diameter of veins, arterioles, and arteries changes SVR. When SVR is increased, the heart must work harder to pump against the increased pressure. In other words, the pressure in the LV must be higher than the pressure being exerted on the opposite side of the aortic valve by systemic vascular pressure. The ventricular pressure must overcome the aortic pressure for contraction and ventricular emptying to occur. When the myocardium works against an elevated systemic pressure for a prolonged period of time, the LV will enlarge, and HF may ensue.

Risk Factors

There are both modifiable and nonmodifiable risk factors associated with the development of HTN. Modifiable risk factors include obesity, a sedentary lifestyle, tobacco use, a diet high in sodium, dyslipidemia, excessive alcohol consumption, stress, sleep apnea, and diabetes. Age, race, and family history are nonmodifiable risk factors.

Treatment

First-line treatments include lifestyle changes and pharmacologic therapy.

Initial therapy includes diuretics, CCBs, ACE inhibitors, and ARBs. Diuretics decrease fluid volume. CCBs decrease myocardial contractility. Both ACE inhibitors and ARBs interfere with the RAAS by preventing the normal mechanism that retains fluids and narrows blood vessels. The result is decreased volume and SVR.

Hypertensive Crisis/Emergency

A **hypertensive crisis** is defined as a BP higher than 180/120 mmHg. BP must be lowered quickly to prevent end organ damage. Pregnancy, an acute MI, a dissecting aortic aneurysm, and an intracranial hemorrhage are associated with a hypertensive crisis. The therapeutic goal is to reduce the BP by 25 percent within the first hour of treatment with a continual reduction over the following 2 to 6 hours and an ongoing reduction to the target goal over a period of days. Short-acting antihypertensive medications administered intravenously is the primary treatment.

Summary

The astute nurse will conduct an in-depth patient interview to identify prescribed and illicit drug use, alcohol and tobacco use, family history, sleep patterns, and dietary habits. Patient education should include information about the Dietary Approach to Stop Hypertension (DASH) diet and alcohol in moderation with a limit of one to two drinks per day. Aerobic exercise and resistance training three to four times weekly for an average of 40 minutes is recommended. Information about prescribed hypertensive medications should also be reviewed with the patient.

Pericardial Tamponade

Cardiac tamponade, or pericardial tamponade, is a syndrome caused by the excessive accumulation of blood or fluid in the pericardial sac, resulting in the compression of the myocardium and reduced ventricular filling. It is a medical emergency with complications of pulmonary edema, shock, and death, if left untreated.

The pericardium, or outer layer of the heart wall, is a two-layer membrane that forms the pericardial sac, which envelops the heart. The parietal (outer) layer of the pericardium is made of tough, thickened fibrous tissue. This layer is attached to the mid-diaphragm and to the back of the sternum. These attachments keep the heart in place during acceleration or deceleration. The fibrous nature of the parietal layer prevents cardiac distention into the mediastinal region of the chest.

The visceral (inner) layer of the pericardium is a double-layered membrane. One layer is affixed to the heart. The second layer lines the inside of the parietal (outer) layer. The small space between the parietal and visceral layers is the pericardial space. The space normally contains between 15 and 50 milliliters of pericardial fluid. The pericardial fluid lubricates the membranes and allows the two layers to slide over one another as the heart beats.

A pericardial effusion develops when excess blood or fluid accumulates in the pericardial sac. If the effusion progresses, a pericardial tamponade will ensue. Because the fibrous parietal layer prevents cardiac distention, the pressure from the excessive blood or fluid is exerted inward, compressing the myocardium and reducing space for blood to fill the chambers. The normally low-pressure right ventricle and atrium are the first structures to be impacted by tamponade. Therefore, signs of right-sided HF such as jugular vein distention, edema, and hepatomegaly may be present.

Symptoms of a pericardial tamponade are dyspnea, chest tightness, dizziness, tachycardia, muffled heart sounds, and restlessness. Pulsus paradoxus is an important clinical finding in tamponade; it represents an abnormal BP variation during the respiration cycle and is evidenced by a decrease of 10 mmHg or more in systolic BP during inspiration. Pulsus paradoxus represents decreased diastolic ventricular filling and reduced volume in all four chambers of the heart. The clinical signs associated with tamponade are distended neck veins, muffled heart sounds, and hypotension. These clustered symptoms are known as **Beck's triad**.

Removal of the pericardial fluid via pericardiocentesis is the definitive therapy. A pericardiectomy or pericardial window may be performed to remove part of the pericardium. Fluid removed during the procedure is analyzed to determine the cause of the effusion. Malignancies, metastatic disease, and trauma are major causes of the development of pericardial effusions.

Identification and treatment of a tamponade requires emergent medical intervention. A rapid focused assessment of heart sounds and BP, including assessing for pulsus paradoxus, is a critical first step. An in-depth medical and surgical history can aid in identifying the etiology.

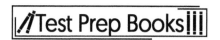

Pericarditis

Pericarditis is inflammation of the pericardium, which forms the pericardial sac that surrounds the heart.

Look at this graphic again for reference:

Layers of the Heart Wall

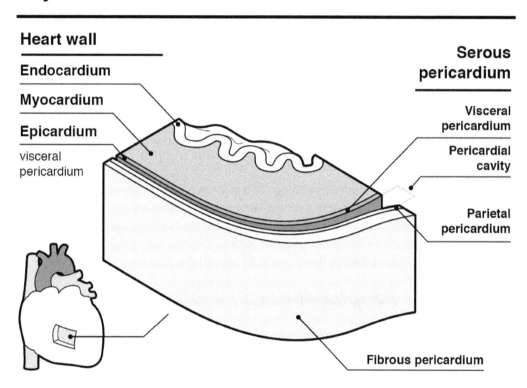

The fibrous attachments between the pericardium the mid-diaphragm and to the back of the sternum keep the heart in place during acceleration or deceleration. The fibrous nature of the parietal layer prevents cardiac distention into the mediastinal region of the chest. It separates the heart from the surrounding structures, and it protects the heart against infection and inflammation from the lungs. The pericardium contains pain receptors and mechanoreceptors, both of which prompt reflex changes in the BP and HR.

Pericarditis can be either acute or chronic in presentation. Causes are varied and include an acute MI; bacterial, fungal, and viral infections; certain medications; chest trauma; connective tissue disorders such as lupus or rheumatic fever; metastatic lesions from lung or breast tumors; and a history of radiation therapy of the chest and upper torso. Frequent or prolonged episodes of pericarditis can lead to thickening and scarring of the pericardium and loss of elasticity. These conditions limit the heart's ability to fill with blood, and therefore limit the amount of blood being pumped out to the body. The result is a decrease in CO. Pericarditis can also cause fluid to accumulate in the pericardial cavity, known as **pericardial effusion**.

A characteristic symptom of pericarditis is chest pain. The pain is persistent, sharp, pleuritic, felt in the mid-chest, and aggravated by deep inhalation. Pericarditis may also cause ST elevation, thereby mimicking an acute MI, or it may be asymptomatic.

A pericardial friction rub is diagnostic of pericarditis. It is a creaky or scratchy sound heard at the end of exhalation. The rub is best heard when the patient is sitting and leaning forward. Stethoscope placement should be at the left lower sternal border in the fourth intercostal space. The rub is audible on auscultation and synchronous to the heartbeat. A pericardial friction rub is differentiated from a pleural friction rub by having patients hold their breath. The pericardial friction rub will remain constant with the heartbeat. Other presenting symptoms include a mild fever, cough, and dyspnea. Common laboratory findings are elevated white blood cell (WBC), ESR, or CRP levels.

The diagnosis of pericarditis is based on history, signs, and symptoms. Treatment goals are to determine the cause, administer therapy for treatment and symptom relief, and detect signs of complications. A thorough medical and surgical history will identify patients at risk for developing pericarditis. The physical assessment should evaluate the reported pain level during position changes, inspiration, expiration, coughing, swallowing, and breath holding. In addition, flexion, extension, and rotation of the neck and spine should be assessed for their influence on reported pain.

In patients not showing signs of any specific etiology or a poor prognosis, a one-week trial of NSAIDs with follow-up is recommended for patients with acute pericarditis. Physical activity in non-athletic patients should be restricted to regular daily activity until symptoms resolve, and a three-month minimal restriction on activity for athletes. In patients with moderate risk not responding ideally to NSAIDs, an etiological search is advised to diagnose and manage the specific form of pericarditis.

Peripheral Vascular Disease

Peripheral vascular disease (PVD) refers to diseases of the blood vessels that are outside the heart and brain. The term PVD is used interchangeably with **peripheral arterial disease** (PAD). It is the narrowing of peripheral vessels caused by atherosclerosis. The narrowing can be compounded by emboli or thrombi. Limb ischemia due to reduced blood flow can result in loss of limb or life. The primary factor for the development of PVD is atherosclerosis.

PVD encompasses several conditions: atherosclerosis, Buerger's disease, chronic venous insufficiency, deep vein thrombosis (DVT), Raynaud's phenomenon, thrombophlebitis, and varicose veins.

Risk Factors

Coronary artery disease, atrial fibrillation, cerebrovascular disease (stroke), and renal disease are common comorbidities. Risk factors include smoking, phlebitis, injury, surgery, and hyperviscosity of the blood. Autoimmune disorders and hyperlipidemia are also common factors. The two major complications of PVD are limb complications or loss and the risk for stroke or heart attack.

Symptoms

Intermittent claudication (cramping pain in the leg during exercise) may be the sole manifestation of early symptomatic PVD. It occurs with exercise and stops with rest. Physical findings during examination may include the classic five Ps: pulselessness, paralysis, paresthesia, pain, and pallor of the extremity.

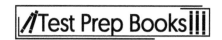

The most critical symptom of PVD is critical limb ischemia (CLI), which is pain that occurs in the affected limb during rest. Manifestations of PVD may include the following symptoms:

- Feet that are cool or cold to the touch
- Aching or burning in the legs that is relieved by sitting
- Pale color when legs are elevated
- Redness when legs are in a hanging-down (dependent) position
- Brittle, thin, or shiny skin on the legs and feet
- Loss of hair on feet
- Nonhealing wounds or ulcers over pressure points
- Loss of muscle or fatty tissue
- Numbness, weakness, or heaviness in muscles
- Reddish-blue discoloration of the extremities
- Restricted mobility
- Thickened, opaque toenails

Diagnostics

The ankle-brachial index (ABI) should be measured. The ABI is the systolic pressure at the ankle, divided by the systolic pressure at the arm. It is a specific and sensitive indicator of peripheral artery disease (PAD). The Allen test looks for an occlusion of either the radial or ulnar arteries. A Doppler ultrasonography flow study can determine the patency of peripheral arteries.

The patient should be assessed for heart murmurs, and all peripheral pulses should be evaluated for quality and bruit. An ECG may reveal an arrhythmia. Because the presence of atherosclerosis initiates an inflammatory response, inflammatory markers such as the D-dimer, CRP, interleukin 6, and homocysteine may be present. Blood urea nitrogen (BUN) and creatinine levels may provide indications of decreased organ perfusion. A lipid profile may reveal the risk for atherosclerosis. A stress test or angiogram may be necessary.

Treatment

The two main goals for treatment of PVD are to control the symptoms and halt the progression to lower the risk of heart attack and stroke. Specific treatment modalities depend on the extent and severity of the disease, the patient's age, overall medical history, clinical signs, and his or her preferences. Lifestyle modifications include smoking cessation, improved nutrition, and regular exercise. Aggressive treatment of comorbidities can also aid in stopping the progression. Pharmacotherapy may include anticoagulants and vasodilators.

Summary

The primary factor in PVD is atherosclerosis. Prevention should begin early and be centered on balanced nutrition and exercise, alcohol in moderation, and smoking cessation. Once diagnosed, management of PVD will include preventive measures and the incorporation of pharmacotherapeutics. Providing patient education about proper diet and exercise should occur during every patient encounter. The conscientious nurse will take advantage of an encounter to improve patient outcomes through education and referral.

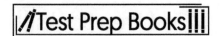

Thromboembolic Disease

In simplest terms, a **thrombus** is a blood clot that forms in a vein. Clots can be caused by either a fat globule, gas bubble, amniotic fluid, or any foreign material that gets into the bloodstream. A DVT usually forms in the leg. A thrombus becomes an **embolus** when a fragment dislodges and travels through the circulatory system. The embolus will remain in the circulatory system until it reaches a vessel too narrow for its passage. An **embolism** occurs when the embolus lodges and prevents blood flow. In the cardiac cycle, veins begin at the capillary bed and get progressively larger as they return deoxygenated blood to the right side of the heart. From the right side of the heart, blood flows to the lungs.

A **pulmonary embolism** (PE) occurs when the embolus, or a fragment of the embolus, becomes lodged in the pulmonary circulation. A DVT frequently results in a PE. A **fat embolism** may form when fat globules pass into the small vessels and damage the endothelial lining. As the fat breaks down to free fatty acids, it causes toxic damage. When the damage occurs in the lungs, acute respiratory failure ensues.

Mechanism

A strong clinical link exists between clot formation and atherosclerosis, PAD, diabetes, and other factors contributing to heart disease. Anything that damages a vein's endothelial lining may cause a DVT to form. Damage to vessel lining can occur from smoking, cancer, chemotherapy, injury, or surgery. In addition to a damaged endothelial layer, increased age, dehydration, and viscous or slow-flowing blood increase the risk of DVT formation. Factors that slow blood flow are prolonged bed rest, sitting for extended periods, smoking, obesity, and HF. In the presence of atrial fibrillation, the atria do not empty adequately. Blood pools in the upper chambers, increasing the risk for clots to form.

Closed long-bone fractures carry a high risk for a fat embolism to develop because when the bone marrow is exposed as a result of a fracture, its particles can enter the bloodstream. Orthopedic procedures, a bone marrow biopsy, massive soft tissue injury, and severe burns are also associated with the development of an embolus. In addition, there are nontraumatic conditions associated with a fat embolism, such as prolonged corticosteroid therapy, pancreatitis, liposuction, fatty liver, and osteomyelitis.

Women who are pregnant or taking oral contraceptives are at risk for the development of an embolus. Estrogen increases plasma fibrinogen, some coagulation factors, and platelet formation, which lead to the hypercoagulability of the blood. During pregnancy, the expanding uterus can slow blood flow in the veins. The combined effects of hypercoagulability and slowed blood flow exacerbate the risk. During delivery, an embolus can form from the amniotic fluid and travel through maternal circulation. Therefore, during pregnancy and the subsequent postpartum period, women are at increased risk for DVT formation.

Symptoms

Swelling of the leg below the knee is a common symptom of a DVT. There may also be redness, tenderness, or pain over the area around the clot, but a DVT may be asymptomatic. When a DVT becomes a PE, the patient may experience difficulty breathing and a rapid HR. Reported symptoms may include chest pain, coughing up blood, fainting, and low BP. There is a 24- to 72-hour latent period from injury to onset in the development of a fat embolism.

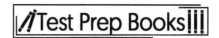

Diagnosis and Treatment

The clinician will consider presenting signs and symptoms, the patient's and family's medical history, and an ultrasound to evaluate blood flow to identify a DVT. The differential diagnoses are pneumonia and a thrombus. A vena cava filter may be placed in the inferior vena cava to capture a clot or fragments. In life-threatening situations such as a PE, an IV thrombolytic may be used to break up the clot. Indications for thrombolytic therapy are chest pain lasting longer than 20 minutes, ST elevation in two leads, and less than 6 hours from the pain's onset. However, thrombolytic medications are absolutely contraindicated in a patient with active bleeding. Prior to the administration of a thrombolytic, the international normalized ration (INR) must be calculated to determine clotting time. In healthy people, an INR of 1.1 or below is considered normal. An INR range of 2.0 to 3.0 is an effective acceptable therapeutic range for people taking warfarin.

For long-term management, patient education should include anticoagulant medication therapy, the use of compression stockings, and avoidance of tight clothing. Patients should be instructed to regularly elevate their feet, avoid prolonged periods of sitting, and increase their exercise to counteract slowed blood flow.

Trauma

The causes of trauma can be categorized into three types, according to their potential degree of injury: penetrating injuries, blunt nonpenetrating injuries, and medical injuries that occur during an invasive procedure. **Penetrating injuries** are associated with knife and gunshot wounds. **Blunt nonpenetrating injuries** are most commonly due to automobile accidents. **Medical injuries** may occur during the implantation of a medical device, an endomyocardial biopsy, the placement of a Swan-Ganz catheter, and cardiopulmonary resuscitation (CPR).

Trauma is evaluated according to a prioritized systematic assessment approach that starts with the **primary survey** and proceeds to the **secondary survey**. The findings gathered during the surveys in conjunction with the type of injury identified will direct the treatment approach.

Types of Injuries

A penetrating injury is categorized by the mechanism of injury as low, medium, or high velocity. A knife wound is low velocity, disrupting just the surface penetrated. A handgun wound, or medium-velocity injury, damages more than the penetrated surface, but less than a high-velocity injury. A high-velocity injury is related to rifles and military weapons.

Penetrating chest trauma comprises a broad spectrum of injury and severity. Any structure within the thoracic cavity may be impacted, such as the heart and great vessels, the tracheobronchial tree, the esophagus, the diaphragm, and surrounding bony structures.

The following conditions may result from penetrating chest trauma: hemothorax, pneumothorax, or pneumomediastinum. These conditions compromise oxygenation and ventilation. A diaphragmatic rupture, pulmonary contusion, rib or sternal fractures, and esophageal or thoracic tears may be present.

A blunt nonpenetrating injury can also affect any of the components of the thoracic cavity. The major damage from both penetrating and nonpenetrating injuries involves derangement in the flow of air, blood, or both. If esophageal perforations are present, alimentary contents may leak into the bloodstream, causing sepsis. Blunt injuries can be further categorized according to the area of impact.

- Chest wall fractures, dislocations, or diaphragmatic injuries
- The pleural lining, the lungs, and upper digestive tract
- The heart, great arteries, veins, and lymphatics

Trauma Survey

The **primary survey** begins with the ABCDE resuscitation system: *a*irway, *b*reathing, *c*irculation, *d*isability or neurological status, and *e*xposure. Adjuncts to the primary survey are x-rays, an EKG, laboratory testing, and the focused assessment with sonography in trauma (*FAST*) examinations.

Trauma patients may not be able to provide a historical account, or verbalize symptoms. Injuries within the thoracic cavity can quickly become life-threatening. Hypoxia and hypoventilation are the major causes of death in chest trauma. Therefore, the FAST examinations can provide a timely diagnosis when compared to older methods of assessment. Blood and fluid tend to pool in dependent areas within the body. The primary FAST examination includes the hepatorenal recess (Morison pouch), the perisplenic view, the subxiphoid pericardial window, and the suprapubic window (Douglas pouch). The extended version (E-FAST) incorporates additional views of the thoracic cavity to assess for hemothorax and pneumothorax. These specific views can rapidly identify injuries and bleeding in the pericardial, pleural, and peritoneal areas. The ease and noninvasiveness of the FAST approach allows for serial examinations to observe changes and monitor progression.

The **secondary survey** incorporates the physical assessment beginning with the **ample history** acronym. *A*llergies, *m*edication, *p*ast illnesses, *l*ast meal, and *e*vents, environment, or mechanism of injury are assessed. The head-to-toe physical assessment should be done using inspection, auscultation, percussion, and palpation, as appropriate.

The head, face, and neck are first assessed for injury. The presence of Battle's sign or raccoon's eyes may indicate intracranial bleeding. Central nervous system function is evaluated using the Glasgow Coma Scale (GCS). Motor, verbal, and eye responses are graded from total paralysis (3) to normal strength (15). Next, the chest, abdomen, pelvis, perineal, rectal, and genital areas are assessed for injury. Finally, the neurovascular status of the musculoskeletal system is evaluated.

In addition to sonographic and physical assessments, trauma scoring systems are used by clinicians to identify the severity of the trauma and to guide treatment, ensure continuous quality improvement, and direct future research.

Severity Scoring

Scoring the level of injury in a trauma patient has several applications, and there are a variety of tools available for use. **Field trauma** scoring can guide prehospital triage decisions, reduce time of transfer and treatment, and maximize resources. It also serves as a quality assurance measure between facilities and during transfer.

Trauma scoring tools are categorized according to the data points they evaluate as either **physiologic, anatomical,** or **combined**.

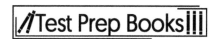

Physiologic Scoring Tools

The **Revised Trauma Score** (RTS) is the most common physiologic scoring tool in use. The RTS combines three parameters: the GCS, systolic blood pressure (SBP), and respiratory rate (RR). The best motor or eye-opening response can be substituted for the GCS in the presence of central nervous system influences such as drugs or alcohol.

Revised Trauma Score			
Coded Value	**GCS**	**Systolic Blood Pressure (mmHg)**	**Respiratory Rate (breaths per minute)**
0	3	0	0
1	4-5	< 50	< 5
2	6-8	50-75	5-9
3	9-12	76-90	> 30
4	13-15	> 90	10-30

The **Acute Physiology and Chronic Health Evaluation** (APACHE II) scoring tool incorporates the chronic health evaluation and comorbid conditions with the Acute Physiology Score (APS).

The **Emergency Trauma Score** (EMTRAS) uses patient data that is quickly available, and it does not require knowledge of anatomic injuries. EMTRAS comprises patient age, GCS, base excess, and prothrombin time (PT) to accurately predict mortality.

Anatomic and Combined Scoring Tools

The **Injury Severity Score** (ISS) tool is based on the Abbreviated Injury Scale (AIS). The ISS uses an anatomical scoring system to give an overall score for patients who have sustained multiple injuries, each of which is assigned an AIS score. Only the highest AIS score for each of six different body regions (head, face, chest, abdomen, extremities and pelvis, and external) is used. The ISS tool grades the severity of injury from minor injury (1) to lethal injury (6); the three most severely injured body regions have their score squared and added together to produce the ISS score. The Trauma and Injury Severity Scoring (**TRISS**) tool combines ISS, RTS, and the age of the patient to grade severity and predict mortality.

Summary

Regardless of the cause or degree of injury, the astute clinician begins the assessment with the primary survey. The secondary survey focusing on the head-to-toe physical assessment also includes evaluation of the FAST examination, x-rays, laboratory testing, and severity scoring tools. Although there is no universally accepted tool for scoring the severity of trauma, there are many valid tools. Coupled with clinician judgment, the assessment findings and severity scoring tools can improve and predict mortality.

Shock

Cardiogenic Shock

The clinical definition of cardiogenic shock is decreased CO and evidence of tissue hypoxia in the presence of adequate intravascular volume. It is a medical emergency and the most severe expression of

LV failure. It is the leading cause of death following an MI with mortality rates between 70 and 90 percent without aggressive treatment. When a large area of the myocardium becomes ischemic, the heart cannot pump effectively. Therefore, SV, CO, and BP drastically decline. The result is end-point hypoperfusion and organ failure. Characteristics of cardiogenic shock include ashen, cyanotic, or mottled extremities; distant heart sounds; and rapid, faint peripheral pulses. Additional signs of hypoperfusion such as altered mental status and decreased urine output may be present.

Work-Up/Treatment

The key to survival in cardiogenic shock is rapid diagnosis, supportive therapy, and coronary artery revascularization. Diagnosis is based on clinical presentation, cardiac and metabolic laboratory studies, chest x-ray, ECG, echocardiogram, and invasive hemodynamic monitoring. Treatment is the restoration of coronary blood flow and correction of electrolyte and acid-base abnormalities.

Obstructive Shock

Obstructive shock occurs when the heart or the great vessels are mechanically obstructed. A cardiac tamponade or massive PE is a frequent cause of obstructive shock. Systemic circulatory collapse occurs because blood flow in or out of the heart is blocked. Generalized treatment goals for shock are to identify and correct the underlying cause. In the case of obstructive shock, the goal is to remove the obstruction.

Treatment begins simultaneously with evaluation. Stabilization of the airway, breathing, and circulation are primary, followed by fluid resuscitation to increase BP. Vital signs, urine flow, and mental status using the GCS should be monitored. Shock patients should be kept warm. Serial measurements of renal and hepatic function, electrolyte levels, and ABGs should be monitored.

Summary

Shock is characterized by organ blood flow that is inadequate to meet the oxygen demands of the tissue. The management goal for shock is to restore oxygen delivery to the tissues and reverse the perfusion deficit. This is accomplished through fluid resuscitation, increasing CO with inotropes, and raising the SVR with vasopressors.

Practice Questions

1. A 44-year-old male patient presents to the emergency department with a complaint of chest pain and shortness of breath. Examination by the nurse reveals distended neck veins and muffled heart sounds. The patient's blood pressure is 80/55. The nurse should suspect which of the following?
   a. Cardiac tamponade
   b. Abdominal aortic aneurysm (AAA)
   c. Cardiopulmonary arrest
   d. Cardiogenic shock

2. The nurse is caring for a patient who presents to the emergency department with an exacerbation of congestive heart failure (CHF). Which clinical manifestation should be most concerning to the nurse?
   a. An oxygenation level of 92 percent
   b. Dyspnea on exertion
   c. New onset of peripheral edema
   d. Elevated BNP levels

3. A patient brought in to the emergency department by the paramedics is complaining of chest pain. Which of the following actions should the nurse anticipate as part of the MONA protocol?
   I. IV administration of magnesium sulfate
   II. IV administration of morphine sulfate
   III. IV administration of nitroglycerine
   IV. IV administration of acetaminophen

   a. Choices I and II
   b. Choices I, III, and IV
   c. Choices II and III
   d. Choices II, III, and IV

4. Which of the following statements made by the patient would cause the nurse to suspect an abdominal aortic aneurysm (AAA)?
   a. "I have indigestion when I lie down."
   b. "I often have a pulsating sensation in my abdomen."
   c. "I get fatigued and short of breath on exertion."
   d. "I have extreme pain radiating down my left arm."

5. The patient is admitted with a diagnosis of heart failure. Which assessment finding supports the diagnosis of left-sided heart failure?
   a. Pitting edema
   b. Ascites
   c. Fatigue
   d. Tachycardia

6. The patient with primary hypertension is being treated with medications to reduce blood volume and lower systemic vascular resistance. Which of the following medication combinations should the nurse anticipate for the patient?

    a. A diuretic and a calcium channel blocker (CCB)

    b. A diuretic and an angiotensin-converting enzyme (ACE) inhibitor

    c. An angiotensin II receptor blocker (ARB) and morphine

    d. A diuretic and a beta-blocker

7. Which of the following is a contraindication for thrombolytic therapy?

    a. Current anticoagulant therapy

    b. Over age 75

    c. Severe hepatic disease

    d. INR of 3.5

8. A patient is admitted with a diagnosis of heart block. The nurse is aware that the pacemaker of the heart is which of the following?

    a. AV node

    b. Purkinje fibers

    c. SA node

    d. Bundle of His

9. During an ECG, the nurse observes an abnormally lengthened PR interval (greater than 0.3). The nurse recognizes this finding as a characteristic of which of the following?

    a. Sinus rhythm

    b. Junctional rhythm

    c. Mobitz type I heart block

    d. Mobitz type II heart block

10. A patient walks into the emergency department and collapses. The nurse identifies the condition as cardiopulmonary arrest, and resuscitation efforts are started. The nurse understands that, in addition to CPR, defibrillation, and the ACLS protocol, the most important factor for patient survival is which of the following?

    a. Administration of oxygen

    b. Establishing IV access

    c. Inserting a Foley catheter

    d. Time between the collapse and the start of resuscitation efforts

11. A patient presents to the emergency department with the complaint of fever and shortness of breath. During the physical examination, the nurse observes a petechial rash on both hands and a recent nipple piercing on the right chest. The patient reports being on a corticosteroid for a respiratory infection. These findings alert the nurse to the possibility of which of the following?

    a. Endocarditis

    b. An autoimmune disease

    c. Pneumonia

    d. Heart failure

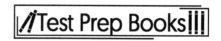

12. A patient with a known history of lupus presents to the emergency department complaining of chest pain. During the physical assessment, the nurse identifies a scratchy, squeaky sound at the end of exhalation. Which *next* action by the nurse indicates an understanding of the patient's presenting symptoms?

a. The nurse requests a breathing treatment for the patient.
b. The nurse auscultates at the left lower sternal border in the fourth intercostal space with the patient in the seated position.
c. The nurse establishes IV access.
d. The nurse auscultates at the left lower sternal border in the fourth intercostal space with the patient lying on his or her right side.

13. A patient is being discharged from the emergency department with the diagnosis of peripheral vascular disease with intermittent claudication. Which of the following information should be discussed with the patient prior to discharge?
    I. Avoid tight clothing.
    II. Wear compression stockings.
    III. Avoid airplane travel.
    IV. Minimize exercise.

a. Choices I and II
b. Choices I and III
c. Choices I, II, and III
d. All of the above

14. A patient involved in a motor vehicle accident (MVA) has sustained blunt nonpenetrating trauma to the chest. Upon arrival in the emergency department, the nurse observes asymmetrical chest rise. Which action(s) by the nurse indicate(s) an understanding of the presenting symptom?
    I. Preparation for placement of a chest drain.
    II. Assessment of oxygenation.
    III. Administration of pain medication.
    IV. Collection of a detailed medical history.

a. Choices II and III
b. Choices II, III, and IV
c. Choices I and III
d. Choices I and II

15. A patient who has sustained multiple trauma has arrived at the emergency department. Which of the following are the first two priority assessments, in the correct order?
    I. Respiratory rate and breath sounds
    II. Level of consciousness
    III. Airway patency

a. Choice I, then II
b. Choice I, then III
c. Choice III, then I
d. Choice III, then II

16. The patient with decreased level of consciousness is brought to the emergency department by EMS. During the assessment, the nurse observes mottled extremities and distant heart sounds. The nurse demonstrates an understanding of the physician's diagnosis of cardiogenic shock by anticipating which of the following?
    a. Arterial blood gas (ABG)
    b. Chest x-ray
    c. Angiogram
    d. Doppler study of the lower extremities

17. The nurse is receiving reports at the beginning of the shift. One of the patients has been admitted to the hospital and is awaiting transfer to the ICU with an admitting diagnosis of obstructive shock. Which of the following findings are characteristic of obstructive shock?
    a. Jugular vein distention, peripheral edema, and pulmonary congestion
    b. Decreased urine output, increased BUN, and increased creatinine
    c. Chest pain, fatigue, and lightheadedness
    d. Problems with coordination, blurred vision, and partial paralysis

18. The nurse understands that which of the following is the most concerning symptom associated with peripheral vascular disease (PVD)?
    a. Faint peripheral pulses
    b. Restricted mobility
    c. Critical limb ischemia
    d. Pale feet when elevated

19. A patient has had three separate blood pressure readings of 138/88, 132/80, and 135/89, respectively. The nurse anticipates the patient to be categorized by the physician as which of the following?
    a. Prehypertensive
    b. Normal
    c. Stage 1 hypertension
    d. Stage 2 hypertension

20. Which of the following patients is NOT at increased risk for the development of an embolism?
    a. A 24-year-old with a broken femur
    b. An 85-year-old female with a history of a stroke
    c. A 62-year-old male with first-degree heart block
    d. A 19-year-old female two weeks postpartum

Answer Explanations

1. A: Beck's triad of muffled heart sounds, distended neck veins, and hypotension are cardinal signs of cardiac tamponade. Chest pain and back pain are the most common presenting symptoms with an AAA. Heart function, breathing, and consciousness are not evident in cardiopulmonary arrest. Cardiogenic shock includes ashen, cyanotic, or mottled extremities; distant heart sounds; and rapid and faint peripheral pulses.

2. C: New onset of peripheral edema may be signaling decompensation by the right side of the heart and progressive heart failure. Oxygenation levels for CHF patients are generally lower but tolerated well. Ninety-two percent is an acceptable oxygen saturation level for this patient. Dyspnea upon exertion is not an unusual finding during a CHF exacerbation. Elevated BNP levels, although abnormal, are anticipated with CHF.

3. C: Morphine is part of the MONA protocol given for pain relief, while nitroglycerine is a vasodilator that reduces preload in the presence of chest pain. Magnesium sulfate is administrated for the Torsade de pointes dysrhythmia and is not part of the MONA protocol. Acetaminophen is not part of the MONA protocol.

4. B: An abdominal aneurysm may present or be found on examination as a pulsating mass in the abdomen. Indigestion when lying down is associated with gastrointestinal reflux disease (GERD) and is not indicative of an AAA. Fatigue and shortness of breath on exertion may be indicative of coronary artery or pulmonary disease. It is not directly associated with an AAA. Pain radiating down the left arm is a classic sign of a myocardial infarction (MI).

5. D: Symptoms of left-sided heart failure are tachycardia, shortness of breath, and the expectoration of frothy pink sputum. Pitting edema is symptomatic of right-sided heart failure and increased venous pressure that backs up into the tissues, causing edema. Ascites is a result of diffuse congestion in the liver caused by the increased venous pressure that characterizes right-sided heart failure. Fatigue is a generalized symptom not associated with the diagnosis of either right- or left-sided heart failure.

6. B: The diuretic reduces blood volume, and the ACE inhibitor reduces SVR by interfering with the RAAS. A CCB works by increasing myocardial contractility; therefore, Choice *A* is incorrect. Choice *C* is incorrect because an ARB reduces systemic vascular resistance, but morphine is used to treat pain. Choice *D* is also incorrect because a beta-blocker increases myocardial contractility.

7. D: An INR of 3.5 is elevated and will cause bleeding complications if thrombolytic therapy is initiated before the INR returns to the normal level of less than or equal to 1.1.

8. C: The SA, or sinoatrial, node is the heart's natural pacemaker. The AV node, which is positioned between the atria and ventricle, receives the impulse from the SA node. The Purkinje fibers are the end points of the conduction system. These fibers spread out across the ventricles after receiving the impulse through the Bundle of His. The Bundle of His receives the impulse from the AV node.

9. C: In second-degree heart block, specifically Mobitz type I, the PR interval is lengthened and greater than 0.20. The PR interval for a normal sinus rhythm is 0.12–0.20. In a junctional rhythm, the impulse is starting at the AV node, so the P wave is absent. In Mobitz type II second-degree heart block, the P waves are not followed by the QRS complex. The atria and ventricles are asynchronously contracting.

10. D: Time between the collapse and the start of resuscitation efforts is the most important factor in patient survival. Administering supplemental oxygen and establishing IV access are essential components of resuscitation efforts. Inserting a Foley catheter to drain the urinary bladder is not related to survival.

11. A: Fever and petechial rash are signs of endocarditis. Body piercings and corticosteroids are among the risk factors for developing endocarditis. Autoimmune conditions vary, but the most frequent presenting symptoms are fatigue and body aches. Pneumonia presents with fever, chills, and cough. Heart failure (HF) is not associated with a petechial rash or a fever.

12. B: A pericardial friction rub is a scratchy, squeaky sound heard at the end of exhalation. It is indicative of pericarditis. It is best heard at the left lower sternal border in the fourth intercostal space while the patient is seated. The best *next* action for the nurse to take is to reposition the patient and the stethoscope. A breathing treatment is needed when oxygen saturations are low and in the presence of wheezing. The nurse needs more information to confirm the suspicion of a pericarditis. Establishing IV access is important but not the next action to be taken. A pericardial friction rub is best heard when the patient is seated, not lying down.

13. A: Avoiding tight clothing and wearing compression stockings are appropriate. Although prolonged sitting should be avoided, airplane travel itself is not contraindicated. Exercise should be continued with frequent rest periods as needed. The occurrence and severity of claudication can be decreased with regular exercise.

14. D: Hypoventilation and hypoxia are the primary causes of death in chest trauma. Assessing oxygenation and preparing for placement of a chest drain to alleviate a possible hemothorax or pneumothorax are the correct first actions. Pain medication is secondary to ensuring airway, breathing, and circulation. A medical history is important, but it is secondary to the lifesaving interventions.

15. C: For the ABCD of primary survey, airway patency is the first priority assessment, followed by respiration rate and breath sounds. Assessing the level of consciousness is secondary to establishing and maintaining a patent's airway.

16. C: An angiogram to restore coronary blood flow is the priority treatment for cardiogenic shock. ABGs, a chest x-ray, and a Doppler study are not treatments; they are diagnostic tools.

17. A: Jugular vein distention, peripheral edema, and pulmonary congestion are characteristics of blood volume backing up due to an obstruction. Decreased urine output, increased BUN, and increased creatinine are signs of renal failure. Chest pain, fatigue, and lightheadedness are signs of an MI. Problems with coordination, blurred vision, and paralysis are symptomatic of a stroke.

18. C: Critical limb ischemia (CLI) is the most concerning symptom of PVD. It is indicative of decreased circulation even at rest. Faint peripheral pulses may be a finding associated with PVD, but are not the most concerning symptom. Restricted mobility may be a sequela to PVD, but it is also not the most concerning. Feet that become pale when elevated are a symptom of PVD, but this is not the most concerning symptom.

19. A: Prehypertension is defined as systolic pressures ranging between 120 and 139 mmHg or diastolic pressures between 80 and 89 mmHg. Normal blood pressure is less than 120/80 mmHg. Stage 1 hypertension ranges from 140 to 159 mmHg systolic or 90 to 99 mmHg diastolic. Stage 2 hypertension is greater than or equal to 160 mmHg systolic or greater than or equal to 100 mmHg diastolic.

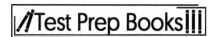

20. C: A first-degree heart block is NOT a direct risk factor for the development of an embolus. Women during pregnancy and in the postpartum period, individuals with a history of a previous stroke, and patients with fractures that involve long bones are all at risk for the development of am embolus.

Respiratory Emergencies

Aspiration

There are four types of respiratory aspiration that can result in aspiration pneumonitis, pneumonia, or an acute respiratory emergency. The aspiration of gastric contents often causes a chemical pneumonitis. Infective organisms from the oropharynx can result in aspiration pneumonia. Depending on its size and composition, the aspiration of a foreign body can result in a respiratory emergency or bacterial pneumonia. Rarely, aspiration of mineral or vegetable oil can cause an exogenous lipoid pneumonia.

Aspiration Pneumonitis/Pneumonia

Respiratory aspiration is the abnormal entry of foreign substances (such as food, drink, saliva, or vomitus) into the lungs as a person swallows. This is normally prevented by the epiglottis, a flap of cartilage that pulls forward and forces substances into the esophagus and digestive tract. If inoculum is inhaled into the lungs, it can (depending on the amount) lead to aspiration pneumonitis/pneumonia. Aspiration pneumonia often results from a primary bacterial infection, while aspiration pneumonitis (which is non-infectious) results from aspiration of the acidic gastric contents.

Risk factors for aspiration pneumonitis/pneumonia are altered or reduced consciousness and a poor gag reflex. These risk factors are associated with the following conditions:

- Excessive alcohol and/or drugs
- Stroke
- Seizures
- Dysphagia
- Head trauma
- General anesthesia
- Critical illness
- Dementia
- Intracranial mass lesion
- Multiple sclerosis
- Pseudobulbar palsy
- Myasthenia gravis
- Gastroesophageal reflux disease (GERD)
- Use of H_2 antagonists, H_2 blockers, or proton pump inhibitors
- Bronchoscopy
- Endotracheal intubation
- Tracheostomy
- Upper endoscopy
- Nasogastric (NG) tube
- Feeding tubes

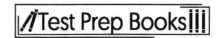

Signs and symptoms of aspiration pneumonitis/pneumonia include:

- Fever
- Cyanosis
- Wheezing
- Dyspnea
- Tachypnea
- Tachycardia
- Rales
- Hypoxia
- Altered mental status
- Hypotension
- Decreased breath sounds
- Fatigue
- Cough with discolored phlegm
- Chest pain
- Hypothermia (possible in older patients)
- Pleuritic chest pain

The diagnosis of aspiration pneumonitis/pneumonia is based upon: a chest x-ray revealing pulmonary infiltrates; an arterial blood gas (ABG) analysis consistent with hypoxemia; a complete blood count (CBC) with an elevated white blood cell count (WBC) with neutrophils predominating; and other clinical findings. Infiltrates are most commonly found in the right, lower lobe of the lung, but can be found in other lobes, depending on an individual's position at the time of aspiration. If possible, a sputum specimen for culture, sensitivity, and gram stain should be collected before beginning antibiotic therapy. In addition, blood cultures should be obtained, as indicated.

Treatment of aspiration pneumonitis/pneumonia includes:

- Suctioning of the upper airway as needed to remove the aspirate
- Oxygen supplementation
- Pulse oximetry
- Cardiac monitoring
- Antibiotics (only if symptoms fail to resolve within 48 hours)
- Supportive care with intravenous fluids (IVFs) and electrolyte replacement
- For those with severe respiratory distress, possible intubation and mechanical ventilation
- NG drainage to avoid gastric distention (in the ventilated patient)

Foreign Body Aspiration

Foreign body aspiration is a respiratory emergency. A foreign body can lodge in the larynx or trachea causing varying degrees of airway obstruction. Complete airway obstruction can quickly lead to asphyxia and death. The most commonly aspirated object is food. Other frequently aspirated objects include nuts, nails, seeds, coins, pins, small toys, needles, bone fragments, and dental appliances. In children and adolescents, aspirated foreign bodies are found with equal frequency on either side of the lungs. In adults, they are most often found in the right lung because of the acute angle of the right mainstem bronchus.

Signs and symptoms of foreign body aspiration include:

- Coughing
- Wheezing
- Decreased breath sounds
- Dyspnea
- Choking
- Cyanosis
- Hemoptysis
- Chest pain
- Asphyxia (with complete airway obstruction)
- Inability to speak (with complete airway obstruction)

As more time elapses, local inflammation and edema can worsen the airway obstruction. This also makes removing the foreign body more difficult and the lung more likely to bleed with manipulation.

Foreign body aspiration can be diagnosed using a chest x-ray or a computed tomography (CT) scan. Less than 20% of all aspirated foreign bodies are radiopaque. A CT scan can provide information about the anatomic location, composition, shape, size, and extent of edema associated with the aspirated foreign body. ABG analysis can reveal hypoxemia. Bronchoscopy (rigid or flexible) can be diagnostic as well as therapeutic.

Treatment of foreign body aspiration can include:

- Heimlich maneuver for acute choking with total airway obstruction by foreign body
- Foreign body extraction via bronchoscopy (rigid or flexible)
- Surgical bronchotomy or segmental lung resection (rarely required)
- Antibiotics for secondary pneumonia or other respiratory infection
- Oxygen supplementation
- Symptomatic respiratory support

Since the likelihood of complications increases after 24 to 48 hours, prompt extraction of the foreign body is critical. Complications can include mediastinitis, atelectasis, pneumonia, tracheoesophageal fistulas, or bronchiectasis.

Asthma

Status Asthmaticus

Status asthmaticus is an acute episode of worsening asthma that's unresponsive to treatment with bronchodilators. Even after increasing their bronchodilator use to every few minutes, individuals still experience no relief. Status asthmaticus represents a respiratory emergency that can lead to respiratory failure. Airway inflammation, bronchospasm, and mucus plugging highlight the condition. Common triggers include exposure to an allergen or irritant, viral respiratory illness, and exercise in cold weather. Status asthmaticus is more common among individuals of low socioeconomic status, regardless of race.

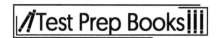

The main symptoms of status asthmaticus are wheezing, cough, and dyspnea; however, severe airway obstruction can result in a "silent chest" without audible wheezes. This can be a sign of impending respiratory failure. Other signs and symptoms of status asthmaticus include:

- Chest tightness or pain
- Tachypnea
- Tachycardia
- Cyanosis
- Use of accessory respiratory muscles
- Inability to speak more than one or two words at a time
- Altered mental status
- Pulsus paradoxus >20mm Hg
- Syncope
- Hypoxemia
- Hypercapnia
- Retractions and the use of abdominal muscles to breathe
- Hypertension
- Seizures (late sign)
- Bradycardia (late sign)
- Hypotension (late sign)
- Agitation (late sign)

Useful tests for the diagnosis of status asthmaticus include:

- Chest x-ray (for the exclusion of pneumonia, pneumothorax, and CHF)

- ABG analysis can be diagnostic as well as therapeutic (tracking response to treatment measures). Assess cost/benefit for children due to pain associated with ABG sampling.

- CBC with differential can reveal an elevated WBC count with left shift (possible indication of a microbial infection)

- Peak flow measurement can be diagnostic as well as therapeutic (tracking response to treatment measures)

- Pulse oximetry provides continuous measurement of O_2 saturation. Reading is affected by decreased peripheral perfusion, anemia, and movement.

- Blood glucose levels, stress, and therapeutic medications can lead to hyperglycemia. Younger children may exhibit hypoglycemia.

- Blood electrolyte levels (therapeutic medications can lead to hypokalemia)

Intubation and mechanical ventilation should be used with extreme caution in individuals with status asthmaticus. It's usually considered a therapy of last resort due to its inherent dangers: air trapping leading to an increased risk for barotrauma (especially pneumothorax); decreased cardiac output; and increasing bronchospasm. Mechanical ventilation of individuals with status asthmaticus often requires controlled hypoventilation with low tidal volumes, prolonged exhalation times, low respiratory rates, and tolerance of permissive hypercapnia. The majority of individuals needing mechanical ventilation can be extubated within 72 hours.

Supportive Treatment

- O_2 therapy to maintain O_2 saturation > 92%; non-rebreathing mask can deliver 98% O_2
- Hydration
- Correction of electrolyte abnormalities
- Antibiotics only with evidence of concurrent infective process

Pharmacological Agents Used for Acute Asthma

Various classes of pharmacological agents are used for the treatment and control of status asthmaticus. The following discussion concentrates on pharmacological agents to treat and control acute asthma rather than chronic asthma. Urgent care of asthma can include the following:

Beta-2 Adrenergic Agonists (Beta-2 Agonists)

Short-acting preparations of Beta-2 agonists are the first line of therapy for the treatment of status asthmaticus. These medications relax the muscles in the airways, resulting in bronchodilation (expanding of the bronchial air passages) and increased airflow to the lungs. It is important to remember that one of the underlying factors in asthma is bronchoconstriction. Albuterol is the most commonly used short-acting Beta-2 agonist. Dosing for acute asthma is 2.5 mg to 5 mg once, then 2.5 mg every twenty minutes for 3 doses via nebulizer, and finally 2.5 mg to 10 mg every one to four hours as needed.

Adverse effects of albuterol include tachycardia, tremors, and anxiety. Another short-acting Beta-2 agonist used to treat acute asthma is levalbuterol (Xopenex™). This medication is related to albuterol and has the same result, but without the adverse effects. Dosage for acute asthma is 1.25 mg to 2.5 mg every twenty minutes for 3 doses, then 1.25 mg to 5 mg every one to four hours as needed. However, it must be noted that the frequent use of adrenergic agents prior to receiving emergency care can decrease a patient's response to these medications in a hospital setting.

Anticholinergics

These medications block the action of the neurotransmitter acetylcholine which, in turn, causes bronchodilation. Anticholinergics can also increase the bronchodilating effects of short-acting Beta-2 agonists. The most commonly used anticholinergic is ipatroprium (Atrovent™), which is used in combination with short-acting Beta-2 agonists for the treatment of status asthmaticus. Dosing for acute asthma is 2.5 mL (500 mcg) every twenty minutes for 3 doses via nebulizer, then as needed. Adverse effects can include dry mouth, blurred vision, and constipation.

Corticosteroids

Corticosteroids are potent anti-inflammatory medications that fight the inflammation accompanying asthma. Corticosteroids commonly used in the treatment of status asthmaticus include prednisone, prednisolone, and methylprednisolone. Methylprednisolone (Solu-Medrol™) is administered once in doses of 60 mg to 125 mg intravenously (IV) in cases of status asthmaticus and then followed by a taper of oral prednisone over seven to ten days. The intravenous administration of corticosteroids is equal in effectiveness to oral corticosteroid administration. Corticosteroids have numerous adverse effects, and they should not be used for more than two weeks. Adverse effects of long-term corticosteroid use can include weight gain, osteoporosis, thinning of skin, cataracts, easy bruising, and diabetes. Therefore, it is

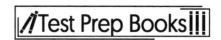

necessary to monitor blood glucose routinely and use regular insulin on a sliding scale. Electrolytes (particularly potassium) must also be monitored.

Methylxanthines

These medications are used as bronchodilators and as adjuncts to Beta-2 agonists and corticosteroids in treating status asthmaticus. The primary methylxanthines are theophylline and aminophylline. At therapeutic doses, methylxanthines are much weaker bronchodilators than Beta-2 agonists. The adverse effects of methylxanthines can include nausea, vomiting, tachycardia, headaches, and seizures. As a result, therapeutic monitoring is mandatory. Therapeutic levels of theophylline range from 10 mcg/mL to 20 mcg/mL. Dosing of theophylline is a loading dose of 6 mg/kg, followed by a maintenance dose of 1 mg/kg/h IV. Methylxanthines aren't frequently used to treat status asthmaticus because of their possible adverse effects and the need for close monitoring of drug blood levels.

Magnesium Sulfate

Magnesium sulfate is a calcium antagonist that relaxes smooth muscle in the lung passages leading to bronchodilation. Clinical studies indicate it can be used as an adjunct to Beta-2 agonist therapy during status asthmaticus. A dose of 30 mg/kg to 70 mg/kg is administered by IV over 20 to 30 minutes. It is given slowly to prevent adverse effects such as bradycardia and hypotension. The use of magnesium sulfate is controversial.

Leukotriene Inhibitors

These medications target inflammation related to asthma. Typically used for the long-term control of asthma, a minority of individuals with status asthmaticus may respond to this class of medication. The primary leukotriene inhibitors used in the treatment of asthma are zafirlukast (Accolate™) and zileuton (Zyflo™). Zafirlukast can be administered orally in doses of 10 mg to 20 mg twice daily. Zileuton can be administered in a dose of 600 mg four times daily. Adverse effects of leukotriene inhibitors include headache, rash, fatigue, dizziness, and abdominal pain.

Heliox

Heliox, administered via face mask, is a mixture of helium and oxygen that can help relieve airway obstruction associated with status asthmaticus. Benefits of heliox include decreased work of breathing, decreased carbon dioxide production, and decreased muscle fatigue. It can only be used in individuals able to take a deep breath or while on mechanical ventilation. The 80/20 mixture of helium to oxygen has been the most effective in clinical trials. One limitation to using heliox is the amount of supplemental oxygen required by an individual suffering from status asthmaticus. Heliox loses its clinical efficacy when the fraction of inspired oxygen (FiO_2) is greater than 40%. No significant adverse effects have been reported with heliox.

Chronic Obstructive Pulmonary Disease (COPD)

Chronic Obstructive Pulmonary Disease (COPD) is characterized by an airflow obstruction that's not fully reversible. It's usually progressive and is associated with an abnormal inflammatory response in the lungs. The primary cause of COPD is exposure to tobacco smoke, and is one of the leading causes of death in the United States. COPD includes chronic bronchitis, emphysema, or a combination of both. Though asthma is part of the classic triad of obstructive lung diseases, it is not part of COPD. However, someone with COPD can have an asthma component to their disease. Chronic bronchitis is described as a chronic productive cough for three or more months during each of two consecutive years. Emphysema is the abnormal enlargement of alveoli (air sacs) with accompanying destruction of their walls. Signs and symptoms of COPD can include:

- Dyspnea
- Wheezing
- Cough (usually worse in the morning and that produces sputum/phlegm)
- Cyanosis
- Chest tightness
- Fever
- Tachypnea
- Orthopnea
- Use of accessory respiratory muscles
- Elevated jugular venous pressure (JVP)
- Barrel chest
- Pursed lip breathing
- Altered mental status

A diagnosis of COPD can be made through pulmonary function tests (PFTs), a chest x-ray, blood chemistries, ABG analysis, or a CT scan. A formal diagnosis of COPD can be made through a PFT known as spirometry, which measures lung function. PFTs measure the ratio of forced expiratory volume in one second over forced vital capacity (FEV_1/FVC) and should normally be between 60% and 90%. Values below 60% usually indicate a problem. The other diagnostic tests mentioned are useful in determining the acuity and severity of exacerbations of the disease. In acute exacerbations of COPD, ABG analysis can reveal respiratory acidosis, hypoxemia, and hypercapnia. Generally, a pH less than 7.3 indicates acute respiratory compromise. Compensatory metabolic alkalosis may develop in response to chronic respiratory acidosis. A chest x-ray can show flattening of the diaphragm and increased retrosternal air space (both indicative of hyperinflation), cardiomegaly, and increased bronchovascular markings. Blood chemistries can suggest sodium retention or hypokalemia. A CT scan is more sensitive and specific than a standard chest x-ray for diagnosing emphysema.

Treatment for acute exacerbations of COPD can include oxygen supplementation, short-acting Beta-2 agonists, anticholinergics, corticosteroids, and antibiotics. Oxygen should be titrated to achieve an oxygen saturation of at least 90%. Short-acting Beta-2 agonists (albuterol or levalbuterol) administered via nebulizer can improve dyspnea associated with COPD. The anticholinergic medication ipratroprium, administered via nebulizer, can be added as an adjunct to Beta-2 agonists. Short courses of corticosteroids can be given orally or intravenously. In clinical trials, the administration of oral corticosteroids in the early stage of a COPD exacerbation decreased the need for hospitalization. Also in clinical trials, the use of antibiotics was found to decrease the risk of treatment failure and death in individuals with a moderate to severe exacerbation of COPD.

Infections

Bronchiolitis

Bronchiolitis is inflammation of the bronchioles (the small airways in the lungs) and is most commonly caused by respiratory syncytial virus (RSV). It typically affects children under the age of two, with a peak onset of three to six months of age. The disease is spread through direct contact with respiratory droplets. Bronchiolitis results in hospitalization of approximately 2% of children, the majority of which

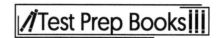

are under six months of age. Criteria for hospitalization can include prematurity, under three months of age, diagnosis of a congenital heart defect, respiratory rate >70-80 bpm, inability to maintain oral hydration, and cyanosis.

Signs and symptoms of bronchiolitis include:

- Difficulty feeding
- Fever
- Congestion
- Cough
- Dyspnea
- Tachypnea
- Nasal flaring
- Tachycardia
- Wheezing
- Fine rales
- Hypoxia
- Retractions
- Apnea

A diagnosis of bronchiolitis is usually established through a clinical examination. The most common diagnostic tests for the disease are: a rapid, viral antigen test of nasopharyngeal secretions for RSV; white blood cell (WBC) count with differential; ABG analysis; a chest x-ray; and a test of C-reactive protein (a marker of inflammation).

Although highly contagious, the disease is self-limiting and typically resolves without complication in one to two weeks. Treatment of bronchiolitis is supportive and can include oxygen supplementation, maintenance of hydration, fever reducers, nasal and oral suctioning, and intubation and mechanical ventilation.

Croup and Other Infections

Acute Laryngotracheobronchitis

Acute laryngotracheobronchitis, or classic croup, is a common viral illness in children. It results in inflammation of the larynx, trachea, and occasionally the bronchi. As a result, croup can be life-threatening in some children. Croup is primarily a disease of infants and toddlers, peaking between the ages of six months and three years. It rarely occurs after age six. The most common cause of croup is the parainfluenza viruses (types 1, 2, and 3), accounting for approximately 80% of the diagnosed cases. Other viral causes include adenovirus, rhinovirus, RSV, enterovirus, coronavirus, echovirus, and influenza A and B.

Croup is the most common pediatric ailment that causes stridor, an abnormal, high-pitched breath sound indicating partial or complete airway obstruction. Other signs and symptoms of the disease can include:

- Barking cough
- Pharyngitis
- Rhinorrhea
- Wheezing
- Tachypnea
- Tachycardia
- Fever
- Cyanosis
- Agitation
- Hypoxemia
- Respiratory failure

Croup is primarily a clinical diagnosis that relies on clues from the patient history and physical examination. In children, a chest x-ray occasionally reveals the "steeple sign," which indicates airway narrowing at the level of the glottis.

Treatment of croup can include:

- Corticosteroids, especially dexamethasone administered intravenously (IV), intramuscularly (IM), or orally (PO)

- Nebulized racemic epinephrine (typically reserved for hospital use; effects last only one and a half to two hours and require observation for at least three hours after dose)

- Cool mist (once the mainstay of treatment, but little evidence supports its clinical utility)

- Intubation and mechanical ventilation (for severe cases)

Acute Epiglottitis

Acute epiglottitis (also known as supraglottitis) is inflammation of the epiglottis. The epiglottis is the small piece of cartilage that's pulled forward to cover the windpipe when a person swallows. The cause of the condition is usually bacterial, with **Haemophilus influenzae** type B being the most common. Other bacterial causes include **Streptococcus pneumoniae**, **Streptococcus** groups A, B, and C, and non-typeable **Haemophilus influenzae**. The disease is most commonly diagnosed in children, but can be seen in adolescents and adults. A decline in the number of cases of acute epiglottitis has been noted since the introduction of the **Haemophilus influenzae** type B (Hib) vaccine in the 1980s.

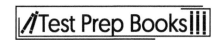

Acute epiglottitis is usually accompanied by the classic triad of symptoms: dysphagia, drooling, and respiratory distress. Other signs and symptoms can include:

- Fever
- Sore throat
- Inability to lay flat
- Voice changes (can be muffled or hoarse)
- Tripod breathing position (a position said to optimize the mechanics of breathing where an individual sits up on their hands, head leaning forward, and tongue protruding)
- Tachypnea
- Hypoxia
- Agitation
- Cyanosis

Direct visualization of the epiglottis via a nasopharyngoscopy/laryngoscopy is the gold standard for diagnosing acute epiglottitis since an infected epiglottis has a cherry red appearance.

Acute epiglottitis is a potentially life-threatening medical emergency and should be treated promptly. It can quickly progress to total obstruction of the airway and death. Treatment of the condition can include:

- IV antibiotics (after blood and epiglottic cultures have been obtained)

- Analgesic-antipyretic agents such as aspirin, acetaminophen, and nonsteroidal anti-inflammatory drugs (NSAIDs), such as ibuprofen

- Intubation with mechanical ventilation, tracheostomy, or needle-jet insufflation (options for immediate airway management, if needed)

- Racemic epinephrine, corticosteroids, and Beta-2 agonists are also sometimes used; however, they have yet to been proven as useful treatments

Acute Tracheitis

A rare condition, acute tracheitis, is the inflammation and infection of the trachea (windpipe). The majority of cases occur in children under the age of sixteen. The etiology of acute tracheitis is predominantly bacterial, with **Staphylococcus aureus** being the leading cause. Community-associated, methicillin-resistant **Staphylococcus aureus** (CA-MRSA) has recently emerged as an important causative agent. Other bacterial causes of acute tracheitis include **Streptococcus pneumoniae**, **Haemophilus influenzae**, and **Moraxella catarrhalis**.

Acute tracheitis is often preceded by an upper respiratory infection (URI). Signs and symptoms of acute tracheitis can include:

- Bark-like cough
- Dyspnea
- Fever
- Tachypnea
- Respiratory distress
- Stridor
- Wheezing
- Hoarseness
- Nasal flaring
- Cyanosis

The only definitive means of diagnosis is the use of a laryngotracheobronchoscopy to directly visualize mucopurulent membranes lining the mucosa of the trachea. Additional tests can include pulse oximetry, blood cultures, nasopharyngeal and tracheal cultures, and neck x-rays.

Treatment of acute tracheitis should be prompt because of the increased likelihood of complete airway obstruction leading to respiratory arrest and death. Treatment can include:

- IV antibiotics (if living in an area with high or increasing rates of CA-MRSA, the addition of vancomycin should be considered)

- Intubation and mechanical ventilation or tracheostomy (rarely needed) are options if immediate airway management is needed

- Fever reducers

Viral Pneumonia

Viral pneumonia is more common at the extremes of age (young children and the elderly). It accounts for the majority of cases of childhood pneumonia. Cases of viral pneumonia have been increasing over the past decade, mostly as a result of immunosuppression (weakened immune system). Common causes of viral pneumonia in children, the elderly, and the immunocompromised are the influenza viruses (most common), RSV, parainfluenza virus, and adenovirus.

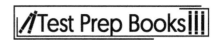

Signs and symptoms of viral pneumonia largely overlap those of bacterial pneumonia and can include:

- Cough (nonproductive)
- Fever/chills
- Myalgias
- Fatigue
- Headache
- Dyspnea
- Tachypnea
- Tachycardia
- Wheezing
- Cyanosis
- Hypoxia
- Decreased breath sounds
- Respiratory distress

Viral pneumonia is diagnosed via a chest x-ray and viral cultures. The chest x-ray usually reveals bilateral lung infiltrates, instead of the lobar involvement commonly seen in bacterial causes. Viral cultures can take up to two weeks to confirm the diagnosis. Rapid antigen testing and gene amplification via polymerase chain reaction (PCR) have been recently incorporated into the diagnostic mix to shorten the diagnosis lag.

Treatment of viral pneumonia is usually supportive and can include:

- Supplemental oxygen
- Rest
- Antipyretics
- Analgesics
- Intravenous fluids
- Parenteral nutrition
- Intubation and mechanical ventilation

Specific causes of viral pneumonia can benefit from treatment with antiviral medications. Influenza pneumonia can be treated with oseltamivir (Tamiflu®) or zanamivir (Relenza®). Ribavirin® is the only effective antiviral agent for the treatment of RSV pneumonia.

Acute Respiratory Tract Infections

Acute Bronchitis
Acute bronchitis is inflammation of the bronchial tubes (bronchi), which extend from the trachea to the lungs. It is one of the top five reasons for visits to healthcare providers and can take from ten days to three weeks to resolve. Common causes of acute bronchitis include respiratory viruses (such as influenza A and B), RSV, parainfluenza, adenovirus, rhinovirus, and coronavirus. Bacterial causes include **Mycoplasma** species, **Streptococcus pneumoniae**, **Chlamydia pneumoniae**, **Haemophilus influenzae**, and **Moraxella catarrhalis**. Other causes of acute bronchitis are irritants such as chemicals, pollution, and tobacco smoke.

Signs and symptoms of acute bronchitis can include:

- Cough (most common symptom) with or without sputum
- Fever
- Sore throat
- Headache
- Nasal congestion
- Rhinorrhea
- Dyspnea
- Fatigue
- Myalgia
- Chest pain
- Wheezing

Acute bronchitis is typically diagnosed by exclusion, which means tests are used to exclude more serious conditions such as pneumonia, epiglottitis, or COPD. Useful diagnostic tests include a CBC with differential, a chest x-ray, respiratory and blood cultures, PFTs, bronchoscopy, laryngoscopy, and a procalcitonin (PCT) test to determine if the infection is bacterial.

Treatment of acute bronchitis is primarily supportive and can include:

- Bedrest
- Cough suppressants, such as codeine or dextromethorphan
- Beta-2 agonists, such as albuterol for wheezing
- Nonsteroidal anti-inflammatory drugs (NSAIDs) for pain
- Expectorants, such as guaifenesin

Although acute bronchitis should not be routinely treated with antibiotics, there are exceptions to this rule. It's reasonable to use an antibiotic when an existing medical condition poses a risk of serious complications. Antibiotic use is also reasonable for treating acute bronchitis in elderly patients who have been hospitalized in the past year, have been diagnosed with congestive heart failure (CHF) or diabetes, or are currently being treated with a steroid.

Pneumonia

Pneumonia is an infection that affects the functional tissue of the lung. Microscopically, it is characterized by consolidating lung tissue with exudate, fibrin, and inflammatory cells filling the alveoli (air sacs). Pneumonia can represent a primary disease or a secondary disease (e.g., post-obstructive pneumonia due to lung cancer), and the most common causes of pneumonia are bacteria and viruses. Other causes of pneumonia include fungi and parasites.

Pneumonia can be categorized according to its anatomic distribution on a chest x-ray or the setting in which it is acquired. Pneumonia categorized according to its anatomic distribution on chest x-ray can be:

- Lobar: Limited to one lobe of the lungs. It can affect more than one lobe on the same side (multilobar pneumonia) or bilateral lobes ("double" pneumonia).

- Bronchopneumonia: Scattered diffusely throughout the lungs

- Interstitial: Involving areas between the alveoli

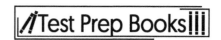

- Pneumonia categorized according to the setting in which it is acquired can be:

- Community-Acquired Pneumonia (CAP): Pneumonia in an individual who hasn't been recently hospitalized, or its occurrence in less than 48 hours after admission to a hospital.

- Hospital-Acquired (Nosocomial) Pneumonia: Pneumonia acquired during or after hospitalization for another ailment with onset at least 48 hours or more after admission.

- Aspiration Pneumonia: Pneumonia resulting from the inhalation of gastric or oropharyngeal secretions.

Community-Acquired Pneumonia (CAP)

Common causes of community-acquired pneumonia (CAP) include:

- *Streptococcus pneumoniae*

- *Haemophilus influenzae*

- *Moraxella catarrhalis*

- Atypical organisms (such as *Legionella* species, *Mycoplasma pneumoniae*, and *Chlamydia pneumoniae*)

- *Staphylococcus aureus*

- Respiratory viruses

Streptococcus Pneumoniae

Streptococcus pneumoniae (also known as **S. pneumoniae** or pneumococcus) is a gram-positive bacterium and the most common cause of CAP. Due to the introduction of a pneumococcal vaccine in 2000, cases of pneumococcal pneumonia have decreased. However, medical providers should be aware there is now evidence of emerging, antibiotic-resistant strains of the organism. Signs and symptoms of pneumococcal pneumonia can include:

- Cough productive of rust-colored sputum (mucus)
- Fever with or without chills
- Dyspnea
- Wheezing
- Chest pain
- Tachypnea
- Altered mental status
- Tachycardia
- Rales over involved lung
- Increase in tactile fremitus
- E to A change
- Hypotension
- Lung consolidation

Diagnosis of pneumococcal pneumonia can include:

- CBC with differential
- Chest x-ray
- CT scan (if underlying lung cancer is suspected)
- Sputum gram stain and/or culture
- Blood cultures
- Procalcitonin and C-reactive protein blood level tests
- Sputum, serum, and/or urinary antigen tests
- Immunoglobulin studies
- Bronchoscopy with bronchoalveolar lavage (BAL)

Treatment of pneumococcal pneumonia can include:

- Antibiotics, such as ceftriaxone plus doxycycline, or azithromycin

- Respiratory quinolones, such as levofloxacin (Levaquin®), moxifloxacin (Avelox®), or gemifloxacin (Factive®)

- Supplemental oxygen

- Beta-2 agonists, such as albuterol via nebulizer or metered-dose inhaler (MDI), as needed for wheezing

- Analgesics and antipyretics

- Chest physiotherapy

- Active suctioning of respiratory secretions

- Intubation and mechanical ventilation

Mycoplasma Pneumoniae

Mycoplasma pneumoniae, also known as **M. pneumoniae**, is a bacterium that causes atypical CAP. It is one of the most common causes of CAP in healthy individuals under the age of forty. The most common symptom of mycoplasmal pneumonia is a dry, nonproductive cough. Other signs and symptoms can include diarrhea, earache, fever (usually ≤ 102 °F), sore throat, myalgias, nasal congestion, skin rash, and general malaise. Chest x-rays of individuals with mycoplasmal pneumonia reveal a pattern of bronchopneumonia. Cold agglutinin titers in the blood can be significantly elevated (> 1:64). Polymerase chain reaction (PCR) is becoming the standard confirmatory test for mycoplasmal pneumonia, though currently it is not used in most clinical settings. Other diagnostic tests for **M. pneumoniae** are usually nonspecific and therefore do not aid in its diagnosis.

Treatments for mycoplasmal pneumonia are no different than for CAP, except for antibiotic choices, which include:

- Macrolide antibiotics, such as erythromycin, azithromycin (Zithromax®), clarithromycin (Biaxin®, Biaxin XL®)

- Doxycycline (a tetracycline antibiotic derivative)

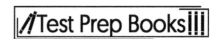

Methicillin-Resistant Staphylococcus Aureus

Community-Acquired Methicillin-Resistant **Staphylococcus aureus** (CA-MRSA) has emerged as a significant cause of CAP over the past twenty years. It also remains a significant cause of hospital-acquired pneumonia. The majority (up to 75%) of those diagnosed with CA-MRSA pneumonia are young, previously healthy individuals with influenza as a preceding illness. Symptoms are usually identical to those seen with other causes of CAP. Chest x-ray typically reveals multilobar involvement with or without cavitation/necrosis. Gram staining of sputum and/or blood can reveal gram-positive bacteria in clusters. Other diagnostic tests are nonspecific and do not aid in the diagnosis of CA-MRSA pneumonia.

Treatment of CA-MRSA should be prompt as it has a high mortality rate. Supportive measures are needed as in other cases of CAP. CA-MRSA is notoriously resistant to most antibiotics with the exception of the following:

- Vancomycin: The mainstay and only treatment for CA-MSRA pneumonia for many years (unfortunately with a disappointing cure rate). A loading dose of 25 mg/kg (max 2,000 mg) is needed with a maintenance dose based on creatinine clearance and body weight (in kg). Vancomycin trough should be drawn prior to fourth dose with a target goal of 15-20 mcg/mL (mg/L).

- Linezolid: An alternative to vancomycin and quickly becoming the agent of choice for the treatment of CA-MRSA pneumonia. It is administered 600 mg PO/IV every twelve hours.

Inhalation Injuries

Gases and vapors are the most common causes of lung inhalation injuries. This is because inhaled substances cause direct injury to respiratory epithelium. Exposure to accidental chemical spills, fires, and explosions can all lead to lung inhalation injuries. Some of the more common pulmonary irritants and gases include smoke, ozone, chlorine (Cl_2), hydrogen chloride (HCl), ammonia (NH_3), hydrogen fluoride (HF), sulfur dioxide (SO_2), and nitrogen oxides. The degree of inhalation injury is dependent on such factors as:

- Specific gas or substance inhaled
- Presence of soot
- Degree of exposure
- Presence of underlying lung disease
- Inability to flee the area

Inhalation injuries can even occur when there are no skin burns or other visible, external signs of exposure. Therefore, medical professionals should maintain a high level of suspicion when it comes to inhalation injuries, watching for signs and symptoms that can include:

- Tachypnea
- Dyspnea
- Facial burns
- Cough productive of carbonaceous sputum
- Wheezing
- Rhinitis
- Retractions
- Decreased breath sounds
- Hoarseness
- Blistering or swelling involving the mouth
- Singed nasal hairs
- Headache
- Vomiting
- Dizziness
- Change in mental status
- Coma

The best diagnostic tools for inhalation injuries are clinical presentation and findings from a bronchoscopy (the gold standard for diagnosing inhalation injuries). Other useful tests include:

- Chest x-ray
- CT scan
- Pulse oximetry
- ABG analysis
- Blood carboxyhemoglobin levels (for all fire and explosion victims)
- Pulmonary function tests (PFTs)

Inhalation injuries have an excellent prognosis since more than 90% of those affected make complete recoveries with no long-term pulmonary complications. However, depending on the injury source,

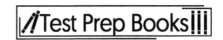

medical providers should be aware that respiratory function can deteriorate up to 36 hours post-injury. Treatment of inhalation injuries is largely supportive care, which can include:

- Supplemental oxygen (usually 100% humidified oxygen)
- IV fluids, especially in individuals with burns
- Inhaled bronchdilators for bronchospasm, such as albuterol
- Gentle respiratory suctioning
- Close observation of developing edema around the head and neck
- Mucolytic agents such as N-acetylcysteine (NAC)
- Hyperbaric oxygen therapy (specifically for carbon monoxide poisoning)
- Hydroxocobalamin (Cyanokit®) (preferred agent), sodium thiosulfate, or sodium nitrite for hydrogen cyanide (HCN) poisoning/toxicity
- Intubation and mechanical ventilation, tidal volume of 6 mL/kg recommended to reduce likelihood of barotrauma
- Monitoring for the onset of secondary pneumonia (commonly caused by *Staphylococcus aureus* and *Pseudomonas aeruginosa*)

Obstruction

Obstruction is a blockage in any part of the respiratory tract. The upper respiratory tract consists of the nose, paranasal sinuses, throat, and larynx. The lower respiratory tract consists of the trachea, bronchi, and lungs. Obstructions can be categorized as upper airway obstructions or lower airway obstructions. Obstructions can be partial (allowing some air to pass) or complete (not allowing any air to pass), and they can also be acute or chronic. This discussion focuses on acute upper airway obstruction.

The most common causes of acute upper airway obstruction are anaphylaxis, croup, epiglottitis, and foreign objects. These are all considered respiratory emergencies. Anaphylaxis is a severe allergic reaction usually occurring within minutes of exposure to an allergen. During anaphylaxis, the airways swell and become blocked. Bee stings, penicillin (an antibiotic), and peanuts are the most common allergens that cause anaphylaxis.

Signs and symptoms of acute upper airway obstruction can include:

- Dyspnea
- Agitation/panic
- Wheezing
- Cyanosis
- Drooling
- Decreased breath sounds
- Tachypnea
- Tachycardia
- Swelling of the face and tongue
- Choking
- Confusion
- Unconsciousness

Diagnosis of acute upper airway obstruction can entail imaging studies (x-rays of the neck and chest; CT scans of the head, neck, or chest), pulse oximetry, blood tests and cultures, and bronchoscopy/laryngoscopy. Treatment depends on the etiology of the obstruction and can include:

- Heimlich maneuver (if choking on a foreign object)
- Epinephrine, antihistamines, and anti-inflammatory medications (if anaphylaxis)
- Supplemental oxygen
- Tracheostomy or cricothyrotomy (to bypass a total obstruction)
- CPR (if unconsciousness and unable to breathe)

Pleural Effusion

A pleural effusion is an abnormal accumulation of fluid in the pleural space. The pleural space is located between the parietal and visceral pleurae of each lung. The parietal pleura covers the inner surface of the chest cavity, while the visceral pleura surrounds the lungs. Approximately 10 milliliters of pleural fluid are maintained by oncotic and hydrostatic pressures and lymphatic drainage and is necessary for normal respiratory function. Pleural effusions can be categorized as transudates or exudates. Transudates result from an imbalance between oncotic and hydrostatic pressures, so they are characterized by low protein content. The transudates are often the result of congestive heart failure (CHF), cirrhosis, low albumin blood levels, nephrotic syndrome, and peritoneal dialysis. Exudates result from decreased lymphatic drainage or inflammation of the pleura, so they are characterized by high protein content. The exudates are often the result of malignancy, pancreatitis, pulmonary embolism, uremia, infection, and certain medications.

The main symptoms of a pleural effusion include dyspnea, cough, and chest pain. Diagnosis of a pleural effusion can include chest x-ray, chest CT scan, ultrasonography, and thoracentesis. Thoracentesis can provide pleural fluid for analysis such as LDH, glucose, pH, cell count and differential, culture, and cytology. Pleural fluid should be distinguished as either transudate or exudate. Exudative pleural effusions are characterized by:

- Ratio of pleural fluid to serum protein > 0.5
- Ratio of pleural fluid to serum LDH > 0.6
- Pleural fluid LDH > 2/3 of the upper limit of normal blood value

Treatment of a pleural effusion is usually dictated by the underlying etiology; however, the treatment of a very large pleural effusion can include:

- Thoracentesis
- Chest tube (also known as tube thoracostomy)
- Pleurodesis (instillation of an irritant to cause inflammation and subsequent fibrosis to obliterate the pleural space)
- Indwelling tunneled pleural catheters

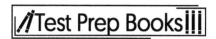

Pneumothorax

Pneumothorax is the abnormal presence of air in the pleural cavity, which is the space between the parietal and visceral pleurae. Pneumothorax can be categorized as:

- Spontaneous Pneumothorax: This can be classified as either primary or secondary. Primary spontaneous pneumothorax (PSP) occurs in individuals with no history of lung disease or inciting event. Those at risk for PSP are typically eighteen to forty years old, tall, thin, and smokers. There's also a familial tendency for primary spontaneous pneumothorax. Secondary spontaneous pneumothorax occurs in individuals with an underlying lung disease such as COPD, cystic fibrosis, asthma, tuberculosis (TB), or lung cancer.

- Traumatic Pneumothorax: This occurs as a result of blunt or penetrating trauma to the chest wall. The trauma disrupts the parietal and/or visceral pleura(e). Examples of inciting events include: gunshot or stab wounds; air bag deployment in a motor vehicle accident; acute respiratory distress syndrome (ARDS); and medical procedures such as mechanical ventilation, lung biopsy, thoracentesis, needle biopsy, and chest surgery.

- Tension Pneumothorax: This is the trapping of air in the pleural space under positive pressure. It causes a mediastinal shift toward the unaffected lung and a depression of the hemidiaphragm on the side of the affected lung. Shortly after, the event is followed by severe cardiopulmonary compromise. Tension pneumothorax can result from any of the conditions or procedures listed for Spontaneous and Traumatic Pneumothorax.

Signs and symptoms of pneumothorax depend on the degree of lung collapse (partial or total) and can include:

- Chest pain
- Dyspnea
- Cyanosis
- Tachypnea
- Tachycardia
- Hypotension
- Hypoxia
- Anxiety
- Adventitious breath sounds
- Unilateral distant or absent breath sounds
- Jugular venous distention (JVD)
- Tracheal deviation away from the affected side (with tension pneumothorax)

Diagnosis of pneumothorax is primarily clinical (based on signs and symptoms), but can involve an upright posteroanterior chest x-ray, chest CT scan (the most reliable imaging for diagnosis), ABG analysis, and ultrasonography of the chest. Treatment of a pneumothorax depends on the severity of the condition and can include:

- Supplemental oxygen

- The standard of treatment for all large, symptomatic pneumothoraces is a tube thoracostomy (chest tube).

- Observation (a reasonable option for small asymptomatic pneumothorax; multiple series of chest x-rays are needed until resolution)

- Simple needle aspiration (an option for small, primary spontaneous pneumothorax)

- Because they can quickly cause life-threatening cardiopulmonary compromise, the standard of treatment for all tension pneumothoraces is an emergent needle thoracostomy.

Pulmonary Edema, Noncardiogenic

Pulmonary edema can be categorized as cardiogenic or noncardiogenic in origin. Cardiogenic pulmonary edema is the most common type, while noncardiogenic pulmonary edema is the least common. This discussion focuses on noncardiogenic pulmonary edema. Direct injury to the lungs, followed by subsequent inflammation, leads to the development of noncardiogenic pulmonary edema. The inflammation causes lung capillaries in the alveoli to leak and fill with fluid, resulting in impaired oxygenation. Common causes of noncardiogenic pulmonary edema include:

- Acute respiratory distress syndrome (ARDS)
- High altitudes
- Nervous system conditions (especially head trauma, seizures, or subarachnoid hemorrhage)
- Pulmonary embolism
- Kidney failure
- Illicit drug use (especially cocaine and heroin)
- Medication side effects (such as aspirin overdose or chemotherapy)
- Inhaled toxins (such as ammonia, chlorine, or smoke)
- Pneumonia
- Near drowning

Signs and symptoms of noncardiogenic pulmonary edema can include:

- Dyspnea (most common symptom)
- Wheezing
- Respiratory distress
- Cough
- Anxiety
- Hypoxia
- Tachypnea
- Altered mental status
- Fatigue
- Lung crackles
- Headache
- Cyanosis

There is no single test to determine whether the cause of the pulmonary edema is cardiogenic or noncardiogenic. Diagnosis of noncardiogenic pulmonary edema can include chest x-ray, blood tests, pulse oximetry, ABG analysis, electrocardiogram (ECG), echocardiogram, cardiac catheterization with coronary angiogram, and pulmonary artery catheterization. For pulmonary artery catheterization, a pulmonary artery wedge pressure <18 mmHg is consistent with pulmonary edema of noncardiogenic

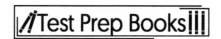

origin. Most of these tests help to differentiate between cardiogenic and noncardiogenic causes of pulmonary edema.

Treatment of noncardiogenic pulmonary edema is directed toward its underlying cause and can include:

- Supplemental oxygen (first-line treatment)
- Hyperbaric oxygen chamber
- Intubation and mechanical ventilation
- Morphine (can be used to allay anxiety)

Pulmonary Embolism

A pulmonary embolism (PE) is the abnormal presence of a blood clot, or thrombus, causing a blockage in one of the lungs' pulmonary arteries. It is not a specific disease, but rather a complication due to thrombus formation in the venous system of one of the lower extremities, which is termed **deep venous thrombosis** (DVT). Other rarer causes of PEs are thrombi arising in the veins of the kidneys, pelvis, upper extremities, or the right atrium of the heart. Occasionally, other matter besides blood clots can cause pulmonary emboli, such as fat, air, and septic (infected with bacteria) emboli. PE is a common and potentially fatal condition.

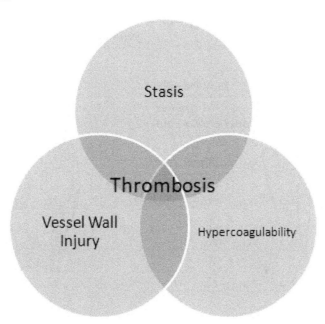

The primary influences on the development of DVT and PE are shown in Virchow's triad: blood hypercoagulability, endothelial injury/dysfunction, and stasis of blood.

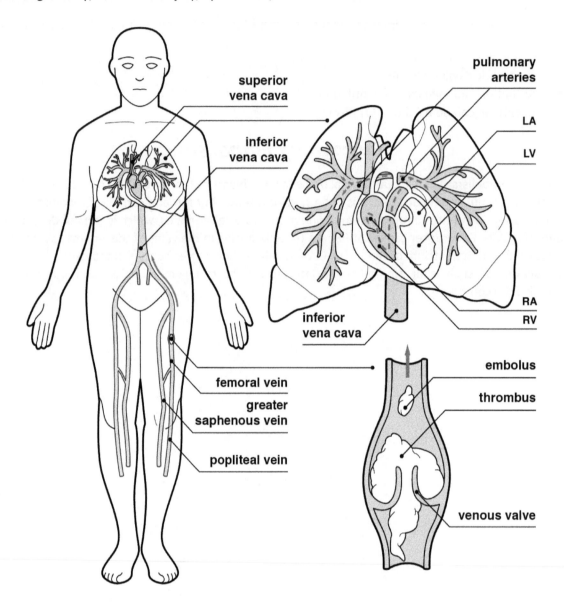

Risk factors for DVT and PE include:

- Cancer
- Heart disease, especially congestive heart failure (CHF)
- Prolonged immobility (such as prolonged bedrest or lengthy trips in planes or cars)
- Surgery (one of the leading risk factors, accounting for up to 15% of all postoperative deaths)
- Overweight/obesity
- Smoking
- Pregnancy
- Supplemental estrogen from birth control pills or estrogen replacement therapy (ERT)

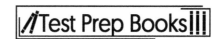

The signs and symptoms of PE are nonspecific, which often presents a diagnostic dilemma and a delay in diagnosis. Nearly half of all individuals with PE are asymptomatic. The signs and symptoms of PE can vary greatly depending on the size of the blood clots, how much lung tissue is involved, and an individual's overall health. Signs and symptoms of PE can include:

- Pleuritic chest pain
- Dyspnea
- Cough
- Tachypnea
- Hypoxia
- Fever
- Diaphoresis
- Rales
- Cyanosis
- Unilateral lower extremity edema (symptom of DVT)

The diagnosis of PE can be a difficult task. Many clinicians support determining the clinical probability of PE before proceeding with diagnostic testing. This process involves assessing the presence or absence of the following manifestations:

- Pulmonary Signs: Tachypnea, rales, and cyanosis

- Cardiac Signs: Tachycardia, S3 - S4 gallop, attenuated second heart sound, and cardiac murmur

- Constitutional Signs: Fever, diaphoresis, signs and symptoms of thrombophlebitis, and lower extremity edema

Once the clinical probability of PE has been determined, diagnostic testing ensues. Duplex ultrasonography is the standard for diagnosing a DVT. A spiral computed tomography (CT) scan with or without contrast has replaced pulmonary angiography as the standard for diagnosing a PE. If spiral CT scanning is unavailable or if individuals have a contraindication to the administration of intravenous contrast material, ventilation-perfusion (V/Q) scanning is often selected. Magnetic resonance imaging (MRI) is usually reserved for pregnant women and individuals with a contraindication to the administration of intravenous contrast material. A D-dimer blood test is most useful for individuals with a low or moderate pretest probability of PE, since levels are typically elevated with PE. Arterial blood gas (ABG) analysis usually reveals hypoxemia, hypocapnia, and respiratory alkalosis.

A chest x-ray, though not diagnostic for PE since its findings are typically nonspecific, can exclude diseases that mimic PE, as can an echocardiography. Electrocardiography is also useful because it can assess right ventricular heart function and be prognostic, since there's a 10% death rate from PE with right ventricular dysfunction. Lastly, transesophageal echocardiography (TEE) can reveal central PE.

Treatment of PE should begin immediately to prevent complications or death. PE treatment is focused on preventing an increase in size of the current blood clots and the formation of new blood clots. Supportive care treatment of PE can include:

- Supplemental oxygen to ease hypoxia/hypoxemia
- Dopamine (Inotropin®) or dobutamine (Dobutrex®) administered via IV for related hypotension
- Cardiac monitoring in the case of associated arrhythmias or right ventricular dysfunction
- Intubation and mechanical ventilation

Medications involved in treatment can include: thrombolytics or clot dissolvers (such as tissue plasminogen activator (tPA), alteplase, urokinase, streptokinase, or reteplase). These medications are reserved for individuals with a diagnosis of acute PE and associated hypotension (systolic BP < 90 mm Hg). They are not given concurrently with anticoagulants. Anticoagulants or blood thinners may also be used. The historical standard for the initial treatment of PE was unfractionated heparin (UFH) administered via IV or subcutaneous (SC) injection, which requires frequent blood monitoring. Current treatment guidelines recommend low-molecular weight heparin (LMWH) administered via SC injection over UFH IV or SC as it has greater bioavailability than UFH and blood monitoring is not necessary. Fondaparinux (Arixtra®) administered via SC injection is also recommended over UFH IV or SC; blood monitoring is not necessary.

Warfarin (Coumadin®), an oral anticoagulant was the historical standard for the outpatient prevention and treatment of PE. It is initiated the same day as treatment with UFH, LMWH, or fondaparinux. It is recommended INR of 2-3 with frequent blood monitoring, at which time IV or SC anticoagulant is discontinued. Alternatives to Warfarin include oral factor Xa inhibitor anticoagulants such as apixaban (Eliquis®), rivaroxaban (Xarelto®), and edoxaban (Savaysa®), or dabigatran (Pradaxa®), an oral direct thrombin inhibitor anticoagulant. Blood monitoring is not necessary with these medications. The most significant adverse effect of both thrombolytics and anticoagulants is bleeding.

An embolectomy (removal of emboli via catheter or surgery) is reserved for individuals with a massive PE and contraindications to thrombolytics or anticoagulants. Vena cava filters (also called inferior vena cava (IVC) filters or Greenfield filters) are only indicated in individuals with an absolute contraindication to anticoagulants, a massive PE who have survived and for whom recurrent PE will be fatal, or documented recurrent PE.

Respiratory Distress Syndrome

Acute respiratory distress syndrome (ARDS) is the widespread inflammation of the lungs and capillaries of the alveoli and results in the rapid development of pulmonary system failure. It can occur in both adults and children and is considered the most severe form of acute lung injury. Presence of the syndrome is determined by:

- Timing: Onset of symptoms within one week of inciting incident
- Chest x-ray: Bilateral lung infiltrates not explained by consolidation, atelectasis, or effusions
- Origin of Edema: Not explained by heart failure or fluid overload
- Severity of Hypoxemia

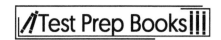

It should be noted that the severity of hypoxemia is based on PaO_2/FiO_2 ratio while on 5 cm of continuous positive airway pressure (CPAP). PaO_2 is the partial pressure of oxygen, while FiO_2 is the fraction of inspired oxygen. Categories are:

- Mild (PaO_2/FiO_2 = 200–300)
- Moderate (PaO_2/FiO_2 = 100–200)
- Severe ($PaO_2/FiO_2 \leq$ 100)

ARDS has a high mortality rate (30–40%), which increases with advancing age. It also leads to significant morbidity because of its association with extended hospital stays, frequent nosocomial (hospital-acquired) infections, muscle weakness, significant weight loss, and functional impairment. The most common cause of ARDS is sepsis, a life-threatening bacterial infection of the blood. Other common causes include:

- Severe pneumonia
- Inhalation of toxic fumes
- Trauma (such as falls, bone fractures, motor vehicle accidents, near drowning, and burns)
- Massive blood transfusion

It should also be noted that, for one in five patients with ARDS, there will be no identifiable risk factors. Therefore, the cause of ARDS may not be evident.

The onset of ARDS symptoms is fairly rapid, occurring 12 to 48 hours after the inciting incident. Many of the signs and symptoms of ARDS are nonspecific. Signs and symptoms of ARDS can include:

- Dyspnea (initially with exertion, but rapidly progressing to occurring even at rest)
- Hypoxia
- Tachypnea
- Tachycardia
- Fever
- Bilateral rales
- Cyanosis
- Hypotension
- Fatigue

The diagnosis of ARDS is clinical since there's no specific test for the condition. Diagnosing ARDS is done by exclusion, ruling out other diseases that mimic its signs and symptoms. Tests used to diagnose ARDS can include:

- Chest x-ray, which, by definition, should reveal bilateral lung infiltrates
- ABG analysis (usually reveals extreme hypoxemia and respiratory alkalosis or metabolic acidosis)
- CBC with differential (can reveal leukocytosis, leukopenia, and/or thrombocytopenia)
- Plasma B-type natriuretic peptide (BNP), a level < 100 pg/mL favors ARDS rather than CHF
- CT scan
- Echocardiography, which is helpful in excluding CHF (cardiogenic pulmonary edema)
- Bronchoscopy with bronchoalveolar lavage (BAL), which is helpful in excluding lung infections

Numerous medications, such as corticosteroids, synthetic surfactant, antibody to endotoxin, ketoconazole, simvastatin, ibuprofen, and inhaled nitric oxide, have been used for the treatment of

ARDS, but none have proven effective. Therefore, treating the underlying symptoms of ARDS and providing supportive care are the most crucial components of therapy. The only therapy found to improve survival in ARDS is intubation and mechanical ventilation using low tidal volumes (6 mL/kg of ideal body weight). Because sepsis, an infection, is the most common etiology of ARDS, early administration of a broad-spectrum antibiotic is crucial.

Treatment also includes fluid management and nutritional support. For individuals with shock secondary to sepsis, initial aggressive fluid resuscitation is administered, followed by a conservative fluid management strategy. It is best to institute nutritional support within 48 to 72 hours of initiation of mechanical ventilation.

Important preventative measures include DVT prophylaxis with enoxaparin, stress ulcer prophylaxis with sucralfate or omeprazole, turning and skin care to prevent decubitus ulcers, and elevating the head of the bed and using a subglottic suction device to help prevent ventilator-associated pneumonia.

Trauma

Chest trauma is a significant factor in all trauma deaths. There are two general categories of chest traumas: blunt chest traumas and penetrating chest traumas.

Pulmonary Contusion

A pulmonary contusion is a deep bruise of the lung secondary to chest trauma. Associated swelling and blood collecting in the alveoli of the lung lead to loss of structure and function. It is estimated that 50% to 60% of individuals with pulmonary contusions develop ARDS. Motor vehicle accidents, sports injuries, explosive blast injuries, work injuries, serious falls, or crush injuries can cause blunt chest trauma. Signs and symptoms of a pulmonary contusion typically develop 24 to 48 hours after the inciting event. Signs and symptoms can include:

- Dyspnea
- Hypoxia
- Cyanosis
- Tachypnea
- Tachycardia
- Hemoptysis
- Chest pain
- Hypotension

Diagnosis of a pulmonary contusion relies on physical examination and diagnostic tests. A chest x-ray is useful in the diagnosis of most significant pulmonary contusions; however, it often underestimates the extent of the injury, which is sometimes not apparent for 24 to 48 hours after event. CT scans are more accurate than chest x-rays for identifying of a pulmonary contusion; they can also accurately assess and reflect the extent of lung injury. ABG analysis is used to assess the extent of hypoxemia, and pulse oximetry is used to assess the extent of hypoxia.

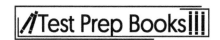

Treatment for a pulmonary contusion is primarily supportive, and no treatment is known to accelerate its resolution. These treatments can include:

- Supplemental oxygen to relieve hypoxia
- Analgesics (as needed for pain)
- Conservative fluid management to reduce the likelihood of fluid overload and PE
- Aggressive suction of pulmonary secretions to reduce likelihood of pneumonia
- Incentive spirometry to reduce the likelihood of atelectasis, which can lead to pneumonia
- Intubation and mechanical ventilation (in severe cases)

Hemothorax

Hemothorax, the presence of blood in the pleural space, is most commonly the result of blunt or penetrating chest trauma. The pleural space lies between the parietal pleura of the chest wall and the visceral pleura of the lungs. A large accumulation of blood in the pleural space can restrict normal lung movement and lead to hemodynamic compromise. Common signs and symptoms of hemothorax include chest pain, dyspnea, and tachypnea. When there is substantial systemic blood loss, tachycardia and hypotension can also be present.

Diagnosis of hemothorax primarily involves a chest x-ray, which reveals blunting of the costophrenic angle on the affected side of the lung. A helical CT scan has a complementary role in the management of hemothorax, and it can localize and quantify the retention of blood or clots within the pleural space.

Small hemothoraces usually require no treatment, but need close observation to ensure resolution. Tube thoracostomy drainage is the mainstay of treatment for significant hemothoraces. Needle aspiration has no place in the management of hemothorax. Blood transfusions can be necessary for those with significant blood loss or hemodynamic compromise. Complications from hemothorax can include empyema (secondary bacterial infection of a retained clot) or fibrothorax (fibrosis of the pleural space which can trap lung tissue and lead to decreased pulmonary function).

Flail Chest

Flail chest is clinically defined as the paradoxical movement of a segment of the chest wall caused by at least two fractures per rib (usually anteriorly and posteriorly) in three or more ribs while breathing. The ribs are then free to float away from the chest wall and produce paradoxical breathing, which is the flail area contracting on inspiration and relaxing on expiration. The flail area of the chest disrupts the normal mechanics of breathing. Variations include anterior flail segments, posterior flail segments, and flail affecting the sternum and fractures of the ribs bilaterally. Flail chest requires a tremendous amount of blunt force trauma to the thorax in order to fracture multiple ribs in multiple places. This type of trauma can be produced by motor vehicle accidents, serious falls, crush injuries, rollover injuries, and physical assaults.

The diagnosis of flail chest is visual. It is seen in individuals with a history of blunt chest trauma by the presence of paradoxical chest wall motion while spontaneously breathing. The rib fractures can be verified with chest x-ray. A CT scan of the chest provides very little additional information and isn't usually indicated in the initial assessment of a chest wall injury. In flail chest, the lungs cannot expand properly, which can lead to varying degrees of respiratory compromise. Treatment of flail chest can include:

- Supplemental oxygen (to relieve hypoxia, if present)

- Analgesia (for relief of pain secondary to multiple rib fractures, usually via patient-controlled administration (PCA) or continuous epidural infusion)

- External fixation and stabilization of rib fractures (once the historical standard for treatment, it has been replaced by intubation and mechanical ventilation)

- Intubation and mechanical ventilation (usually needed for the treatment of an underlying disease such as pulmonary contusion; addition of positive pressure provides stabilization of the chest wall and helps improve oxygenation and ventilation)

- Operative fixation of ribs (reserved for individuals requiring a thoracotomy for underlying lung injuries)

Common complications of flail chest include hemothorax, pneumothorax, pulmonary contusion, and pneumonia. Hemothorax or pneumothorax would require concomitant tube thoracostomy drainage. Hemothorax and pneumothorax can both be identified by quiet or absent breath sounds in the affected lung along with reduced chest wall movement. Chest physiotherapy and aggressive pulmonary hygiene should be implemented to reduce the likelihood of complicating pneumonia.

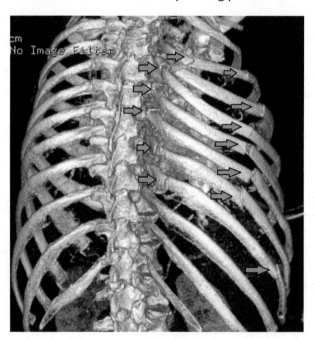

Fractured Ribs

A fracture is a crack or splinter in a bone. Simple rib fractures are the most common injury after sustaining blunt chest trauma. Only 10% of individuals admitted with a diagnosis of blunt chest trauma have multiple rib fractures. Causes of rib fractures include falls from an elevation or from standing (most common in the elderly), motor vehicle accidents (most common in adults), and recreational and athletic

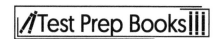

activities (most common in children). Rib fractures can also be pathologic, or related to cancers that have undergone metastasis such as prostate, renal, and breast.

Ribs four through nine (4–9) are the most commonly fractured ribs. Other rib fractures and possible underlying injuries are:

- Ribs 1–2: Tracheal, bronchus, or great vessels can be injured
- Right-sided ≥ rib 8: Liver trauma
- Left-sided ≥ rib 8: Spleen trauma

Common signs and symptoms of rib fractures include tenderness on palpation, chest wall deformities, and crepitus. Other signs and symptoms can include cyanosis, dyspnea, tachycardia, agitation, tachypnea, retractions, and use of accessory respiratory muscles.

Laboratory blood tests are of no use in the diagnosis of fractured ribs. A chest x-ray can be used to diagnose rib fractures and other underlying injuries such as hemothorax, lung contusion, pneumothorax, atelectasis, and pneumonia. A chest CT scan is more sensitive than a chest x-ray for the detection of rib fractures. A bone scan of the chest wall is the preferred diagnostic imaging study for the diagnosis of rib stress fractures.

The treatment of rib fractures is primarily supportive. Younger individuals with rib fractures have a better prognosis than older individuals (age ≥ 65 years) who have higher rates of serious lung complications. Therapies for rib fractures can include:

- Supplemental oxygen
- Incentive spirometry (to avoid complications such as atelectasis and pneumonia)
- Pain control, which is essential and usually provided by NSAIDs and/or other analgesics

Tracheal Perforation/Injury

Tracheal perforation/injury is a tear in the trachea or bronchial tubes, which are major airways leading to the lungs. Common causes of tracheal perforation/injury include trauma (gunshot wounds and motor vehicle accidents), infections, and ulcerations secondary to foreign objects. Common signs and symptoms of tracheal perforation/injury can include hemoptysis, dyspnea, subcutaneous emphysema, and respiratory distress. Diagnosis may include chest x-rays, a chest CT scan, and MRI. A CT scan is the preferred imaging method for diagnosing a tracheal perforation/injury. Treatment should be prompt and depends on the etiology and the extent of the damage to the area. Surgical repair of the tear is often needed, and other measures to manage a tracheal perforation/injury include:

- Intubation and mechanical ventilation
- Tube thoracostomy drainage
- Rigid or fiberoptic bronchoscopy (to extract foreign objects)
- Antibiotics (as indicated)

Ruptured Diaphragm

The diaphragm separates the thoracic (chest) cavity and the abdominal cavity. Rupture of the diaphragm is rare and usually the result of a blunt or penetrating trauma. The majority of blunt traumas causing ruptures of the diaphragm are the result of motor vehicle accidents. Gunshot and knife injuries are the most common causes of a traumatic diaphragmatic rupture. A ruptured diaphragm can lead to significant ventilatory compromise, and difficulty breathing is a common symptom. A chest x-ray is the most important diagnostic tool in diagnosing a ruptured diaphragm. It can reveal elevation of a hemidiaphragm, a nasogastric (NG) tube being present in chest (rather than in the abdomen), or the abnormal presence of bowel in the chest. Abnormalities such as widening of the mediastinum can also be observed on a chest x-ray. Treatment of a ruptured diaphragm requires surgical repair. The prognosis is excellent with the emergent repair of the diaphragmatic rupture.

Practice Questions

1. A 25-year-old male presents to the Emergency Department (ED) after accidentally inhaling a dime. He can speak and recounts that the incident occurred eight hours ago. His only complaints are a cough and wheezing. Upon bronchoscopy, where would the ED physician likely find the dime?
   a. Left lung
   b. Trachea
   c. Larynx
   d. Right lung

2. An 18-year-old female presents to the Emergency Department (ED) complaining of worsening wheezing, shortness of breath, and a cough over the past twelve hours. She has a history of asthma and has been using her albuterol metered-dose inhaler (MDI) every ten minutes for the past two hours. She's given supplemental oxygen, both albuterol and ipratropium (Combivent®) via nebulizer, and methylprednisolone IV in quick succession. Shortly afterwards, she complains of anxiety, develops hand tremors, and her pulse increases from 80 to 120 beats per minute (bpm). Which treatment is most likely responsible for her anxiety, tremors, and tachycardia?
   a. Supplemental oxygen
   b. Albuterol
   c. Ipratropium
   d. Methylprednisolone

3. A 65-year-old ex-smoker presents with a complaint of increasing shortness of breath over the past 24 hours. He has a medical history conducive of chronic obstructive pulmonary disease (COPD). He is administered supplemental oxygen, albuterol via nebulizer, methylprednisolone IV, and a dose of azithromycin IV. Which of these therapies has been clinically proven to decrease the risk of treatment failure and death?
   a. Supplemental oxygen
   b. Albuterol
   c. Methylprednisolone
   d. Azithromycin

4. A 55-year-old male presents with a cough producing rust-colored sputum, a fever (102 °F), and shortness of breath. A complete blood count (CBC) reveals an elevated white blood cell count with predominant neutrophils. A chest x-ray reveals consolidation of the left, lower lobe of the lung. Blood cultures reveal gram-positive diplococci. What is the most likely cause of this patient's pneumonia?
   a. *Haemophilus influenzae*
   b. *Moraxella catarrhalis*
   c. *Streptococcus pneumoniae*
   d. *Staphylococcus aureus*

5. A 66-year-old female with type 2 diabetes mellitus presents with a nonproductive cough, nasal congestion, wheezing, and occasional shortness of breath for the last ten days. She reports that her symptoms are worse at night. A chest x-ray, complete blood count (CBC), and comprehensive metabolic panel (CMP) are all unremarkable, except for an elevated blood glucose level of 150 mg/dL. What is the most appropriate course of management?
    a. Bronchoscopy with bronchoalveolar lavage (BAL)
    b. Sputum gram stain and culture
    c. Arterial blood gas (ABG) analysis
    d. Doxycycline 100 mg BID for seven days

6. A 25-year-old male presents to the Emergency Department (ED) complaining of shortness of breath, coughing, and wheezing for two days. His cough is productive, and he reports seeing black material mixed in with his phlegm. Visual examination reveals carbonaceous sputum. At this point in the examination, he develops severe respiratory distress and is subsequently intubated and placed on mechanical ventilation. What is the mostly likely diagnosis for this patient?
    a. Acute bronchitis
    b. Inhalation injury
    c. Community-acquired pneumonia
    d. Hemothorax

7. A 7-year-old male presents with hypoxia, hoarseness, fever, agitation, dysphagia, drooling, and complaints of a sore throat. What is the most likely diagnosis for this patient?
    a. Laryngotracheobronchitis
    b. Acute tracheitis
    c. Acute epiglottitis
    d. Bronchiolitis

8. A 55-year-old male presents with dyspnea, cough, and chest pain. A chest x-ray reveals a large pleural effusion. Thoracentesis is performed and pleural fluid analysis reveals a ratio of pleural fluid to serum LDH > 0.6. What is the most likely diagnosis for this patient?
    a. Malignancy
    b. Congestive heart failure (CHF)
    c. Cirrhosis
    d. Nephrotic syndrome

9. A 25-year-old male arrives at the Emergency Department (ED) after blunt chest trauma. On initial evaluation, he has absent breath sounds over the right lung and tracheal deviation to the left. A chest x-ray reveals mediastinal shift to the left and depression of the right hemidiaphragm. What is the most likely diagnosis?
    a. Secondary spontaneous pneumothorax
    b. Bronchiolitis
    c. Tension pneumothorax
    d. Acute respiratory distress syndrome (ARDS)

10. Which of the following test results is consistent with pulmonary edema of a non-cardiogenic origin?
    a. Chest x-ray with bilateral pulmonary infiltrates
    b. Elevated blood levels of B-type natriuretic peptide (BNP)
    c. ABG analysis revealing hypoxemia
    d. A pulmonary artery wedge pressure of 12 mmHg

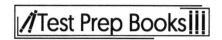

11. All EXCEPT which of the following are components of Virchow's triad?
    a. Heart disease
    b. Hypercoagulability
    c. Endothelial injury/dysfunction
    d. Hemodynamic changes such as stasis or turbulence

12. Which of the following is an indication for the placement of a vena cava filter to prevent pulmonary embolism (PE)?
    a. Pregnancy
    b. Documented recurrent PE
    c. Active smoking history
    d. Age > 65 years

13. All EXCEPT which of the following help define acute respiratory distress syndrome (ARDS)?
    a. Timing
    b. Origin of edema
    c. Pulmonary artery wedge pressure
    d. Severity of hypoxemia

14. A 30-year-old female presents to the Emergency Department (ED) after penetrating chest trauma. She complains of chest pain and shortness of breath. On examination, she's found to have tachypnea, tachycardia, and hypotension. A chest x-ray reveals blunting of the left costophrenic angle. What's the most likely diagnosis for this patient?
    a. Flail chest
    b. Myocardial contusion
    c. Inhalation injury
    d. Hemothorax

15. A 40-year-old policeman presents to the Emergency Department (ED) after being physically assaulted by a suspect. He complains of shortness of breath and right-sided rib pain. A chest x-ray reveals fractures of ribs 4, 5, and 6 on the left. Physical examination reveals paradoxical movement of the area while breathing. What is the most likely diagnosis for this patient?
    a. Ruptured diaphragm
    b. Flail chest
    c. Tracheal perforation
    d. Pulmonary embolism (PE)

16. Which of the following is the best antibiotic treatment for pneumonia caused by community-acquired methicillin-resistant *Staphylococcus aureus* (CA-MRSA)?
    a. Azithromycin
    b. Doxycycline
    c. Vancomycin
    d. Levofloxacin

Answer Explanations

1. D: This scenario depicts a foreign body aspiration in an adult. Since the patient can speak, it's a partial obstruction of the airways. The foreign body should be promptly extracted as the likelihood of complications increases after 24 to 48 hours. Bronchoscopy (rigid or flexible) can be diagnostic as well as therapeutic. Due to the acute angle of the right mainstem bronchus, aspirated foreign bodies in an adult are most commonly found in the right lung.

2. B: The scenario depicts an episode of status asthmaticus. Common pharmacological agents used to treat this condition include albuterol (short-acting Beta-2 agonist), ipratropium (anticholinergic), and methylprednisolone (corticosteroid). Her new symptoms (anxiety, tremors, and tachycardia) are all common side effects which can be attributed to albuterol. Anticholinergics can induce side effects such as dry mouth, blurred vision, and constipation. Corticosteroids (if used for longer than two weeks) can have side effects such as weight gain, osteoporosis, thinning of skin, cataracts, easy bruising, and diabetes. She should be switched to the short-acting Beta-2 agonist levalbuterol because it's as effective as albuterol but without the alarming side effects.

3. D: This scenario depicts a moderate to severe acute exacerbation of COPD. Azithromycin is a macrolide antibiotic. In clinical trials, the use of antibiotics in individuals with a moderate to severe exacerbation of COPD diminishes the risk of treatment failure and death. Oxygen and albuterol target dyspnea. In clinical trials, the administration of oral corticosteroids fairly early in the midst of a COPD exacerbation decreased the need for hospitalization.

4. C: This scenario depicts a case of community-acquired pneumonia (CAP), specifically pneumococcal pneumonia. The most common cause of CAP is *Streptococcus pneumoniae*, or pneumococcus. It's a gram-positive bacterium, usually occurring in pairs (diplococci). The other bacteria (*Haemophilus influenzae*, *Moraxella catarrhalis*, and *Staphylococcus aureus*) are less common causes of CAP.

5. D: This scenario depicts a case of acute bronchitis. The most common causes of acute bronchitis are respiratory viruses (such as influenza A and B), respiratory syncytial virus (RSV), parainfluenza, adenovirus, rhinovirus, and coronavirus. Acute bronchitis should not be routinely treated with antibiotics, but there are exceptions to this rule. It's reasonable to use antibiotics if an existing medical condition poses a risk of serious complications. Antibiotic treatment of acute bronchitis is also reasonable in individuals older than 65 years of age with a hospitalization in the past year, those being currently treated with a steroid, and those diagnosed with congestive heart failure or diabetes.

6. B: This scenario depicts an inhalation injury. Although the patient's history is limited, the fact that he produced carbonaceous sputum makes an inhalation injury the most likely diagnosis (specifically smoke inhalation). This scenario emphasizes the point that medical professionals should maintain a high level of suspicion when it comes to inhalation injuries. Treatment of inhalation injuries is largely supportive with an excellent prognosis for complete recovery.

7. C: This scenario depicts the classic triad of symptoms of acute epiglottitis, including hypoxia, drooling and dysphagia. Acute epiglottitis is most often caused by *Haemophilus influenzae* type B. Direct visualization reveals that the epiglottis appears cherry red in color. Treatment includes antibiotic therapy, analgesic-antipyretic agents, and emergency airway management. Laryngotracheobronchitis (classic croup) is a common viral illness that primarily affects children and toddlers from six months to three years of age. The parainfluenza viruses (types 1, 2, and 3) account for 80% of all cases. Presenting

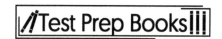

symptoms include a barking cough, wheezing, tachypnea, and tachycardia. Treatment is symptomatic and includes corticosteroids, racemic epinephrine, and mechanical ventilation. Tracheitis is the inflammation of the trachea caused most commonly by *Staphylococcus aureus*. Children under the age of fifteen are most commonly affected. Antibiotic therapy and anti-pyretic medications are used. Mechanical ventilation is rarely necessary. Bronchiolitis is an inflammation of the bronchioles caused by the respiratory syncytial virus. It most commonly affects children under the age of two. Its diagnosis is based on clinical examination and the disease is self-limiting.

8. A: This scenario depicts the diagnosis of pleural effusion. Pleural effusions can be categorized as transudates or exudates. The pleural effusion is exudative, which can be characterized by the following:

- Ratio of pleural fluid to serum protein > 0.5
- Ratio of pleural fluid to serum LDH > 0.6
- Pleural LDH > 2/3 of the upper limit of normal blood value

Causes of exudative pleural effusions include malignancy, pancreatitis, pulmonary embolism, uremia, infection, and certain medications. Causes of transudative pleural effusions include CHF, cirrhosis, nephrotic syndrome, low blood levels of albumin, and peritoneal dialysis.

9. C: This scenario depicts the diagnosis of a right-sided tension pneumothorax. The triad of tracheal deviation (to opposite side), mediastinal shift (to opposite side), and depression of the hemidiaphragm (on affected side) is pathognomonic for tension pneumothorax. Medical professionals must be quick and decisive in their treatment of tension pneumothorax. The condition is life-threatening and valuable time is often wasted waiting around for the results of imaging studies. Definitive treatment of a tension pneumothorax is emergent needle thoracostomy.

10. D: Pulmonary edema can be of cardiogenic or non-cardiogenic origin. There is no single test to differentiate whether the cause of pulmonary edema is cardiac or noncardiac. Bilateral pulmonary infiltrates and hypoxemia are nonspecific symptoms and can occur in both. A pulmonary artery wedge pressure < 18 mmHg is consistent with pulmonary edema of non-cardiogenic origin.

11. A: Virchow's triad identifies factors that contribute to the thrombotic process associated with deep venous thrombosis (DVT) and pulmonary embolism (PE). The triad consists of hypercoagulability, endothelial injury/dysfunction, and hemodynamic changes such as stasis and turbulence. Heart disease is a risk factor for DVT and PE, but it is not part of Virchow's triad.

12. B: Vena cava filters are also known as inferior vena cava (IVC) filters or Greenfield filters. They are used to prevent a pulmonary embolism (PE). Indications for the placement of a vena cava filter include:

- An absolute contraindication to anticoagulants
- Survival after a massive PE and a high probability that a recurrent PE will be fatal
- Documented recurrent PE

13. C: Acute respiratory distress syndrome (ARDS) is defined by the timing, a chest x-ray, the origin of the edema, and the severity of hypoxemia. In terms of timing, the onset of symptoms in ARDS is within one week of inciting incident. A chest x-ray should reveal bilateral lung infiltrates not explained by consolidation, atelectasis, or effusions. The edema origin is not explained by heart failure or fluid overload, and the severity of hypoxemia is based on the PaO_2/FiO_2 ratio while on 5 cm of continuous positive airway pressure (CPAP).

14. D: This scenario depicts the presentation of hemothorax, which is usually a consequence of a blunt or penetrating chest trauma. Blunting of the costophrenic angle on the affected side is pathognomonic for hemothorax. Chest tube drainage is the mainstay of treatment for hemothorax.

15. B: This scenario depicts a case of flail chest, which is clinically defined as the paradoxical movement of a segment of the chest wall caused by at least two fractures per rib (usually anteriorly and posteriorly) in three or more ribs while breathing. Flail chest requires a tremendous amount of blunt force trauma to the thorax in order to fracture multiple ribs in multiple places. This type of trauma can be produced by motor vehicle accidents, serious falls, crush injuries, rollover injuries, and physical assaults.

16. C: Community-associated, methicillin-resistant *Staphylococcus aureus* (CA-MRSA) is notoriously resistant to most antibiotics, except vancomycin and linezolid, with linezolid quickly becoming the agent of choice for the treatment of CA-MRSA pneumonia.

Neurological Emergencies

Dementia/Alzheimer's Disease

Dementia

Dementia is a general term used to describe a state of general cognitive decline. Although Alzheimer's disease accounts for up to 80 percent of all cases of dementia in the United States, the remaining two million cases may result from any one of several additional causes. The destruction of cortical tissue resulting from a stroke, or more commonly from multiple small strokes, often results in altered cognitive and physical function, while repetitive head injuries over an extended period also potentially result in permanent damage, limiting normal brain activity. Less common causes of dementia include infection of the brain by prions (abnormal protein fragments) as in Creutzfeldt-Jakob disease or the human immunodeficiency virus (HIV) as in AIDS, deposition of Lewy bodies in the cerebral cortex as in Parkinson's disease, and reversible conditions such as vitamin B-12 deficiency and altered function of the thyroid gland. The onset and progression of the disease relate to the underlying cause and associated patient comorbidities.

Alzheimer's Disease

Alzheimer's disease is a chronic progressive form of dementia with an insidious onset that is caused by the abnormal accumulation of amyloid-β plaque in the brain. The accumulation of this plaque eventually interferes with neural functioning, which is responsible for the progressive manifestations of the disease. Although the exact etiology is unknown, environmental toxins, vascular alterations due to hemorrhagic or embolic events, infections, and genetic factors have all been proposed as the triggering mechanism for the plaque formation. The progression of the disease and the associated manifestations are specific to the individual; however, in all individuals, there is measurable decline over time in cognitive functioning, including short-term and long-term memory, behavior and mood, and the ability to perform activities of daily living (ADLs).

The diagnosis is based on the patient's presenting history and manifestations, imaging studies of the brain, protein analysis of the cerebrospinal fluid (CSF), and cognitive assessment with measures such as the Mini-Mental State Exam. Current treatments are only supportive, although cholinesterase inhibitors and *N*-Methyl-D-aspartate receptor antagonists may slow the progression of the manifestations for a limited period if administered early in the course of the disease. All patients will suffer an eventual decline in all aspects of cognitive functioning, with the average survival rate dependent on the presence of comorbidities and the level of care and support available to the patient.

Experiencing a fall with or without a resulting fracture, somatic illnesses, and caregiver strain are the most common reasons for emergency department visits in this population. The nursing care of the patient with Alzheimer's disease in the emergency department must focus on patient safety because the usual chaotic environment of the department is disorienting to the confused patient. Safeguards against increased confusion and wandering, which is a common behavior in this patient population, should be implemented. In addition, the entire family unit should be assessed by the interdisciplinary health team to identify any alterations of family process or additional resources that are required for adequate patient care after discharge from the emergency department or the acute care facility.

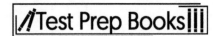

Chronic Neurological Disorders

Multiple Sclerosis

Multiple sclerosis (MS) is a chronic disease manifested by progressive destruction of the myelin sheath and resulting plaque formation in the central nervous system (CNS). The precipitating event of this autoimmune disease is the migration of activated T cells to the CNS, which disrupts the blood-brain barrier. Exposure to environmental toxins is considered to be the likely trigger for this immune response. These alterations facilitate the antigen-antibody reactions that result in the demyelination of the axons. The onset of this disease is insidious, with symptoms occurring intermittently over a period of months or years. Sensory manifestations may include numbness and tingling of the extremities, blurred vision, vertigo, tinnitus, impaired hearing, and chronic neuropathic pain. Motor manifestations may include weakness or paralysis of limbs, trunk, and head; diplopia; scanning speech; and muscle spasticity. Cerebellar manifestations include nystagmus, ataxia, dysarthria, dysphagia, and fatigue.

The progress of the disease and presenting clinical manifestations vary greatly from one individual to another; however, there are common forms of the disease that relate to the expression of the clinical manifestations or disability and the disease activity over time. An initial episode of neurological manifestations due to demyelination that lasts for at least 24 hours is identified as a clinically isolated episode of MS. The potential for progression of the disease to the relapsing-remitting form of MS is predicted by magnetic resonance imaging (MRI) studies indicating the presence or absence of plaque formation.

The remaining forms of MS are all associated with increasing disability related to the disease over time. The relapsing-remitting form is common to 85 percent of all patients diagnosed with MS and presents a variable pattern of active and inactive disease. The manifestations may resolve, decrease in severity, or become permanent after a relapse. In the primary-progressive form of MS that affects 10 percent of patients diagnosed with MS, the disease is constantly active without periods of remission. The secondary- progressive form of MS is identified as the progression of the relapsing-remitting form to a state of permanently active disease without remission.

Acute exacerbations of MS are treated with interferon or another of several disease-modifying drugs (DMDs), which are used to decrease the frequency of relapses and slow the progression of the disease. Research indicates that the medications are most effective when therapy is begun as soon as the diagnosis is confirmed. Other treatments are symptomatic and may treat conditions such as bladder infections, gastrointestinal (GI) disorders, and muscle spasticity. Patients with MS most commonly

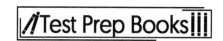

access care in the emergency department for non-neurological conditions, including GI disorders, falls, and bladder infections, and management of the manifestations associated with acute relapses.

Forms of Multiple Sclerosis

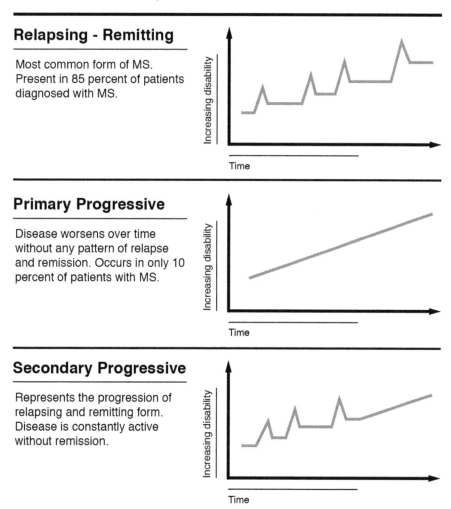

Relapsing - Remitting

Most common form of MS. Present in 85 percent of patients diagnosed with MS.

Primary Progressive

Disease worsens over time without any pattern of relapse and remission. Occurs in only 10 percent of patients with MS.

Secondary Progressive

Represents the progression of relapsing and remitting form. Disease is constantly active without remission.

Myasthenia Gravis

Myasthenia gravis is also an autoimmune disease of the CNS that is manifested by severe muscle weakness resulting from altered transmission of acetylcholine at the neuromuscular junction due to antibody formation. Relapses and remissions are common, and these relapses may be triggered by infection, increases in body temperature due to immersion in hot water, stress, and pregnancy. Subjective manifestations include weakness, diplopia, dysphagia, fatigue on exertion, and bowel and bladder dysfunction. Objective manifestations include unilateral or bilateral ptosis of the eye, impaired respiratory function, impaired swallowing, and decreased muscle strength. Tensilon testing and electromyography, which measures muscle activity over time, are used to diagnose this disorder, while anticholinesterase agents and immunosuppressant agents are the mainstays of treatment. Additional treatments include plasmapheresis to decrease circulating antibodies and removal of the thymus gland to slow T-cell production.

Patients in myasthenic crisis due to a lack of cholinesterase may present in the emergency department with hypertension and severe muscle weakness that requires mechanical ventilation. Tensilon therapy may temporarily reduce the symptoms of myasthenic crisis, not cholinergic crisis; consequently, return of normal heart function on an ECG, after being administered Tensilon, indicates myasthenic crisis as the cause. Patients in cholinergic crisis due to an excess of cholinesterase exhibit hypotension, hypersecretion, and severe muscle twitching, which eventually results in respiratory muscle fatigue requiring ventilatory support. Atropine is used to control manifestations of this complication.

Guillain-Barré Syndrome

The most common form of Guillain-Barré syndrome (GBS) is acute immune-mediated demyelinating polyneuropathy. This rare syndrome may develop two to four weeks after a bacterial or viral infection of the respiratory or GI systems or following surgery. The most common causative organisms are **C. jejuni** and **Cytomegalovirus** that may produce a subclinical infection that occurs unnoticed by the patient prior to the development of the acute onset of GBS. Other causative agents that are associated with GBS include the Epstein-Barr virus, **Mycoplasma pneumoniae**, and varicella-zoster virus. There is also an association between GBS and HIV. Current research is focused on investigating any association between the Zika virus and GBS; however, to date, there is little evidence of that relationship because there are few laboratories in the United States with the technology needed to identify the virus. The incidence of GBS has also been associated with vaccine administration; however, accumulated data does not support these claims.

The manifestations present as an acute onset of progressive, bilateral muscle weakness of the limbs that begins distally and continues proximally. The syndrome is the result of segmental demyelination of the nerves with edema, resulting from the inflammatory process. Additional presenting manifestations include pain, paresthesia, and abnormal sensations in the fingers. The progressive muscle weakness peaks at four weeks and potentially involves the arms, the muscles of the core, the cranial nerves, and the respiratory muscles. Involvement of the cranial nerves may result in facial drooping, diplopia, dysphagia, weakness or paralysis of the eye muscles, and pupillary alterations. Alterations in the autonomic nervous system also may result in orthostatic hypotension, paroxysmal hypertension, heart block, bradycardia, tachycardia, and asystole. Respiratory manifestations include dyspnea, shortness of breath, and dysphagia. In addition, as many as 30 percent of patients will progress to respiratory failure requiring ventilatory support due to the demyelination of the nerves that innervate the respiratory muscles.

The syndrome is diagnosed by the patient's history and laboratory studies to include electrolytes, liver function analysis, erythrocyte sedimentation rate (ESR), pulmonary function studies, and the assessment of CSF for the presence of excess protein content. In addition, electromyography and nerve conduction studies are used to identify the signs of demyelination, which confirms the diagnosis.

The emergency care of the patient with Guillain-Barré syndrome follows the Airway, Breathing, Circulation (ABC) protocol. Intubation with assisted ventilation is indicated in the event of hypoxia or decreasing respiratory muscle function as evidenced by an ineffective cough or aspiration. Cardiac manifestations vary according to the progression of the disease and are treated symptomatically. Placement of a temporary cardiac pacemaker may be necessary to treat second- or third-degree heart block. Treatment with plasmapheresis to remove the antibodies and intravenous (IV) immunoglobulin (Ig) to interfere with the antigen expression must be initiated within two to four weeks of the onset of symptoms to induce progression to the recovery phase of the syndrome. Care of the patient in the recovery phase must also address the common complications of immobility. Emergency care providers

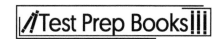

often make the initial diagnosis of this rare disease and therefore must be alert for the presenting manifestations that can progress rapidly to respiratory failure.

Headaches and Head Conditions

Temporal Arteritis

Temporal arteritis, also known as **giant cell arteritis,** is an inflammatory disorder of unknown origin that manifests as inflammatory changes in the intima, media, and adventitia layers of the artery as well as scattered accumulations of lymphocytes and macrophages that result in ischemic changes distal to the damaged areas. The condition is more common in women over fifty years of age, and current research indicates that infection and genetics also may be related to the development of the disease. The onset may be acute or insidious, and common signs and symptoms include head pain, neck pain, jaw claudication (jaw pain caused by ischemia of the maxillary artery), visual disturbances, shoulder and pelvic girdle pain, and general malaise and fever. The condition is diagnosed by a patient history of the onset of the headaches or the change in the characteristics of the headache in patients with chronic headaches, elevated ESR, and temporal artery biopsy that confirms the diagnosis. The condition is immediately treated with steroids if possible, or alternatively with cyclosporine, azathioprine, or methotrexate.

The onset of ophthalmic alterations requires emergency care because any loss of vision before treatment is initiated will be irreversible. In addition, if treatment is delayed beyond two weeks after the onset of the initial vision loss, vision in the unaffected eye will be lost as well. Additional complications are related to steroid therapy and include stroke, myocardial infarction, small-bowel infarction, vertebral body fractures, and steroid psychoses. Even with successful treatment that prevents irreversible vision alterations, the patient with temporal arteritis has a lifelong risk of inflammatory disease of the large vessels.

Migraine

Migraine headaches are often preceded by an aura, which may be visual or sensory. The pulsatile pain associated with migraine headaches is described as throbbing and constant and most often localizes to one side of the head. Other manifestations include photophobia, sound sensitivity, nausea and vomiting, and anorexia. The pain increases over a period of one to two hours and then may last from 4 to 72 hours. The exact cause of the migraine headache syndrome is not well understood; however, there is strong evidence of a genetic link and some support for the role of alterations in neurovascular function and neurotransmitter regulation. Risk factors include elevated C-reactive protein and homocysteine levels, increased levels of TNF-alpha and adhesion molecules (systemic inflammation markers), increased body weight, hypertension, impaired insulin sensitivity, and coronary artery disease. The diagnosis is determined by the patient's history, laboratory testing for inflammatory markers, and imaging studies and lumbar puncture, as indicated by the severity of the patient's condition.

The treatment for migraine headaches may be preventive, therapeutic, or symptomatic. Medications used to prevent migraine headaches are used for those patients with chronic disease who have fourteen or more headaches per month. Antiemetics are used to lessen nausea and vomiting, while opioids may be prescribed even though their use in migraine management is not recommended. The emergency care of the patient with a migraine headache is focused on establishing the differential diagnosis and correcting fluid volume alterations that may result from vomiting. Although most patients who seek

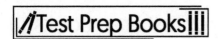

emergency care are diagnosed with migraine headaches, the importance of early intervention for temporal arteritis, stroke, or brain tumor requires a prompt diagnosis.

Increased Intracranial Pressure

Under normal circumstances, there is a dynamic equilibrium among the bony structure of the cranium, brain tissue, and extracellular fluid that comprise approximately 85 percent of the intracranial volume; the blood volume that comprises 10 percent of the volume; and the CSF that occupies the remaining 5 percent of the volume of the cranium. If any one of these volumes increases, there must be a compensatory decrease in one or more of the remaining volumes to maintain normal intracranial pressure (ICP) and optimal cerebral perfusion pressure (CPP). The CPP represents the pressure gradient for cerebral perfusion and is equal to the difference between the mean arterial pressure (MAP) and the ICP ($MAP - ICP = CPP$).

The process of autoregulation maintains optimal CPP by dilation and constriction of the cerebral arterioles; however, if the MAP falls below 65 millimeters of mercury or rises above 150 millimeters of mercury, autoregulation is ineffective, and cerebral blood flow is dependent on blood pressure (BP). Once this mechanism fails, any increase in volume potentially will cause an increase in the ICP. For instance, normal ICP may be maintained in the presence of a slow-growing tumor; however, a sudden small accumulation of blood will cause a sharp increase in the ICP. Eventually, all autoregulatory mechanisms will be exhausted in either circumstance, and the ICP will be increased. In an adult in the supine position, the normal ICP is 7 to 15 millimeters of mercury, while an ICP greater than 15 millimeters of mercury is considered abnormal, and pressures greater than 20 millimeters of mercury require intervention.

Conditions associated with increased ICP include space-occupying lesions such as tumors and hematomas; obstruction of CSF or hydrocephalus; increased production of CSF due to tumor formation; cerebral edema resulting from head injuries, strokes, infection, or surgery; hyponatremia; hepatic encephalopathy; and idiopathic intracranial hypertension. Early manifestations of increased ICP include blurred vision with gradual dilation of the pupil and slowed pupillary response, restlessness, and confusion with progressive disorientation as to time, then to place, and finally to person. Later signs include initially ipsilateral pupillary dilation and fixation, which progresses to bilateral dilation and fixation; decorticate or decerebrate posturing; and Cushing's triad of manifestations that include bradycardia, widening pulse pressure, and Cheyne-Stokes respirations.

ICP monitoring will be used to assess all patients requiring emergency care for any condition that is potentially associated with increased ICP. Depending on the underlying pathology, common interventions for increased ICP include sedation and paralysis, intubation and hyperventilation to decrease the $PaCO_2$, infusion of mannitol, an osmotic diuretic, and hypertonic saline IV solutions. Emergency providers understand that sustained elevations of ICP are associated with a poor prognosis, and therefore, the underlying cause and manifestations must be treated aggressively.

Meningitis

Meningitis is defined as the infection and resulting inflammation of the three layers of the meninges, the membranous covering of the brain and spinal cord. The causative agent may be bacterial, viral, parasitic, or fungal, which commonly occurs in patients who are HIV positive. The most common bacterial agent is **S. pneumoniae**, while meningococcal meningitis is common in crowded living spaces. However, the development and use of the meningococcal vaccine (MCV 4) has reduced the incidence in college

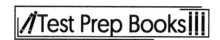

students and military personnel. The **Haemophilus influenzae** type B (Hib) vaccine has decreased the incidence and morbidity of the HI meningitis in infants, and the pneumococcal polysaccharide vaccine (PPSV) is being used to prevent meningitis in at-risk populations, such as immunocompromised adults, smokers, residents in long-term care facilities, and adults with chronic disease.

General risk factors for bacterial infection of the meninges include loss of, or decreased function of, the spleen; hypoglobinemia; chronic glucocorticoid use; deficiency of the complement system; diabetes; renal insufficiency; alcoholism; chronic liver disease; otitis media; and trauma associated with leakage of the CSF. Bacterial meningitis is infectious, and early diagnosis and treatment are essential for survival and recovery.

Emergency providers understand that even with adequate treatment, 50 percent of patients with bacterial meningitis will develop complications within two to three weeks of the acute infection, and long-term deficits are common in 30 percent of the surviving patients. The complications are specific to the causative organism, but may include hearing loss, blindness, paralysis, seizure disorder, muscular deficiencies, ataxia, hydrocephalus, and subdural effusions. In contrast, the incidence of viral meningitis is often associated with other viral conditions such as mumps, measles, herpes, and infections due to arboviruses such as the West Nile virus. The treatment is supportive, and the majority of patients recover without long-term complications; however, the outcome is less certain for patients who are immunocompromised or less than two years old or more than sixty years old.

The classic manifestations of bacterial meningitis include fever, nuchal rigidity, and headache. Additional findings may include nausea and vomiting, photophobia, confusion, and a decreased level of consciousness. Patients with meningococcal meningitis may commonly exhibit a non-blanchable red or purple rash, but rash can occasionally be present in patients with viral meningitis as well. Patients with viral meningitis may report the incidence of fatigue, muscle aches, and decreased appetite prior to the illness. Infants may exhibit a high-pitched cry, muscle flaccidity, irritability, and bulging fontanels.

The diagnosis of meningitis is determined by lumbar puncture; CSF analysis; cultures of the blood, nose, and respiratory secretions and any skin lesions that are present; complete blood count (CBC); electrolytes; coagulation studies; serum glucose to compare with CSF glucose; and procalcitonin to differentiate bacterial meningitis from aseptic meningitis in children. There is a small risk of herniation of the brain when the CSF is removed during the lumbar puncture, and while a computerized tomography (CT) scan may be done to assess the risk, emergency providers understand that effective antibiotic treatment must be initiated as quickly as possible to prevent the morbidity associated with bacterial meningitis. The results of the Gram stain of the CSF and blood will dictate the initial antibiotic therapy, which will be modified when the specific agent is identified. Additional interventions include seizure precautions, cardiac monitoring, and ongoing assessment of respiratory and neurological function. Patients with bacterial meningitis may require long-term rehabilitation.

Seizure Disorders

A **seizure** is defined as a chaotic period of uncoordinated electrical activity in the brain, which results in one of several characteristic behaviors. Although the exact cause is unknown, several possible triggers have been proposed as noted below. The recently revised classification system categorizes seizure activity according to the area of the brain where the seizure initiates, the patient's level of awareness during the seizure, and other descriptive features such as the presence of an aura. The unclassified category includes seizure patterns that do not conform to the primary categories. Seizures that originate in a single area of the brain are designated as **focal** seizures, while seizures that originate in two or more different networks are designated as **generalized** seizures. The remaining seizures in the onset category include seizures without an identified point of onset and seizures that progress from focal seizures to generalized seizures.

Risk factors associated with seizures include genetic predisposition, illnesses with severe temperature elevation, head trauma, cerebral edema, inappropriate use or discontinuance of antiepileptic drugs (AEDs), intracerebral infection, excess or deficiency of sodium and glucose, toxin exposure, hypoxia, and acute drug or alcohol withdrawal. Patients are encouraged to identify any conditions that may be triggers for their seizure activity. Although the triggers vary greatly from one patient to another, commonly identified events include increased physical activity, excessive stress, hyperventilation, fatigue, acute ETOH (ethyl alcohol) ingestion, exposure to flashing lights, and inhaled chemicals, including cocaine.

The tonic phase presents as stiffening of the limbs for a brief period, while the clonic phase is evidenced by jerking motions of the limbs. These manifestations may be accompanied by a decreased level of consciousness, respiratory alterations and cyanosis, incontinence, and biting of the tongue. Absence seizures are manifested by a decreased level of awareness without abnormal muscular activity. The manifestations of the postictal phase include alterations in consciousness and awareness and increased oral secretions. Seizure disorders are diagnosed by serum lab studies to assess AED levels and to identify excess alcohol and recreational drugs, metabolic alterations, and kidney and liver function. Electroencephalography (EEG) and the enhanced magnetoencephalography are used to identify the origin of the altered electrical activity in the brain, and MRI, skull films, and CSF analysis are used to rule out possible sources of the seizure disorder such as tumor formation.

Seizure disorders are treated with AEDs that stabilize the neuron cell membrane by facilitating the inhibitory mechanisms or opposing the excitatory mechanisms. Patients with a chronic seizure disorder, or epilepsy, usually require a combination of medications to minimize seizure activity. Elderly patients respond differently to the AEDs and may require frequent assessment and revision of the care plan. The emergency care of the patient with seizures is focused on patient safety during and after the seizure and the cessation and prevention of the seizure activity. Prolonged seizure activity is defined as **status epilepticus,** which is the occurrence of multiple seizures, each lasting more than 5 minutes over a 30-minute period. This life-threatening condition is commonly the result of incorrect usage of AEDs or the use of recreational drugs. Emergency care of this condition includes the immediate administration of phenytoin and benzodiazepines, in addition to possible general anesthesia if the medication therapy is not effective.

Shunt Dysfunctions

Increased production or decreased absorption and drainage of CSF results in hydrocephalus. This condition develops in infants, due to premature birth, intracranial hemorrhage, and genetic defects such as spina bifida, while in older children and adults, CSF accumulations due to hemorrhagic disease and tumor formation result in a significant increase in ICP due to the presence of a rigid cranium. In any event, emergency care of hydrocephalus is necessary to prevent physical and intellectual deficits.

If tumor formation is responsible for the development of hydrocephalus, removal of the tumor commonly results in an 88 percent reduction in the ICP. Research indicates that medical interventions are only minimally effective, and while surgical interventions have greater efficacy in select patients, 75 percent of patients with hydrocephalus will require the placement of a shunt for long-term drainage of the CSF. A CSF shunt facilitates the flow excess CSF from the ventricle to a distant anatomical site such

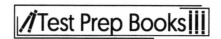

as the peritoneum (the most common site), the atria, and the pleural space. The catheter has a one-way flow pressure valve that limits the rate of flow of the CSF from the cerebral ventricle to the distant absorption site and a reservoir that provides percutaneous access to the shunt. The catheter is positioned in the ventricle and then tunneled subcutaneously to the collection site, allowing the excess CSF to flow from the ventricle to be reabsorbed, thereby decreasing the ICP.

Infections of the shunt manifest with similar signs of increased ICP in addition to possible purulent drainage, skin erosion and erythema, abdominal pain, and signs of peritonitis. Fever may or may not be present and is not necessary to confirm the diagnosis. Noninfectious complications related to the catheter include mechanical failure, migration of the distal catheter due to the patient's growth, and initial mispositioning of the catheter. Obstruction of the catheter accounts for 50 to 80 percent of all shunt failures, with the proximal catheter and shunt valve identified as the most common sites of obstruction due to choroid ingrowth or deposition of blood and cellular debris. Obstruction of the distal catheter, which occurs most often at the abdominal entry site, is less common and may be due to twisting of the catheter or from obstruction by inflammatory cellular debris or pseudocyst formation.

Emergency providers understand that the manifestations of each of these complications are age-dependent, with infants experiencing bulging of the fontanels and increasing head circumference in addition to other expected signs of increased ICP, such as headache, vomiting without nausea, changes in the level of consciousness, irritability, bradycardia, seizures, and visual alterations. Patients and care providers must be alert for these changes to access appropriate emergency care. Previous shunt revision or infection are associated with an increased risk of shunt failure, which typically occurs two to four months after insertion of the catheter. MRI scans, shunt series radiographs and nuclear medicine studies, and ultrasounds are used to assess the integrity and position of the catheter. Emergency management includes initiating a neurosurgical consultation, close observation of all vital signs for the advancement of the increased ICP, identification of the cause of the malfunction, treatment of any infection, and drainage of the excess CSF through the reservoir.

Spinal Cord Injuries

Injuries to the spinal cord are associated with severe and often irreversible neurological deficits and disabilities. Spinal cord injuries (SCIs) may be due to one or a combination of the following types of injury: direct traumatic injuries of the spinal cord, compression of the spinal cord by bone fragments or hematoma formation, or ischemia resulting from damage to the spinal arteries. The anatomical location of the SCI predicts the degree of sensory and motor function that will be lost. In addition, the injury will be labeled as **paraplegia** if the lesion is at the T1 to the T5 level, affecting only the lower extremities, or **tetraplegia** if the lesion is at the C1 to the C7 level, affecting both the upper and lower extremities in addition to respiratory function.

SCIs may be categorized as complete or incomplete depending on the degree of impairment. While complete SCIs are associated with complete loss of sensory-motor function, incomplete lesions are determined by the actual portion of the spinal cord that is affected. Central spinal cord syndrome is an incomplete SCI that involves upper extremity weakness or paralysis with little or no deficit noted in the lower extremities. Anterior spinal cord syndrome is also an incomplete SCI that is associated with loss of motor function, pain, and sensation below the injury; however, the sensations of light touch, proprioception, and vibration remain intact. In addition, Brown-Sequard syndrome is an incomplete lesion of one-half of the spinal cord, which results in paralysis on the side of the injury and loss of pain and temperature sensation on the opposite side of the injury.

Emergency providers understand that the injury to the spinal cord is an evolving process, which means that the level of the injury can rise one to two spinal levels within 48 to 72 hours after the initial insult. An incomplete injury may progress to a complete injury during this time due to the effects of altered blood flow and resulting edema and the presence of abnormal free radicals. Essential interventions aimed at minimizing or preventing this progression include establishing and maintaining normal oxygenation, arterial blood gas (ABG) values, and perfusion of the spinal cord.

SCIs are also associated with three shock syndromes, including hemorrhagic shock, spinal shock, and neurogenic shock. Hemorrhagic shock from an acute or occult source must be suspected in all SCIs below the T6 level that present with hypotension. Spinal shock refers to the loss of sensory-motor function that may be temporary or permanent depending on the specific injury. At the same time, the patient must be monitored for signs of neurogenic shock, which presents with a triad of symptoms that include hypotension, bradycardia, and peripheral vasodilation. This complication is due to alterations in autonomic nervous system function, which causes loss of vagal tone. Most often, it occurs with an injury above the T6 level, resulting in decreased vascular resistance and vasodilation. Neurogenic shock may also be associated with hypothermia due to vasodilation; rapid, shallow respirations; difficulty breathing; cold, clammy, pale skin; nausea; vomiting; and dizziness.

Emergency treatment of neurogenic shock includes IV fluids and inotropic medications to support the BP and IV atropine and/or pacemaker insertion, as needed, to treat the bradycardia. If a patient presents with neurological deficits 8 or more hours after sustaining an SCI, high-dose prednisone may be administered to reverse the manifestations of neurogenic shock.

Emergency management of SCIs is focused on preventing extension of the injury and long-term deficits with immobilization and interventions based on the Airway, Breathing, and Circulation protocol. Cervical SCIs result in an 80 to 95 percent decrease in vital capacity, and mechanical ventilation is often required for lesions at this level. Support of the circulation is addressed in the treatment of neurogenic shock. Other supportive treatment interventions are aimed at minimizing the effects of immobility. Emergency providers are aware that patients with complete SCIs have less than a 5 percent chance of recovery; however, more than 90 percent of all patients with SCIs eventually return home and regain some measure of independence.

Stroke

A **stroke** is defined as the death of brain tissue due to ischemic or hemorrhagic injury. Ischemic strokes are more common than hemorrhagic strokes; however, the differential diagnosis of these conditions requires careful attention to the patient's history and physical examination. In general, an acute onset of neurological symptoms and seizures is more common with hemorrhagic stroke, while ischemic stroke is more frequently associated with a history of some form of trauma. The National Institutes of Health (NIH) Stroke Scale represents an international effort to standardize the assessment and treatment protocols for stroke. The scale includes detailed criteria and the protocol for assessment of the neurological system. The stroke scale items are to be administered in the official order listed and there are directions that denote how to score each item.

Ischemic Stroke

Ischemic strokes result from occlusion of the cerebral vasculature as a result of a thrombotic or embolic event. At the cellular level, the ischemia leads to hypoxia that rapidly depletes the ATP stores. As a result, the cellular membrane pressure gradient is lost, and there is an influx of sodium, calcium, and water into the cell, which leads to cytotoxic edema. This process creates scattered regions of ischemia in

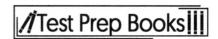

the affected area, containing cells that are dead within minutes of the precipitating event. This core of ischemic tissue is surrounded by an area with minimally-adequate perfusion that may remain viable for several hours after the event. These necrotic areas are eventually liquefied and acted upon by macrophages, resulting in the loss of brain parenchyma. These affected sites, if sufficiently large, may be prone to hemorrhage, due to the formation of collateral vascular supply with or without the use of medications such as recombinant tissue plasminogen activator (rtPA). The ischemic process also compromises the blood-brain barrier, which leads to the movement of water and protein into the extracellular space within 4 to 6 hours after the onset of the stroke, resulting in vasogenic edema.

Nonmodifiable risk factors for ischemic stroke include age, gender, ethnicity, history of migraine headaches with aura, and a family history of stroke or transient ischemic attacks (TIAs). Modifiable risk factors include hypertension, diabetes, hypercholesterolemia, cardiac disease including atrial fibrillation, valvular disease and heart failure, elevated homocysteine levels, obesity, illicit drug use, alcohol abuse, smoking, and sedentary lifestyle. The research related to the occurrence of stroke in women indicates the need to treat hypertension aggressively prior to and during pregnancy and prior to the use of contraceptives to prevent irreversible damage to the microvasculature. In addition, it is recommended that to reduce their risk of stroke, women with a history of migraine headaches preceded by an aura should ameliorate all modifiable risk factors, and all women over seventy-five years old should be routinely assessed for the onset of atrial fibrillation.

Heredity is associated with identified gene mutations and the process of atherosclerosis and cholesterol metabolism. Hypercholesterolemia and the progression of atherosclerosis in genetically-susceptible individuals are now regarded as active inflammatory processes that contribute to endothelial damage of the cerebral vasculature, thereby increasing the risk for strokes. There are also early indications that infection also contributes to the development and advancement of atherosclerosis.

The presenting manifestations of ischemic stroke must be differentiated from other common diseases, including brain tumor formation, hyponatremia, hypoglycemia, seizure disorders, and systemic infection. The sudden onset of hemisensory losses, visual alterations, hemiparesis, ataxia, nystagmus, and aphasia are commonly, although not exclusively, associated with ischemic strokes. The availability of reperfusion therapies dictates the emergent use of diagnostic imaging studies, including CT and MRI scans, carotid duplex scans, and digital subtraction angiography to confirm the data obtained from the patient's history and physical examination. Laboratory studies include CBC, coagulation studies, chemistry panels, cardiac biomarkers, toxicology assays, and pregnancy testing as appropriate.

The emergency care of the patient who presents with an ischemic stroke is focused on the stabilization of the patient's ABCs, completion of the physical examination and appropriate diagnostic studies, and initiation of reperfusion therapy as appropriate, within 60 minutes of arrival in the emergency department. Reperfusion therapies include the use of alteplase (the only fibrinolytic agent that is approved for the treatment of ischemic stroke), antiplatelet agents, and mechanical thrombectomy. Emergency providers must also be alert for hyperthermia, hypoxia, hypertension or hypotension, and signs of cardiac ischemia or cardiac arrhythmias.

Hemorrhagic Stroke

Hemorrhagic strokes are less common than ischemic strokes; however, a hemorrhagic stroke is more likely to be fatal than an ischemic stroke. A hemorrhagic stroke is the result of bleeding into the parenchymal tissue of the brain due to leakage of blood from damaged intracerebral arteries. These hemorrhagic events occur more often in specific areas of the brain, including the thalamus, cerebellum, and brain stem. The tissue surrounding the hemorrhagic area is also subject to injury due to the mass effect of the accumulated blood volume. In the event of subarachnoid hemorrhage, ICP becomes elevated with resulting dysfunction of the autoregulation response, which leads to abnormal vasoconstriction, platelet aggregation, and decreased perfusion and blood flow, resulting in cerebral ischemia.

Risk factors for hemorrhagic stroke include older age; a history of hypertension, which is present in 60 percent of patients; personal history of stroke; alcohol abuse; and illicit drug use. Common conditions associated with hemorrhagic stroke include hypertension, cerebral amyloidosis, coagulopathies, vascular alterations including arteriovenous malformation, vasculitis, intracranial neoplasm, and a history of anticoagulant or antithrombotic therapy.

Although the presenting manifestations for hemorrhagic stroke differ in some respect from the those associated with ischemic stroke, none of these such manifestations is an absolute predictor of one or the other. In general, patients with hemorrhagic stroke present with a headache that may be severe, significant alterations in the level of consciousness and neurological function, hypertension, seizures, and nausea and vomiting. The specific neurological defects depend on the anatomical site of the hemorrhage and may include hemisensory loss, hemiparesis, aphasia, and visual alterations.

Diagnostic studies include CBC, chemistry panel, coagulation studies, and blood glucose. Non-contrast CT scan or MRI are the preferred imaging studies. CT or magnetic resonance angiography may also be used to obtain images of the cerebral vasculature. Close observation of the patient's vital signs, neurological vital signs, and ICP is necessary.

The emergency management of the patient with hemorrhagic stroke is focused on the ABC protocol, in addition to the control of bleeding, seizure activity, and increased ICP. There is no single medication used to treat hemorrhagic stroke; however, recent data suggests that aggressive emergency management of hypertension initiated early and aimed at reducing the systolic BP to less than 140 millimeters of mercury may be effective in reducing the growth of the hematoma at the site, which decreases the mass effect. Beta-blockers and ACE inhibitors are recommended to facilitate this reduction. Endotracheal intubation for ventilatory support may be necessary; however, hyperventilation is not recommended due to the resulting suppression of cerebral blood flow. While seizure activity will be treated with AEDs, there is controversy related to the prophylactic use of these medicines. Increased ICP requires osmotic diuretic therapy, elevation of the head of the bed to 30 degrees, sedation and analgesics as appropriate, and antacids. Steroid therapy is not effective and is not recommended.

Patients who present with manifestations of hemorrhagic stroke with a history of anticoagulation therapy present a special therapeutic challenge due to the extension of the hematoma formation. More than 50 percent of patients taking warfarin who suffer a hemorrhagic stroke will die within thirty days. This statistic is consistent in patients with international normalized ratio (INR) levels within the therapeutic range, with increased mortality noted in patients with INRs that exceed the therapeutic level. Emergency treatment includes fresh frozen plasma, IV vitamin K, prothrombin complex concentrates, and recombinant factor VIIa (rFVIIa). There are administration concerns with each of these therapies that must be addressed to prevent any delays in the reversal of the effects of the warfarin.

Transient Ischemic Attack

A **transient ischemic attack** (TIA) is defined as a short-term episode of altered neurological function that lasts for less than one hour; it may be imperceptible to the patient. The deficit may be related to speech, movement, behavior, or memory and may be caused by an ischemic event in the brain, spinal cord, or retina. The patient's history and neurological assessment according to the NIH Stroke Scale establish the

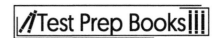

diagnosis. Additional diagnostic studies include CBC, glucose, sedimentation rate, electrolytes, lipid profile, toxicology screen, 12-lead ECG, and CSF analysis. Imaging studies include non-contrast MRI or CT, carotid Doppler exam, and angiography.

Emergency care of the patient with a TIA is focused on the assessment of any neurological deficits and the identification of comorbid conditions that may be related to the attack. Hospital admission is required in the event of an attack that lasts more than one hour, if the patient has experienced more than a single attack in a one-week period, or if the attack is related to a cardiac source such as atrial fibrillation or a myocardial infarction. The $ABCD^2$ stroke risk score calculates the patient's risk for experiencing a true stroke within two days after the TIA based on five factors (see the table below). Interventions aimed at stroke prevention in relation to the risk stratification as calculated by the $ABCD^2$ score are specific to underlying comorbidities; however, treatment with ASA and clopidogrel is commonly prescribed.

$ABCD^2$ Stroke Risk Score		
	1 Point	2 Points
Age	$\geq$ 60 years	
Blood Pressure	SBP $\geq$ 140 mmHg DBP $\geq$ 90 mmHg	
Clinical Features	Speech impairment but no focal weakness	Focal weakness
Duration of Symptoms	$\leq$ 59 minutes	$\geq$ 60 minutes
Diabetes	Diagnosed	
Total Score (denotes risk for stroke (CVA) within 2 days after TIA)	0-3 points = 1% risk 4-5 points = 4.1% risk 6-7 points = 8.1% risk	

Trauma

The Advanced Trauma Life Support protocol is a standardized procedure for the assessment and treatment of trauma patients. Injuries that are immediately fatal or occur minutes to hours after the initial injury are most often due to hemorrhage, cardiovascular collapse, and failed oxygenation, while deaths that occur days to weeks after an injury are commonly due to sepsis and multisystem organ failure.

The primary survey or assessment of a trauma victim follows an ABCDE protocol: *A* refers to airway management; *B* refers to respiratory effort; *C* refers to circulation, including hemorrhage; *D* refers to gross mental status and mobility; and *E* addresses exposure such as hypothermia and environmental conditions. The results of the assessment dictate the interventions, while at the same time, monitoring devices are employed, a nasogastric tube and an indwelling urinary catheter are inserted, and lab samples for type/cross match, glucose, and ABGs are obtained.

The CT scan is the most useful imaging study; however, ultrasound, angiography, and A&P chest and pelvic films are also used. Fluid resuscitation is calculated according to estimated blood loss consistent with a standardized trauma protocol. Once the interventions have been initiated, a second assessment is performed that includes examination of every orifice and body system to identify additional or worsening injuries. Emergency providers understand that the source of any deterioration in a patient's condition after stabilization is most often associated with changes in the airway, breathing, or circulation.

Trauma related to burns, hypothermia, and high-voltage electrical burns require additional consideration. Burn injuries may require chemical neutralization, excision of eschar formation to prevent compartment syndrome, aggressive fluid replacement, and ventilatory support. Resuscitative efforts for patients with hypothermia should not be discontinued until the patient's core temperature has been brought to normal with warm IV solution. Myonecrotic damage due to high-voltage electrical burns may not be visible but can result in direct myocardial injury and life-threatening hyperkalemia due to muscle damage.

Acute care institutions are obligated to provide adequate skilled personnel, equipment, and resources to address the emergency needs of the trauma patient according to the agency's designated trauma care level.

Practice Questions

1. What is the specific pathology responsible for brain damage in Alzheimer's disease?
    a. Invasion of the cortex by infectious prions
    b. Multiple hemorrhagic strokes
    c. Deposition of amyloid-β plaques
    d. Formation of Lewy bodies

2. Which of the following statements correctly identifies the difference between the forgetfulness that is common to the normal aging process and the memory alterations associated with Alzheimer's disease?
    a. The processes are the same; however, memory alterations associated with Alzheimer's disease include only short-term memory loss.
    b. Forgetfulness is progressive and eventually results in the individual's inability to perform ADLs independently.
    c. Memory lapses associated with Alzheimer's disease improve with frequent cueing.
    d. The end stage of memory impairment in Alzheimer's disease is the inability to recognize family members.

3. Tensilon has been administered to treat an acute relapse in a patient with myasthenia gravis. The attached tracing is consistent with the expected response in which form of crisis?

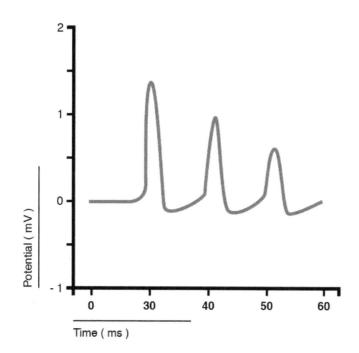

    a. Tensilon is not an effective treatment for either form of crisis.
    b. The tracing is consistent with the Tensilon response in a myasthenic crisis.
    c. The tracing is consistent with the Tensilon response in a cholinergic crisis.
    d. Tensilon will improve the muscle function in both forms of crises.

4. Which of the following statements is true?

    a. Ninety-five percent of the patients diagnosed with multiple sclerosis will potentially advance to a non-remitting disease pattern.

    b. The clinically-isolated incident is a definitive precursor of active MS.

    c. The primary-progressive form of MS is the most common presenting form of the disease.

    d. Prednisone is the medication of choice to slow progression in all forms of MS.

5. A patient arrives in the emergency department complaining of pain, tingling, and weakness in both feet and ankles. Which of the following assessment questions is of the highest priority for this patient?

    a. "When did you first notice the weakness in your feet and ankles?"

    b. "Which activities make the pain better or worse?"

    c. "Have you had a viral or bacterial infection in the last few weeks?"

    d. "Have you ever previously experienced these symptoms?"

6. The emergency care of the patient with temporal arteritis is complex due to the wide range of possible complications that are associated with this condition. Which of the following complications requires immediate intervention to prevent irreversible damage?

    a. Lower extremity claudication

    b. Vertebral body fracture

    c. Early onset of blindness

    d. Infection related to immunosuppression

7. The emergency care provider is developing a care plan for the patient with increased ICP. Which of the following statements is INCORRECT?

    a. Barbiturate coma decreases the cerebral metabolic rate and the cerebral blood volume.

    b. The head of the bed should be elevated to 30 degrees to facilitate venous drainage.

    c. Intravenous mannitol decreases blood viscosity and cerebral parenchymal fluid.

    d. Hyperventilation decreases the $PaCO_2$, leading to arterial vasodilation.

8. Which of the following manifestations is considered to be a late sign of increased ICP?

    a. Mental confusion related to time

    b. Blurred vision

    c. BP of 170/40

    d. HR of 94 bpm

9. The nurse in the emergency department is assessing a nineteen-year-old college student who presents with sudden onset of headache that is associated with neck stiffness and fever. In caring for the patient with meningitis, the nurse understands that which of the following observations is correct?

    a. The presence of a skin rash eliminates the diagnosis of viral meningitis.

    b. Brain herniation after lumbar puncture is more common in immunosuppressed patients.

    c. The CSF protein level is decreased in bacterial meningitis.

    d. The MCV4 vaccine has dramatically decreased the incidence of meningitis in patients in long-term care facilities.

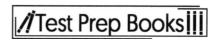

10. The nurse in the emergency department is caring for a patient who had a seizure today for the first time. The patient said that she noticed a strange odor just prior to "not feeling well." Vital signs are BP 120/74, HR 76, and an oral temperature 97.8 °F. The patient has no complaints of pain and no recent history of viral or bacterial illness. A friend witnessed that seizure and stated that the muscular movement lasted about 30 seconds. The patient was incontinent during the seizure but did not suffer any injuries. The patient recovered without any further manifestations of seizure activity. The nurse understands that which of the following interventions is most appropriate for this patient?
   a. Obtain laboratory analysis of recreational drug use.
   b. Institute oral therapy of AEDs.
   c. Prepare the patient for an immediate lumbar puncture for CSF analysis.
   d. Obtain an EEG and an MRI.

11. The nurse in the emergency department is caring for a thirty-year-old male patient with a ventriculoperitoneal shunt who is being assessed for shunt failure. The shunt was inserted four years ago when the patient developed hydrocephalus after a severe closed-head injury, and the patient has exhibited satisfactory control of ICP until 12 hours ago, when the patient complained of a headache, nausea, and tiredness. The patient's vital signs are BP 130/70, HR 82, RR 24, T 98.6 °F, PaO$_2$ 97 percent. Which of the following complications is most likely responsible for the patient's condition?
   a. Choroid ingrowth of the proximal catheter
   b. Migration of the distal catheter to an area that impedes absorption of the CSF
   c. Disconnection of the distal reservoir from the distal catheter tip
   d. Infection of the proximal catheter

12. The nurse is caring for the twenty-five-year-old male patient with an acute spinal cord injury at the C3 to C4 level. Which of the following manifestations is consistent with this injury?
   a. Vital capacity 45 percent of normal, hemoglobin 10.4 g/dL, heart rate 96 beats per minute
   b. Loss of somatic and reflex function, BP 160/90, effective cough effort
   c. Coarse and fine crackles bilaterally, heart rate 56 beats per minute, core temperature 96.7 °F
   d. BP 104/60, urinary output 18 mL over the last 60 minutes, heart rate 120 beats per minute

13. The nurse is caring for a sixty-six-year-old male patient with a history of warfarin therapy who presents with complaints of decreased sensation of the right lower and upper limbs, visual alterations, right hemiparesis, blurred vision, ataxia, nystagmus, and aphasia. The nurse expects to administer which of the following medications?
   a. Mannitol and vitamin K
   b. Warfarin and labetalol
   c. Alteplase and nitroprusside
   d. ASA and enalapril

14. The nurse is caring for a patient with an emerging ischemic stroke. The nurse prepares to administer which of the following fibrinolytic agents?
   a. Urokinase
   b. Streptokinase
   c. Alteplase
   d. Tenecteplase

15. The nurse in the emergency department is providing discharge education for a sixty-six-year-old patient with type 2 diabetes who has had a TIA. Which of the following patient statements indicates that the teaching has been effective?

    a. "There is nothing I can do to change my risk for another episode."

    b. "The best thing I can do is to keep my A1C level below 6.5 like my doctor said."

    c. "I only have type 2 diabetes, so that doesn't affect my blood vessels."

    d. "I'm glad I don't have to take insulin to fix this."

16. The nurse in the emergency department is admitting a patient who has sustained electrical burns 3 hours ago. The patient is awake, alert, and oriented, and vital signs are BP 136/70, HR 86, normal sinus rhythm, T 97.6 °F, pulse oximetry 97 percent, respiratory rate 18. The patient's skin is intact with one area of redness over the anterior chest wall. Two hours after admission, the patient is in cardiac arrest. What is the most likely cause of this complication?

    a. Hypovolemic shock

    b. Pulmonary edema

    c. Myocardial perforation

    d. Myonecrosis of skeletal muscle

Answer Explanations

1. C: The destruction of brain tissue in Alzheimer's disease is the result of amyloid-β plaque formation in the cerebral cortex. Creutzfeldt-Jakob disease is a rare form of dementia that results from tissue damage caused by infectious prions; therefore, Choice *A* is incorrect. Multiple hemorrhagic strokes may be a trigger for the deposition of amyloid-β plaque formation; however, this form of damage can exist without causing Alzheimer's disease. It is not the specific causative process for the disease; therefore, Choice *B* is incorrect. The formation of Lewy bodies is responsible for the damage associated with Parkinson's disease, not Alzheimer's disease; therefore, Choice *D* is incorrect.

2. D: Early manifestations of memory impairment in Alzheimer's disease are associated with short-term memory loss and the inability to assimilate new knowledge, with progressive impairment that affects long-term memory, mood, and independent functioning. The end stage of this process is the inability to recognize family members. The processes are not the same. Memory lapses associated with forgetfulness improve with cueing and do not progress to the inability to recognize family members. Therefore, Choices *A*, *B*, and *C* are incorrect.

3. B: Tensilon is used in myasthenic crisis to improve muscle function affected by deficient cholinesterase inhibitor levels; however, the improvement is temporary. Tensilon administration results in improved muscle function in myasthenic crisis; therefore, Choice *A* is incorrect. Tensilon effectively treats a myasthenic crisis. However, it will not improve a cholinergic crisis and may worsen the symptoms; therefore, Choices *C* and *D* are incorrect.

4. A: Ten percent of MS patients are initially diagnosed with the primary-progressive form of MS, which means that the disease is always active without periods of remission. The relapsing-remitting form of MS accounts for 85 percent of the patients diagnosed with MS, which means that they will eventually progress to the secondary-progressive form; this means that the disease is always active. The potential progression of an isolated incident to MS depends on the presence or absence of plaque formation on MRI scans. The presence of alterations in the myelin sheath is strongly predictive of eventual progression. However, the absence of those lesions does not rule out the possibility of subsequent progression to MS; therefore, Choice *B* is incorrect. Only 10 percent of MS patients present with the primary-progressive form; therefore, Choice *C* is incorrect. Disease-modifying drugs are the preferred agents to treat MS. However, prednisone may be used if a patient is unable to tolerate the DMDs; therefore, Choice *D* is incorrect.

5. C: All of the assessment questions are appropriate for this patient; however, if the patient reports a recent infection, the emergency care providers understand that there is potential for the rapid onset of respiratory failure, which potentially alters the plan of care. Therefore, Choices *A*, *B*, and *D* are incorrect.

6. C: If complete or partial blindness develops in a patient with temporal arteritis prior to therapeutic intervention, the deficit may progress and become irreversible, which constitutes an ophthalmologic emergency. Lower limb claudication due to vasculitis and ischemic changes may occur as the result of the inflammatory process, and the condition does require assessment and monitoring; however, visual alterations remain a higher priority for emergency care. Vertebral body fractures and infection are related to steroid therapy, which may occur during therapy, and both conditions will require assessment and intervention; however, the need to prevent irreversible blindness is a more urgent priority.

10

7. D: Choice *D* states that decreasing the PaCO₂ results in arterial vasodilation, which is incorrect because vasodilation would increase, not decrease, ICP. Decreasing the PaCO₂ results in arterial vasoconstriction; therefore, Choice *D* is the correct answer. Choices *A, B,* and *C* all identify appropriate interventions for increased ICP; therefore, they are incorrect.

8. C: Cushing's triad of manifestations are late signs of increased ICP. Choice *C* is an example of widening pulse pressure: Normal pulse pressure is 40 to 60 mmHg, while the pulse pressure in Choice *C* is 130 mmHg, and thus is the correct choice. Choices *A, B,* and *D* are all early signs of increased ICP and, therefore, are incorrect.

9. B: The risk of brain herniation is higher in patients who are immunosuppressed, over sixty years old, have a history of recent seizure activity, or have a disease of the CNS. A CT scan may be done prior to the lumbar puncture in this patient population; however, instituting antibiotic therapy to prevent morbidity remains the priority intervention. Bacterial meningitis is associated with a characteristic erythematous rash. However, depending on the causative organism, rashes may also be present with viral meningitis; therefore, the presence or absence of the rash cannot differentiate between the two conditions, which means that Choice *A* is incorrect. The protein level of the CSF is elevated, not decreased, in bacterial meningitis. The inflammatory response resulting from the bacterial infection alters the blood-brain barrier, which allows the leakage of protein from the blood into the subarachnoid space, causing marked increase in the protein level of the CSF; therefore, Choice *C* is incorrect. The meningococcal vaccine, MCV4, is effective against meningococcal meningitis and has decreased the incidence of the disease among college students and military personnel who typically reside in close quarters. Residents of long-term care facilities are protected against pneumococcal meningitis by the PPSV; therefore, Choice *D* is incorrect.

10. D: The appropriate response to an initial unprovoked seizure episode—one that is not related to a specific cause such as head trauma—is to identify any abnormal electrical activity of the brain with an EEG and any anatomical lesions in the brain with MRI. There is no indication of substance abuse in the patient's history, which means that this assessment would not be a priority for this patient at this point; therefore, Choice *A* is incorrect. General guidelines indicate that AED therapy should be delayed until a second unprovoked seizure episode occurs and after the initial EEG and MRI studies are completed; therefore, Choice *B* is incorrect. The patient's history does not support the possibility of infection as the precipitating event for this seizure activity, which means performing the invasive lumbar puncture would not be indicated; therefore, Choice *C* is incorrect.

11. A: The most common complication associated with shunts is the obstruction of the proximal catheter. Over a period, the proximal tip of the catheter can become embedded in the choroid, obstructing the catheter and delaying the drainage of the CSF. The shunt valve on the proximal end can also become obstructed with blood cells and other cellular debris. Obstruction of the distal catheter is less common than proximal obstruction but occurs more frequently than infection or dislocation. Migration of the catheter tip is most commonly related to the growth of the patient, which means that this complication occurs in younger children most often. The patient referenced in this scenario was an adult at the time of insertion of the catheter; therefore, this is not a likely cause for his current problem, and Choice *B* is incorrect. Disconnection of the segments of the shunt system is a rare occurrence that is due to a manufacturer's defect or improper installation of the device. When this malfunction does occur, it is readily discovered in the postoperative period; therefore, Choice *C* is incorrect. Infection most commonly occurs during the initial two to four months after the catheter is inserted. Infection is most often associated with overt signs of infection such as erythema, purulent drainage, peritonitis, and abdominal pain; however, fever may or may not be present. The patient included in the scenario has

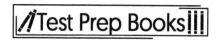

had the shunt in place for four years, which exceeds the common timeline for site infection, and the assessment does not provide any support for a diagnosis of infection; therefore, Choice *D* is incorrect.

12. C: Injuries above the T6 level are associated with neurogenic shock, due to alterations of the autonomic nervous system, resulting in the loss of vagal tone. This manifests as decreased vascular resistance and vasodilation. Injury at this level is also associated with alterations in respiratory function, which results in symptoms such as decreased vital capacity and the presence of adventitious breath sounds. In addition, hypothermia is common; therefore, Choice *C* is correct. A vital capacity level that equals 45 percent of normal is associated with injuries at the T1 level or below, and is an indication of hemorrhagic shock rather than neurogenic shock. A hemoglobin level of 10.4 g/dL in a male patient is also associated with acute or occult blood loss rather than loss of vagal tone, and is indicative of hemorrhagic shock. The patient's level of injury is consistent with neurogenic shock, which is manifested by bradycardia, not tachycardia; therefore, Choice *A* is incorrect. Loss of somatic and reflex function is associated with spinal shock, and hypertension and an effective cough effort are inconsistent with the level of the patient's injury; therefore, Choice *B* is incorrect. The collective manifestations of hypotension, oliguria, and tachycardia are associated with hypovolemic shock rather than neurogenic shock; therefore, Choice *D* is incorrect.

13. A: The patient's manifestations are consistent with a diagnosis of hemorrhagic stroke. Although there is no single therapeutic agent that is specific to the treatment of hemorrhagic stroke, aggressive treatment of hypertension and the use of agents to counteract the anticoagulative effect of warfarin are common interventions. Mannitol is an osmotic diuretic used to decrease intracranial pressure that results from the hematoma formation at the hemorrhagic site. Vitamin K is used to counteract warfarin therapy, and the dose will be titrated to the results of the coagulation studies; therefore, Choice *A* is correct. Warfarin is an anticoagulant that is not recommended for use in hemorrhagic stroke. Labetalol is an antihypertensive agent that might be used for hemorrhagic stroke. However, it would not be ordered with warfarin therapy; therefore, Choice *B* is incorrect. Alteplase is a fibrinolytic agent, and nitroprusside is a potent vasoconstricting agent. Neither of these medications is appropriate in the care of hemorrhagic stroke; therefore, Choice *C* is incorrect. Enalapril is an antihypertensive agent that might be used for hemorrhagic stroke. However, it would not be ordered with ASA, which is an antiplatelet agent; therefore, Choice *D* is incorrect.

14. C: Alteplase is the single fibrinolytic agent approved for the treatment of ischemic stroke because it is associated with fewer adverse effects than the remaining agents. Streptokinase and tenecteplase have been used effectively to treat patients with acute myocardial infarction; however, in patients with ischemic stroke, streptokinase has been associated with an increased risk of intracranial hemorrhage and death. Current evidence for the efficacy and safety of urokinase and tenecteplase does not support their use for the treatment of ischemic stroke. Therefore, Choices *A, B,* and *D* are incorrect.

15. B: The elevated glucose levels associated with both type 1 and type 2 diabetes result in atherosclerosis, or wall thickening of the small arterioles and capillaries, which alters the circulation in the brain, retina, peripheral nerves, and kidneys. These changes are cumulative and irreversible; however, long-term control of the serum glucose level as measured by the A1C can limit the progression of this process. Current research indicates that the optimum A1C level is patient-specific. In this discussion, the patient knows his personal A1C target and understands the association between the elevated glucose levels and the occurrence of the TIA; therefore, Choice *B* is correct. Two of the ABCD[2] score categories are modifiable risk factors. Maintaining the systolic and diastolic blood pressure and blood glucose level as defined by the A1C within normal limits may lower the risk of a repeated attack. The patient should be encouraged to make the necessary lifestyle changes, including smoking cessation, dietary modifications, exercise participation, and compliance with the medication regimen that may include antihypertensive and glucose-lowering agents. Choice A is incorrect. There are differences in the pathophysiology between type 1 and type 2 diabetes; however, the complications are similar. In type 2 diabetes, hyperglycemia and insulin resistance contribute to increased low-density lipoproteins and triglycerides and decreased levels of high-density lipoproteins and alterations in microvasculature; therefore, Choice C is incorrect. To prevent further damage to the vascular system and reduce the risk of recurrent TIAs, the use of insulin may be necessary to control hyperglycemia as evidenced by the A1C level; therefore, Choice D is incorrect.

16. D: Although electrical shock may not result in visible burns on the skin, extensive damage to skeletal muscle tissue can result in myonecrosis of the muscle cells. This damage leads to the release of large amounts of potassium from the cell, resulting in hyperkalemia. Potassium levels in excess of 8.5 mEq/L will cause lethal cardiac arrhythmias; therefore, Choice D is correct. Hypovolemic shock can potentially contribute to cardiac complications. However, there is no evidence of hypovolemia in this discussion; therefore, this is an unlikely cause of the cardiac arrest, and Choice A is incorrect. The patient's oxygenation is normal, and the patient is alert and oriented; therefore, hypoxia is an unlikely cause of the cardiac arrest, so Choice B is incorrect. Cardiac perforation is a possible consequence of electrical burns. However, in this discussion, more than 5 hours has elapsed since the injury, and this lethal consequence is most commonly evident immediately after the injury occurs; therefore, Choice C is incorrect.

Gastrointestinal Emergencies

Acute Abdomen Peritonitis and Appendicitis

An **acute abdomen** is defined as the presence of manifestations associated with nontraumatic intra-abdominal pathology that often requires surgical intervention.

Peritonitis

Peritonitis is an inflammatory process affecting the peritoneum, which is the serosal membrane that lines the abdominal cavity. The normally sterile environment of the peritoneum can become infected by a pathogen, irritated by bile from a perforated gallbladder or lacerated liver, or from secretions from the perforation of the stomach. The onset, severity, and course of the condition vary according to the precipitating event. Presenting manifestations may include abdominal pain, nausea and vomiting, diarrhea, fever and chills, altered peristalsis, abdominal distention, and possible encephalopathy. Diagnosis is based on the patient's history, in addition to the results of routine lab studies and blood cultures; ultrasound, computerized tomography (CT), and x-ray studies of the abdomen; and paracentesis. Emergency care of peritonitis is focused on eliminating the source of infection or irritation, controlling the infection and inflammatory process with aggressive antibiotic therapy as appropriate to prevent progression to generalized sepsis, and maintaining organ function of the abdominal organs.

Appendicitis

Appendicitis is defined as the inflammation of the vermiform appendix, which extends from the cecum at the terminal end of the ileum. The inflammation results from the obstruction of the lumen of the appendix by accumulated fecaliths, bacteria, or parasites. The condition presents a surgical emergency due to the risk of perforation of the wall of the structure with resulting peritonitis and sepsis. The classic presenting symptoms are anorexia and periumbilical pain that evolves to the right lower quadrant, followed by vomiting. The diagnosis is made by the results of the physical examination, routine lab studies, pregnancy testing to rule out ectopic pregnancy, and ultrasound imaging. Emergency care includes antibiotic therapy and appendectomy.

Bleeding

Gastrointestinal (GI) bleeding is defined according to the area of the defect. Upper GI bleeding occurs superiorly to the junction of the duodenum and jejunum. Lower GI bleeding occurs in the large and small intestine. Conditions associated with upper GI bleeding include esophageal varices, gastric and duodenal ulcers, cancer, and Mallory-Weiss tears. Risk factors include age, history of gastroesophageal reflux disorder (GERD), use of nonsteroidal anti-inflammatory drugs (NSAIDs) and steroids, and alcoholism. Acute presenting manifestations include hematemesis, melena, hematochezia, and lightheadedness or fainting. The diagnosis is made by the patient's history and physical examination, routine lab studies including complete blood count (CBC) and coagulation tests, endoscopy, and chest films. Treatment is specific to the cause; e.g., peptic ulcer disease will be treated with the appropriate antibiotic and a proton-pump inhibitor (PPI).

Causative factors for GI bleeding of the lower intestine include anatomical defects such as diverticulosis, ischemic events of the vasculature related to radiation therapy or other embolic events, cancer, and infectious or noninfectious inflammatory conditions. Manifestations that are specific to the cause and location of the hemorrhage include melena, maroon stools or bright red blood, fever, dehydration, possible abdominal pain or distention, and hematochezia. Common diagnostic studies include routine lab studies, endoscopy, radionucleotide studies, and angiography. Treatment is focused on the identification and resolution of the source of the bleeding and correction of any hematologic deficits that resulted from the hemorrhage. Emergency providers are aware that orthostatic hypotension defined as a decrease in diastolic blood pressure (BP) of 10 millimeters of mercury or more is associated with a blood loss of approximately 1000 milliliters. Therefore, the emergency care of massive GI bleeding requires aggressive fluid volume replacement with isotonic crystalloids while the exact source of the bleeding is being confirmed.

Cholecystitis

Cholecystitis is defined as an inflammation of the gallbladder. It is most often due to blockage of the cystic duct by gallstones. The condition may be complicated by the presence of perforation or gangrene of the gallbladder. Common risk factors include increasing age, female gender, obesity or rapid weight loss, and pregnancy. Symptoms include colicky epigastric pain that radiates to the right upper quadrant that may become constant and a palpable gallbladder, jaundice, nausea, vomiting, and fever. Emergency providers understand that the elderly and chronically ill children may present with atypical manifestations of cholecystitis. Presenting symptoms in elderly patients may be limited to vague complaints of localized tenderness; however, the condition can rapidly progress to a more complicated form of cholecystitis due to infection, leading to gangrene or perforation of the gallbladder. This risk is increased in elderly patients with diabetes. Children with sickle cell disease, congenital biliary defects, or chronic illness requiring total parenteral nutrition (TPN) therapy may present with generalized abdominal pain and jaundice.

Diagnostic studies include routine lab tests, liver function tests, and abdominal ultrasounds. Additional imaging studies may be required; however, ultrasound is very sensitive for cholecystitis, does not expose the patient to radiation, and is readily available in the emergency care setting. Treatment options depend on the severity of symptoms. Acalculous cholecystitis may progress quickly to perforation and gangrene of the gallbladder requiring emergency intervention, while uncomplicated cases of acute cholecystitis can be treated with bowel rest, intravenous (IV) fluids, and short-term antibiotic therapy. Emergency providers understand that elective laparoscopic cholecystectomy is the procedure of choice, with the rate of conversion to open cholecystectomy at 5 percent; however, emergency laparoscopic cholecystectomy is associated with a 30 percent conversion rate.

Early recognition and intervention are required due to the rapid progression of acute acalculous cholecystitis to gangrene and perforation.

Cirrhosis

Cirrhosis of the liver is characterized by fibrotic changes that eventually accumulate as scar tissue that replaces functioning liver cells. The manifestations and onset of the disease, which may be gradual or rapid, depend on the exact etiology. Chronic hepatitis due to the hepatitis C virus has replaced alcoholic liver disease as the most common cause of cirrhosis in the United States. Although there are several additional conditions that are associated with the development of cirrhosis as noted below, nonalcoholic fatty liver disease (NAFLD), which is common in patients with diabetes, obesity, and elevated triglyceride levels and is estimated to affect 33 percent of all individuals in the United States, is a growing concern for providers. Cirrhosis is characterized by the abnormal retention of lipids in the cells that worsens as the process of hepatic fibrosis progresses. Other contributing conditions to the development of cirrhosis include sarcoidosis, primary biliary cirrhosis, chronic right-sided heart failure, tricuspid regurgitation, autoimmune hepatitis, and alpha 1 antitrypsin deficiency.

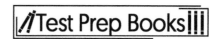

Common symptoms include ascites; abdominal pain; portal hypertension; hepatic encephalopathy with the deterioration of the level of consciousness from normal to somnolence, drowsiness, and coma; hepatorenal disease; fever; anorexia; weight loss; spider angiomas; jaundice; and coagulopathy. Treatment is initially focused on preventing the progression of the precipitating conditions. Hepatitis C is treated with antiviral agents; cardiac conditions are treated with diuretics, beta-blockers, and digoxin; and autoimmune disorders are treated with immunosuppressant agents. Once the fibrotic changes have occurred, symptomatic interventions include treatment of pruritus, zinc deficiency, and osteoporosis. Patients with advanced cirrhosis may be candidates for a liver transplant. The Model for End-Stage Liver Disease (MELD), which is used to allocate donor organs in the United States, calculates the projected patient survival rate following a liver transplant based on patient's age, serum bilirubin, creatinine, prothrombin time international normalized ratio (INR), sodium level, and a history of current or recent renal dialysis.

Diverticulitis

Diverticulitis is the inflammation of the diverticula, which are described as outpouchings or defects in the wall, most commonly located in the rectosigmoid segment of the large intestine. The diverticula are common in people over fifty years old, due to the increased pressure in the lumen of the bowel during defecation; however, most people do not experience diverticulitis. Inflammation of the diverticula occurs when fecaliths and other cellular debris become impacted in the outpouchings, initiating the changes in the mucous lining of the intestine.

Common manifestations of an acute episode include lower left quadrant pain, nausea, vomiting, chills, fever, and tachycardia. The condition must be differentiated from other inflammatory bowel diseases (IBDs), including Crohn's disease and ulcerative colitis, because the underlying pathology and treatment are different. Severe or prolonged manifestations will be treated with bowel rest, IV fluids, antibiotic therapy, and assessment of routine lab studies, including coagulation assay, blood cultures, and nasogastric decompression. More commonly, progressing from a clear liquid diet to a low-fiber diet until symptoms subside, followed by progression to a high-fiber diet is successful in treating the disorder. Repeated episodes with increasingly severe manifestations are associated with possible thinning of the intestinal wall, which increases the risk of perforation of the bowel, resulting in hemorrhage and peritonitis.

Decisions related to surgical intervention may be based on the Hinchey classification criteria, which stage the disease according to the extent of inflammatory changes and the integrity of the bowel wall. The stages of the Hinchey classification are labeled from I to IV. Stage I presents a localized abscess, stage II presents pelvic abscess, stage III with purulent peritonitis, and stage IV with feculent peritonitis. Surgical interventions for diverticulitis may include colectomy, which is the resection of the diseased segment with anastomosis of the normal bowel segments, or the placement of a temporary or permanent colostomy depending on the dimensions of the damage.

Postoperative risks include hemorrhage, altered fluid volume status, infection, delayed wound healing, impaired self-image, and repeated inflammatory attacks.

Diverticulosis and Diverticulitis

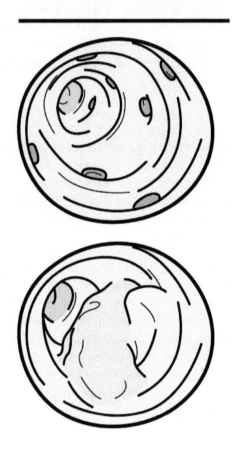

Esophageal Varices

Esophageal varices develop as a compensatory mechanism for the portal hypertension that occurs in liver disease. The superficial veins of the esophagus and the stomach function as a collateral circulation by diverting blood from the portal system to reduce pressure in the vasculature of the liver. Approximately 60 percent of patients with severe cirrhosis will develop esophageal varices at some point because portal hypertension is progressive in these patients. There may be no indication of the presence of esophageal varices until the vessels rupture, which means that all patients with cirrhosis require annual endoscopic screening for the assessment of the presence of varices.

Prophylactic treatment is recommended for varices that are 5 millimeters or more in diameter and/or exhibit longitudinal red streaks or wales along the varices, due to the significant risk of rupture and hemorrhage associated with these findings. Additional risk factors for hemorrhage include a patient history of constipation, vomiting, severe coughing, and alcohol abuse. Beta-blocker therapy is indicated for the prevention of hemorrhage; however, the medications are not effective in delaying the initial

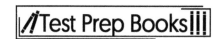

formation of the varices. The therapy is aimed at maintaining the heart at fifty-five beats per minute, and the therapy must be continued indefinitely because the risk of hemorrhage returns if the medication is stopped. Research indicates that as many as one-third of patients with esophageal varices will not respond to this therapy and instead, report fatigue, dyspnea, and bradycardia.

Up to one-third of all patients with esophageal varices will suffer a hemorrhagic episode. The emergency care of this life-threatening condition includes endoscopy with ligation of the varices, vasopressin, placement of a transjugular intrahepatic shunt, and surgery, in addition to aggressive crystalloid and colloid fluid replacement.

Esophagitis

Esophagitis is defined as the inflammation of the mucosal lining of the esophagus that may be caused by chronic GERD, infectious agents such as **Candida,** cytomegalovirus (CMV), human immunodeficiency virus (HIV), herpes, or as the result of chemotherapy or radiation therapy. The condition may be asymptomatic or associated with common manifestations that include heartburn, dyspepsia, dysphagia, hoarseness, and retrosternal chest pain. Symptoms associated with infection may also include nausea, vomiting, fever, and sepsis. Diagnostic tests include CBC to identify signs of neutropenia or alterations in the hematocrit and hemoglobin, fecal occult blood exam, barium studies and endoscopy, ECG to rule out cardiac disease as the cause of the chest discomfort, and testing for autoimmune conditions.

Complications may include anorexia and weight loss, Barrett's esophagus, and rarely, perforation. With Barrett's esophagus, the cells that have been irritated by reflux disease undergo metaplastic transformation and exhibit an increased risk for the development of esophageal adenocarcinoma. Interventions include resolution of the causative agent or condition, pain management, histamine 2 receptor antagonists, PPIs, coating agents, blood component replacement as necessary, and lifestyle changes to alleviate the manifestations of chronic GERD. Corticosteroids may be necessary for esophagitis due to IBD or eosinophilic conditions. Emergency care of this condition involves treatment of bleeding or perforation and elimination of acute cardiac disease as the source of any reported chest pain.

Foreign Bodies

When a foreign body is swallowed accidentally or intentionally, the progress of that object through the GI system is largely dependent on the size of the object. Objects may become lodged in the oropharynx and are either expelled with coughing or advance to the esophagus. Commonly, if an object does not become lodged in the esophagus and reaches the stomach, it will continue through the system and be passed out of the body. Coins may become trapped in the small intestine, objects more than 2 centimeters long may become trapped in the pylorus, and objects more than 6 centimeters long may become lodged in the duodenum. Disc-like or button batteries require emergency care because they cause necrosis of the intestinal wall within 2 hours of contact. Small spherical magnets, which were previously used in some toys that have since been removed from the market, also can adhere to one another with intestinal tissue lodged between them, resulting in ischemia and necrosis of the tissue.

The incidence of intentional or accidental swallowing of foreign bodies is higher in children from eighteen to forty-eight months of age, patients who use dentures, psychiatric patients, and prisoners. The identification of the swallowed object is critical for appropriate treatment and prevention of complications and is often difficult in young children. Radiographs of the entire GI tract are used initially to locate the object and estimate the size. Ultrasound is essential if the patient has respiratory distress and is also preferred if the swallowed object is nonradiopaque or sharp.

Treatment is dependent upon the characteristics of the swallowed object and the patient's resulting condition. The administration of promotility medications and positioning the patient with respiratory manifestations in high Fowler's position are the primary interventions unless there is an apparent need for immediate surgical intervention. Possible complications include gagging, dysphagia, respiratory distress, and possible abdominal symptoms such as gas and bloating. Emergency treatment for the ingestion of button batteries is focused on prevention of complications that may include necrosis, perforation, infection, obstruction, and volvulus.

Gastroenteritis

Gastroenteritis is a general term used to describe GI tract alterations. The characteristic manifestation is diarrhea; however, the exact characteristics of this manifestation are specific to the causative agent. These conditions may be related to osmotic, inflammatory, secretory, or motility alterations. The villi of the small intestine are most commonly affected by these alterations, resulting in fluid loss. Presenting symptoms may be mild to life-threatening, and outbreaks of these infectious conditions can rapidly reach epidemic proportions in susceptible populations. Prolonged diarrhea and vomiting result in severe fluid and electrolyte deficits, which may be associated with hypovolemic shock in high-risk individuals, including children and the elderly.

The norovirus is the causative agent for 50 to 70 percent of all cases of gastroenteritis. The virus is easily transmitted from person to person and is resistant to common cleaning agents. The attacks, manifested by diarrhea, fever, chills, and headache, usually last 36 hours. The rotavirus species may cause severe illness in children. The food-borne **Salmonella** infection is the second most common cause of gastroenteritis and is associated with fever, in addition to abdominal pain, nausea, vomiting, and diarrhea.

Infection caused by **C. difficile** is the leading cause of hospital-acquired GI disease. The elderly population is more commonly affected; however, all patients are susceptible to this infection. The organism exists in the feces and is spread by contact with contaminated surfaces. This condition is commonly associated with broad-spectrum antibiotic therapy that reduces the normal flora of the GI tract. Common manifestations include diarrhea, nausea, vomiting, and abdominal pain. This infection may be complicated by pseudomembranous colitis, toxic megacolon, perforation of the colon, and sepsis. Treatment is aimed at the agent-specific antibiotic therapy, supportive treatment of all manifestations, and possible surgical excision of compromised bowel segments. Emergency care requires restoration of fluid volume and electrolyte homeostasis.

Gastritis

Gastritis may be acute or chronic, and acute gastritis is further differentiated as erosive or nonerosive. Involvement of the entire stomach lining is termed **pangastritis**, while regional involvement is termed **antral gastritis**. Acute gastritis may be asymptomatic or may present with nonspecific abdominal pain, nausea, vomiting, anorexia, belching, and bloating. The most common causes of acute gastritis include use of NSAIDs and corticosteroids and infection by the **H. pylori** bacteria. Acute gastritis may also be associated with alcohol abuse. Double-contrast barium studies, endoscopy, and histological examination of biopsy samples most often confirm the diagnosis and the causative agent. Treatment includes

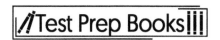

normalization of fluid and electrolyte balance, discontinuance of causative agents such as NSAIDs, and corticosteroids, H$_2$ blockers, PPIs, and appropriate antibiotic therapy in the event of *H. pylori* infection.

Chronic gastritis is an inflammatory state that has not responded to therapy for acute gastritis. Chronic *H. pylori* infection is associated with the development of peptic ulcers, gastric adenocarcinoma, and mucosal-related lymphoid tissue (MALT) lymphoma. In addition to endoscopy and barium studies, gastric biopsy for assessment of antibiotic sensitivity is done because the initial antibiotic therapy was unsuccessful in eradicating the organism.

Autoimmune gastritis is related to vitamin B-12 deficiency due to intrinsic factor deficiency and is associated with megaloblastic anemia and thrombocytopenia. Chemical or reactive gastritis is due to chronic NSAID and steroid use and is manifested by mucosal epithelial erosion, ulcer formation, and mucosal edema and possible hemorrhage. Chronic gastritis is diagnosed by endoscopy, biopsy, and histological studies. Treatment is specific to the causative agent, and in the instance of *H. pylori* infection, a course of three antibiotics will be administered. *H. pylori* infection also requires long-term surveillance for reoccurrence of infection. Emergency care of the patient with acute or chronic gastritis is focused on the assessment for hemorrhage or other potential complications, restoration of fluid volume status, and pain management.

Hepatitis

Hepatitis is an inflammatory condition of the liver, which is further categorized as infectious or noninfectious. Causative infectious agents for hepatitis may be viral, fungal, or bacterial, while noninfectious causes include autoimmune disease, prescription and recreational drugs, alcohol abuse, and metabolic disorders. More than 50 percent of the cases of acute hepatitis in the United States are caused by a virus. Transmission routes include fecal-oral, parenteral, sexual contact, and perinatal transmission. There are four phases of the course of viral hepatitis. During phase 1, which is asymptomatic, the host is infected, and the virus replicates; the onset of mild symptoms occurs in phase 2; progressive symptoms of liver dysfunction appear in phase 3; and recovery from the infection occurs in phase 4. These phases are specific to the causative agent and the individual.

The most common viral agents are hepatitis A (HAV), hepatitis B (HBV), and hepatitis C (HCV). Less commonly, hepatitis D (HDV), hepatitis E (HEV), CMV, Epstein-Barr virus, and adenovirus may cause hepatitis. HAV and HBV often present with nausea, jaundice, anorexia, right upper quadrant pain, fatigue, and malaise. HCV may be asymptomatic or, alternatively, may present with similar symptoms. Approximately 20 percent of acute infections with HBV and HCV result in chronic hepatitis, which is a risk factor for the development of cirrhosis and liver failure. The care of the patient with acute hepatitis due to HAV and HCV is focused on symptom relief, while the antiviral treatment for HBV is effective in decreasing the incidence of adenocarcinoma.

Chronic hepatitis is a complication of acute hepatitis and frequently progresses to hepatic failure, which is associated with deteriorating coagulation status and the onset of hepatic encephalopathy due to alterations in the blood-brain barrier that result in brain cell edema. Emergency care of the patient with hepatic failure is focused on controlling fluid volume, coagulation hemostasis, and reduction of encephalopathy.

Hernia

A hernia is manifested by the displacement or protrusion of a segment of the bowel through an area of weakness in the abdominal wall. This weakness may be an anatomical site, such as the umbilicus, or acquired due to a surgical incision. Hernias are also defined as reversible or irreversible, depending on whether the protruding bowel segment can be repositioned with gentle pressure. An irreversible hernia may become incarcerated or strangulated if the blood supply is compromised for any period of time. Either of these conditions represents a surgical emergency and may be associated with necrosis and perforation of the bowel loop and possible intestinal obstruction.

Manifestations include possible visible protrusion or fullness at the site that increases with any increase in intrabdominal pressure and diffuse pain radiating to the site. Risk factors include male gender, advanced age, increased intra-abdominal pressure related to pregnancy and obesity, and genetic defects. Inguinal hernias in the male account for 75 percent of the 800,000 hernia repairs performed annually in the United States. CT scans and ultrasonography may be used to identify hernias that are not readily identified by the physical examination. A flat plate of the abdomen is useful for identifying free air that may result from bowel perforation secondary to a strangulated hernia. Conservative management of reducible hernias includes modified activity such as no lifting or straining and prevention of constipation. If the manifestations worsen or the protrusion becomes irreversible, surgery is required to prevent incarceration and/or strangulation. Emergency care of the patient with a strangulated hernia is focused on restoration of blood to the bowel segment and prevention of perforation and obstruction.

Inflammatory Bowel Disease

Inflammatory bowel disease (IBD) is an idiopathic disease that results from a harmful immune response to normal intestinal flora. Two types of IBD include Crohn's disease and ulcerative colitis (UC). Crohn's disease is characterized by inflammatory changes in all layers of the bowel. Although the entire length of the GI tract may be involved, the ileum and colon are affected most often. The inflamed areas are commonly interrupted by segments of normal bowel. Endoscopic views reveal the cobblestone appearance of these affected segments. UC is characterized by inflammatory changes of the mucosa and submucosa of the bowel that affect only the colon. There is a genetic predisposition for Crohn's disease, and there is also an increased incidence of cancer in patients with either form of IBD. Additional risk factors include a family history of IBD or colorectal cancer, NSAID and antibiotic use, smoking, and psychiatric disorders. IBD is diagnosed by a patient's history, including details of any recent foreign travel or hospitalization to rule out tuberculosis or **C. difficile** as the precipitating cause, in addition to endoscopy, CT and magnetic resonance imaging (MRI), serum and stool studies, and histologic studies.

Manifestations are nonspecific and are most often associated with the affected bowel segment. Common manifestations of IBD include diarrhea with blood and mucus and possible incontinence; constipation primarily with UC that is associated with progression to obstipation and bowel obstruction; rectal pain with associated urgency and tenesmus; and abdominal pain and cramping in the right lower quadrant with Crohn's disease, and in the umbilical area or left lower quadrant with UC. In addition, anemia, fatigue, and arthritis may be present.

The treatment of IBD focuses on attaining periods of remission and preventing recurrent attacks by modifying the inflammatory response. The stepwise treatment protocol begins with aminosalicylates and progresses to antibiotics, corticosteroids, and immunomodulators. Emergency care of the patient

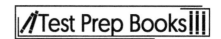

with IBD is focused on assessment and treatment of possible hemorrhage, megacolon, or bowel obstruction.

Intussusception

Intussusception is the abnormal movement of one portion of the bowel that is folded back into the subsequent segment. The condition is most common in infants and appears to be due to altered peristalsis that results in decreased lymphatic and venous drainage, which leads to ischemia and necrosis of the affected bowel segment. Left untreated, the condition is fatal in two to five days. The condition often presents with a history of recent upper respiratory infection, in addition to lethargy, vomiting, colicky abdominal pain that may be severe or intermittent, a palpable abdominal mass, and diarrhea that contains blood and mucus, which is often the initial manifestation of the intussusception.

The contrast enema is used most often to confirm the diagnosis. The treatment is specific to the age of the patient and the precipitating cause. The cause of the condition in infants and children up to three years of age is most often idiopathic, while adhesions, tumor formation, effects of bariatric surgery, and inflammatory changes due to IBD are possible causes of intussusception in older children and adults. Nonoperative reduction with therapeutic enemas is the treatment of choice in infants and young children. Barium, water-based contrast material or air insufflation may be used as the reducing agent. The two contraindications to the nonoperative approach include the presence of peritonitis or perforation of the bowel. The surgical treatment is appropriate for older children, adults, and infants in whom the nonoperative reduction was unsuccessful. A laparoscopic approach is used to manually reduce the intussusception. If reduction is not possible or if there is additional bowel damage such as perforation present, surgical resection and anastomosis of the affected bowel segment are necessary. Emergency care is focused on the identification and immediate intervention of the condition.

Obstructions

There are three anatomical areas of the GI system that are prone to obstruction, including the gastric outlet at the pylorus, the small intestine, and the bowel. The small intestine is the most commonly affected site, and adhesions are responsible for more than 60 percent of all obstructions. These conditions may also be categorized as mechanical or nonmechanical depending on the cause, where mechanical obstructions are due to some extrinsic source such as adhesions, tumor formation, intussusception, or hernias, and nonmechanical obstructions are due to decreased peristalsis, neurogenic disorders, vascular insufficiency, or electrolyte imbalance. The mechanical obstruction of the biliary tract is due to effects of cirrhosis and hepatitis.

The manifestations are specific to the anatomical site of obstruction. The gastric outlet obstruction occurs most commonly in the pylorus and is associated with upper abdominal distention, nausea, vomiting, weight loss, and anorexia. Diagnostic tests include endoscopy and assessment of nutritional deficits, in addition to testing to eliminate *H. pylori* or diabetic gastric paresis as the cause. Obstruction of the small bowel is associated with severe fluid and electrolyte losses, metabolic alkalosis, nausea and vomiting, fever, and tachycardia, and may lead to strangulation of the affected bowel segment. Large-bowel obstruction, most frequently due to tumor formation or stricture resulting from diverticular disease, is manifested by lower abdominal distention, possible metabolic acidosis, cramping abdominal pain, and minimal fluid and electrolyte losses. Common diagnostic studies include endoscopy, common lab studies, flat plate of the abdomen to assess for free air, and CT imaging.

Treatments are specific to the cause and may include tumor excision, antibiotic therapy for *H. pylori*, colectomy to remove the affected bowel segment, and/or colostomy placement. Although some obstructions may be treated with gastric or enteric decompression, bowel rest, and fluids, emergency intervention is usually necessary to prevent complications such as peritonitis and hemorrhage.

Pancreatitis

Pancreatitis has a rapid onset and progression to a critical illness, which is manifested by characteristic abdominal pain, nausea, vomiting, and diarrhea. In addition, fever, tachycardia, hypotension, and abdominal distention and rebound tenderness may be present. The exocrine function of the pancreas is the production and secretion of digestive enzymes.

Pancreatitis exists when one of the causative agents inhibits the homeostatic suppression of enzyme secretion, resulting in excessive amounts of enzymes in the pancreas. This excess of enzymes precipitates the inflammatory response, which results in increased pancreatic vascular permeability and, in turn, leads to edema, hemorrhage, and eventual necrosis of the pancreas. The inflammatory mediators can result in systemic complications that may include sepsis, respiratory distress syndrome, renal failure, and GI hemorrhage. Chronic alcoholism and biliary tract obstruction are the most common causes of pancreatitis; however, as many as 35 percent of the cases of pancreatitis are idiopathic. Pancreatitis can also occur after endoscopic retrograde cholangiopancreatography (ERCP) due to defects in the sphincter of Oddi. Aggressive pre-procedure hydration and rectal indomethacin post procedure are employed to prevent this complication. Less common causes include some antibiotics and chemotherapy agents.

Diagnosis is based on the patient's presenting history and routine lab studies that include amylase P, lipase, metabolic panel, liver panel, C-reactive protein, CBC, and arterial blood gases (ABGs). Imaging studies may be used if the diagnosis is unclear to rule out gallbladder disease. Nonsurgical treatment includes bowel rest with nasogastric decompression, analgesics, and IV fluid administration. Surgical procedures may be open or minimally invasive and are aimed at removing diseased tissue to limit the progression to systemic complications, to repair the pancreatic duct, or to repair defects in the biliary tree. The emergency care of pancreatitis focuses on prompt diagnosis, aggressive fluid management, and treatment of the cause because the disease is associated with the rapid onset of systemic complications.

Trauma

The GI system may be traumatized by blunt or penetrating forces. Penetrating trauma is most commonly due to gunshot or stabbing injuries and usually results in a predictable pattern of injury; however, careful assessment for occult injuries is necessary to prevent catastrophic damage. Presenting manifestations depend on the degree of penetration and the site of the damage but commonly include visible hemorrhage, alterations in level of consciousness, tachycardia, and hypotension. Diagnosis requires a detailed inquiry into all of the facts of the incident, including a description of the weapon, the number of times the patient was stabbed, and an estimation of blood loss at the scene, in addition to the progression of the patient's manifestations during resuscitation and transport. Treatment is aimed at restoring and maintaining fluid volume status with colloids and crystalloids, assessment for and treatment of hemorrhage, prevention of infection, and surgical repair of the damaged structures.

GI injuries due to blunt force trauma often are not immediately apparent, which means that assessment for progression of the original insult is ongoing. Abdominal pain and tenderness and hypotension may

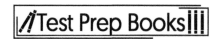

be the only signs of massive internal injuries. Trauma related to automobile accidents may present with a characteristic seatbelt or steering wheel pattern, Cullen's sign due to periumbilical trauma, or an abdominal bruit that may be associated with comorbid vascular disease or acute vascular trauma. Domestic violence must be considered in the event of abdominal blunt force trauma. Diagnosis is based on the history of the event, routine lab studies, ultrasound and CT scanning, peritoneal lavage, and possible exploratory laparotomy. The goals of treatment for blunt trauma are similar to penetrating trauma and include restoring and maintaining fluid volume status with colloids and crystalloids, assessment for and treatment of hemorrhage, prevention of infection, and surgical repair of the damaged structures.

Ulcers

Ulcers of the GI tract are categorized as to the anatomical site of injury. Gastric ulcers are located in the body of the stomach, and peptic ulcers are located in the duodenum. The presenting symptom is abdominal pain 2 to 4 hours after eating for duodenal ulcers, in addition to hematemesis and melena. The defect is due to erosion of the mucosal lining by infectious agents, most commonly *H. pylori,* extreme systemic stress such as burns or head trauma, ETOH abuse, chronic kidney and respiratory disease, and psychological stress. Untreated, the mucosal erosion can progress to perforation, hemorrhage, and peritonitis.

Laboratory studies include examination of endoscopic tissue samples for the presence of the *H. pylori* organism, urea breath test, CBC, stool samples, and metabolic panel. Endoscopy, which is used to obtain tissue samples and achieve hemostasis, and double barium imaging studies made be obtained. The treatment depends on the extent of the erosion and will be focused on healing the ulcerated tissue and preventing additional damage. The treatment protocol for *H. pylori* infection includes the use of a PPI, amoxicillin, and clarithromycin for a minimum of seven to fourteen days. Subsequent testing will be necessary to ensure that the organism has been eradicated. Patients infected with *H. pylori* also must discontinue the use of NSAIDs or continue the long-term use of PPIs. Surgery may be indicated for significant areas of hemorrhage that were not successfully treated by ultrasound, and the procedure will be specific to the anatomical area of ulceration. Emergency care is focused on prompt management of bleeding and identification of the causative agent to guide treatment.

Genitourinary

Foreign Bodies

The emergency care of the male patient who presents with purulent or mucopurulent penile discharge, dysuria, hematuria, or painful intercourse is focused on identifying the cause. Prompt treatment is necessary to prevent renal damage and systemic complications. In addition to obtaining routine lab studies and cultures, the provider will inquire if the patient has a recent history of catheterization of the urethra due to medical intervention or self-induced. Anecdotal reports indicate that insertion of foreign bodies into the urethra for autoerotic purposes is a rare occurrence, and in most cases, is associated with preexisting psychiatric disease.

Depending on the dimensions of the object, a local reaction may not be apparent immediately, which means that any infection may be advanced by the time the patient seeks treatment. The diagnosis is most often identified by the physical examination and patient report. Diagnostic imaging studies and laboratory data are collected to assess the extent of infection and inflammation and to determine the optimal method for retrieval of the foreign body. Common methods of retrieval include endoscopy, surgical removal by suprapubic cystotomy, and urethrotomy. Treatment for localized effects of the existence of the foreign body will include antimicrobial therapy appropriate to results of the cultures and referral for psychiatric care. If the condition has progressed beyond the urethra and bladder, aggressive management is necessary to prevent sepsis.

Infection

Infections of the male genitourinary (GU) tract are considered to be complicated infections because the infective process has overcome the naturally robust defenses of the male urinary tract. Common conditions resulting in infection include the inflammation of the prostate gland, the epididymis, testes, kidney, bladder, urethra; unprotected sexual intercourse; and the use of urinary catheters. Additional contributing factors to the incidence of infection include a history of previous urinary tract infections (UTIs), enlargement of the prostate gland, changes in voiding habits such as the onset of nocturia, comorbid diabetes or HIV infection, immunosuppressive therapy, and previous surgical intervention of the urinary tract. Painful urination, defined as **dysuria**, is the most common presenting manifestation, and complaints of coexisting dysuria, urinary frequency, and urgency are considered to be 75 percent predictive for UTI. Additional manifestations are dependent on the cause but may include fever, tachycardia, flank pain, suprapubic pain, penile discharge, scrotal masses and tenderness, and enlargement of the inguinal lymph nodes.

The diagnosis depends on the patient's history; presenting manifestations and physical examination; cultures of the urine, penile discharge, and blood; and assessment of kidney function. If obstruction of any portion of the urinary tract is suspected, additional diagnostic studies may include ultrasound, CT scans, and IV pyelogram (IVP). The infection will be treated with third-generation antimicrobial therapy, fluid resuscitation, antipyretics, analgesics, and urinary analgesics. The successful treatment of sexually transmitted infections requires adherence to the agent-specific medication regimen and the protocol for the treatment of all sexual partners and follow-up care. Emergency care of the patient with a UTI is focused on prompt identification of any obstructive pathology, treatment of infection and pain, preservation of kidney function, and prevention of systemic disease.

Priapism

Priapism is a urological emergency manifested by the enlargement of the penis that is unrelated to sexual stimulation and is unrelieved by ejaculation. Low-flow priapism is the most common form and is not associated with evidence of trauma but is due to dysfunction of the detumescence mechanism that is responsible for the relaxation of the erect penis. High-flow priapism results from abnormal arterial blood to the penis as a result of trauma to the GU system. The cause of low-flow priapism is most often idiopathic; however, the most common cause of the condition in children is sickle cell disease. Additional conditions that may cause this form of priapism include dialysis, vasculitis, spinal cord stenosis, bladder and renal cancer, and some medications, including heparin, cocaine, and omeprazole. High-flow priapism is due to straddle injuries or, most commonly, injury to the arteries of the penis by the injection of medications into the vasculature of the penis.

Prompt treatment of low-flow priapism within 12 hours of the onset of symptoms is necessary to prevent long-term alterations in erectile function. The primary cause is identified and treated if possible, followed by aspiration of fluid from the corpora cavernosa at the base of the penis, with or without saline irrigation, which is an effective treatment in 30 percent of cases. If aspiration and irrigation are unsuccessful, a vasoconstrictive agent such as phenylephrine can be instilled at 5-minute intervals until the erection is entirely resolved. If these interventions fail to eradicate the priapism, temporary or

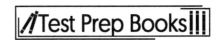

permanent surgical placement of a shunt between the corpus cavernosum and the glans penis or corpus spongiosum is necessary to restore venous drainage. Treatment of high-flow priapism involves cauterization and/or evacuation of areas of bleeding. Emergency treatment is focused on identification of the specific condition and prompt resolution of the erection.

Renal Calculi

Nephrolithiasis is defined as the process of stone or calculi formation in the pelvis of the kidney. The pain associated with this condition is referred to as **renal colic** and most often reflects the stretching and distention of the ureter when the stone leaves the kidney. The most common cause is insufficient fluid intake that concentrates stone-forming substances in the kidney. In order of occurrence, calculi are composed of calcium (75 percent) due to increased absorption of calcium by the GI tract, struvite (15 percent) as a result of repeated UTIs, uric acid (6 percent) due to increased purine intact, and cysteine (1 percent) due to an intrinsic metabolic defect in susceptible individuals. In addition, AIDS medications, some antacids, and sulfa drugs are also associated with stone formation. Renal calculi are more common in men than women, are associated with obesity and insulin resistance, and have a familial tendency.

Diagnosis is based on the patient's history and physical examination. Common lab studies include CBC, coagulation studies, kidney function tests, and C-reactive protein. Imaging studies may include ultrasonography, KUB (kidney, ureter, and bladder) radiographs, and CT scans. Treatment options are based on the likelihood that the stone will be expelled spontaneously from the urinary system, given the size and location of the stone. Common interventions include aggressive fluid management, antimicrobial therapy, and pain management. If necessary, to prevent mechanical damage to the organs or the progression of the condition to urosepsis, the stone may be surgically removed or the patient may undergo extracorporeal shock wave lithotripsy. The emergency care is focused on preventing damage to the urinary tract, restoring fluid volume, managing pain, and preventing progression of the illness to systemic urosepsis. Patient education regarding the essential follow-up care is critical to the prevention of recurrent calculi formation.

Torsion

Torsion refers to the abnormal twisting of the structures of the spermatic cord, which results in ischemia in the ipsilateral testicle that causes irreversible damage to fertility if not relieved within 6 hours. The condition is most common in infants, due to the mobility of the undescended testicles, and in adolescents, due to the abnormal attachment of fascia and muscles to the spermatic cord.

The Testicular Workup for Ischemia and Suspected Torsion (TWIST) is the scoring system used to quantify the risk associated with the condition. The TWIST is used by emergency providers and then validated by the physician, most commonly a urologist, and the score is based on swelling of the testicle, hardened texture of the testicle, absence of the cremasteric reflex, nausea and vomiting, and placement of the testicles at a higher than normal position in the scrotum. The resulting risk factor may be low, intermediate, or high. A low TWIST score may indicate an alternative cause for the patient's manifestations. An intermediate risk requires the use of ultrasound to confirm the diagnosis, while the patient with a high-risk TWIST score requires immediate surgical intervention to prevent long-term dysfunction.

Nonoperative treatments include manual manipulation of the testicle guided by Doppler imaging. If the procedure is successful, surgical stabilization of the spermatic cord structures is required. Immediate surgical repair is required if the procedure is unsuccessful. If the affected testicle is nonviable and is removed, a testicular prosthesis will be inserted after wound healing is complete. Analgesics and antianxiety medications will be included in the treatment plan. Caregivers must be aware that the condition can reoccur. Emergency care of the patient requires immediate intervention based on the calculation of the TWIST score to prevent necrosis of the affected testicle.

Trauma

Organs of the GU tract include the bladder, urethra, and external genitalia, all of which are subject to varied sources of trauma. The bladder is commonly injured by blunt trauma that results from pelvic fractures and is also affected less commonly by penetrating trauma. The different segments of the male urethra can be injured as a result of pelvic fractures, straddle-type injuries, or from penetrating injuries that may be self-inflicted. The penis and scrotum are subject to blunt trauma, often due to sports injuries, and other varied injuries that may be self-inflicted.

The diagnosis depends on the history of the precipitating event and the physical examination. Trauma to the GU tract may not be life-threatening; however, the GU injuries are often secondary to other injuries affecting the pelvis, spine, kidney, and abdomen, which warrant immediate attention. Common lab studies include CBC, prothrombin time, type and cross match, and urinalysis. Ultrasonography and CT scans are used in addition to studies specific to the bladder and testes, which include retrograde urethrogram, retrograde cystogram, and nuclear med studies. Established prehospital trauma care is required. Emergency treatment is aimed at identifying and correcting the underlying injury and preserving the function of the GU tract and includes fluid replacement, antimicrobial therapy, and pain management. Referrals to urologists, orthopedists, and other specialists must be made as necessary. In the event of self-inflicted injuries, psychiatric referrals are also appropriate.

Urinary Retention

Urinary retention may be acute or chronic and is defined as cessation of urination or incomplete emptying of the bladder. It occurs more often in older men, and common causes include prostate gland enlargement, neurogenic bladder due to diabetes or other chronic diseases, urethral strictures and other anatomic abnormalities, and the use of anticholinergic medications. Urinary retention in younger men is most commonly due to pelvic or spinal cord trauma. Unrelieved urinary retention can result in urinary tract infections due to stasis of the urine or renal failure due to the retrograde pressure of the accumulated urine. Common manifestations include suprapubic distension, pain, a history of contributing neurological diseases, and possible systemic signs such as fever and tachycardia. The condition also may be asymptomatic or characterized by urinary frequency or overflow incontinence, with loss of small amounts of urine accompanied by sensations of bladder fullness.

Diagnosis depends on the patient's history, including the presence of causative conditions and physical examination. Common lab studies include CBC, BUN, creatinine, electrolytes, urinalysis, ultrasound, urodynamic testing, and cystoscopy. The emergency treatment of acute urinary retention is aimed at draining the accumulated urine, protecting kidney function, addressing the underlying issue, and preventing systemic effects and recurrence. Urethral or suprapubic catheterization or a percutaneous nephrostomy may be done to drain the urine from the bladder, while urethral catheterization can also be used to obtain urodynamic measurements and to evaluate postvoid volumes after treatment. Clean technique self-catheterization is done by patients with chronic urinary retention due to neurogenic causes. If surgical removal of a portion or all of the bladder is required to repair traumatic damage or to remove malignant tumors, a urinary diversion will be created to maintain kidney function.

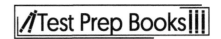

Gynecology

Abnormal Bleeding Dysfunction (Vaginal)

Abnormal or irregular uterine bleeding is defined as episodes of bleeding that are not caused by any specific pathology, systemic illness, or normal pregnancy. It is most often due to alterations in the hormonal stimulation of the endometrium by some source. The bleeding episodes vary widely as to the amount of blood loss and the duration and frequency of the episodes in the same individual. The most common cause of this anovulatory cycle is the presence of an abnormal pregnancy, which may be a threatened or incomplete abortion or an ectopic pregnancy. There are several additional conditions associated with abnormal uterine bleeding, including polycystic ovarian syndrome, thyroid dysfunction, liver dysfunction that affects estrogen metabolism. Endometrial fibroids, polyps, hyperplasia, or cancer can also cause abnormal uterine bleeding. The condition is more common in adolescent women and women over the age of forty.

Once an abnormal pregnancy has been excluded, common diagnostic studies include CBC, Pap smear, thyroid and liver function tests, coagulation studies, and hormonal assays. Routine imaging studies are recommended only if the pelvic examination is unacceptable, as might occur in a patient with morbid obesity. However, pelvic ultrasonography is recommended in all patients who present with abnormal bleeding and are at high risk for cancer. Any identified pathology will be treated first; however, there are general guidelines for idiopathic ovulatory dysfunction, which include age-specific treatment protocols for the use of oral contraceptives as the initial treatment. Oral contraceptives suppress the thickening of the endometrial lining, regulate the menstrual cycle, and decrease menstrual flow, which reduces the risk of iron-deficiency anemia. In the event of the failure of medical treatment, hysterectomy may be recommended. The emergency care of the patient with abnormal bleeding is focused on hemostasis, aggressive fluid replacement, and treatment of the cause, which may require surgical intervention.

Foreign Bodies

Foreign bodies that exceed the dimensions of the female vagina may precipitate an emergency. While this condition is more common in children than adult females, adolescents and adults can present with tampons, condom portions, or other foreign objects that were inserted intentionally or as a form of abuse. Common presenting manifestations include vaginal bleeding and malodorous vaginal discharge and vulvar irritation. In most instances, the effects of the foreign body are limited to the vagina unless the wall of the vagina is penetrated, which can result in abdominal manifestations. Additionally, if the patient is immunocompromised, severe infection may result. Untreated or repeated episodes can result in the formation of fistulae between the vagina and the rectum, bladder, or abdominal cavity; pain with intercourse; and persistent bleeding.

The diagnosis depends on the patient's presenting history and physical examination; however, if the patient is a child or an adolescent, special care is required for both questioning the patient about the precipitating events and in the conduct of the physical examination. Depending on the size and location of the foreign body, sedation and/or anesthesia may be necessary to examine the patient, regardless of age, and to remove the foreign body. CT scans and ultrasonography may be necessary to identify the extent of any injury caused by the object. In most cases, removal of the object is the treatment of choice; however, perforation of the vagina, fistula formation, or infection require additional treatment and a surgical referral. In addition to the removal of the foreign body, emergency care also requires a thorough investigation of any evidence of abuse, consistent with agency policy. Referral to a mental health professional may also be indicated in the event of self-inflicted injury.

Hemorrhage

Hemorrhage in women can be due to abnormal uterine bleeding, hemorrhagic cystitis, trauma to the GU system or the bony pelvic structure, kidney injury or dysfunction, self-inflicted trauma, abuse, complications of pregnancy and childbirth, rupture of an ovarian cyst, or tumor. Manifestations relate to the specific cause but commonly include some degree of vaginal bleeding, flank or suprapubic pain, vital signs indicative of hypovolemia, hematuria, and neurological deficits or crepitus resulting from pelvic trauma. The emergency assessment of the patient with hemorrhage of the gynecologic (GYN) system will be consistent with the Advanced Trauma Life Support protocol. While the diagnosis depends on the history of the precipitating event and the physical examination, prompt use of ultrasonography, CT scanning, pelvic angiography, cystography, and/or retrograde urethrography are required to identify the source of the hemorrhage and to guide treatment. In addition, common lab studies include CBC, coagulation studies, type and screen, electrolytes, ABGs, and urinalysis.

There are several protocols for injury pattern recognition in the patient with pelvic trauma that include treatment recommendations for each category. The emergency treatment of postpartum hemorrhage is discussed in a subsequent section. The initial intervention for these events is the treatment of the underlying condition, in addition to the restoration of hemostasis with aggressive replacement of fluids with crystalloid and colloid solutions and appropriate referrals for all instances of suspected abuse, either self-inflicted or from another source.

Infection

The most common sexually transmitted infective agent in the United States is chlamydia, which is spread by unprotected vaginal, oral, or anal sexual activity. The organism can also be transmitted to an infant delivered vaginally by an infected mother. Risk factors common to all sexually transmitted diseases (STDs) include a history of multiple sexual partners, unprotected sexual intercourse, coinfection with other infective agents, and young age, with most infections occurring in women from fifteen to twenty-four years old. Chlamydial infections may be asymptomatic, which has prompted the U.S. Preventive Services Task Force to recommend routine screening of all females fifteen to twenty-four years of age and all females older than twenty-four who have identifiable risk factors for chlamydia.

Manifestations are specific to the involved organs, as either contained to the vagina and cervix or affecting the uterus, and fallopian tubes and include abnormal vaginal bleeding, rectal and vaginal discharge, and possible infection of the conjunctiva if the patient is pregnant. Diagnostic tests for lower tract infections include Pap smear, pregnancy tests, cultures, and HIV tests, while the diagnosis of infection of the upper GYN tract includes ultrasonography and CT scanning. Untreated infections often result in pelvic inflammatory disease (PID), infertility, and chronic pelvic pain. The treatment of lower tract infection is the administration of a single dose of azithromycin that is witnessed and confirmed by a health care provider to decrease costs of noncompliance. More complicated infections require extended antibiotic therapy to avoid long-term complications.

Gonorrheal infections are associated with risk factors, manifestations, complications, and diagnostic studies, similar to chlamydial infections. Newborns are treated prophylactically for gonorrhea infections; however, emergency care of a child with a gonorrheal infection involves collection of appropriate samples for possible forensic investigation. Untreated gonorrhea can progress to PID, and rarely, to

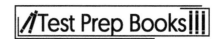

gonococcemia or fatal systemic shock. Typical treatment includes ceftriaxone and azithromycin. Syphilis can progress through four stages if left untreated, with manifestations ranging from the initial chancre at the point of contact to systemic neurological effects, including dementia. Penicillin is the treatment of choice, and the dosage protocol is specific to the stage of the infection when diagnosed.

PID is a potential complication of untreated or recurrent infection by any of the organisms that are sexually transmitted; however, PID most commonly results from chlamydial infection. The infection and inflammation proceed from the vagina through the cervix to the uterus and fallopian tube, with eventual progression to the abdominal cavity. The most common presenting manifestations include lower abdominal pain and possible abnormal vaginal discharge.

Untreated, the condition leads to systemic manifestations that include fever and elevated sedimentation rate. Complaints of upper right quadrant pain may be associated with Fitz-Hugh–Curtis syndrome (perihepatitis), which may present with jaundice and altered liver function studies. Diagnosis is made by the patient's history and physical and the exclusion of pregnancy or other pelvic pathology as the cause of the patient's pain. Treatment is focused on the relief of pain, resolution of the infection, decreasing the risk of long-term effects including sterility and the risk for obstetrical failure, and preventing further transmission of the infective agent. Antibiotic therapy is the treatment of choice and is generally effective in up to 75 percent of cases of PID, with surgery indicated for patients who do not respond to antibiotics.

Ovarian Cysts

An **ovarian cyst** is defined as a discrete accumulation of fluid in an ovary resulting from an alteration in hormonal function. It can form at any point in a female's lifetime. Risk factors for benign ovarian cysts include a history of breast cancer, infertility treatment, smoking, hypothyroidism, and tubal ligation, while malignant cysts are associated with a positive family history, advancing age, Caucasian ethnicity, infertility, nulliparity, early menarche, delayed menopause, and a history of breast cancer. Most cysts are asymptomatic but may be associated with abdominal bloating, early satiety, change in bowel habits, and weight loss and severe abdominal pain if the cysts rupture. Diagnosis is made by the patient's history and physical examination in addition to pelvic ultrasonography, CA-125 measurement, and pregnancy testing. Initial treatment of simple cysts is observation and/or the use of oral contraceptive medications. If cysts grow in size or are associated with increasingly severe manifestations, laparoscopic removal of the cyst and/or the ovary is indicated.

Sexual Assault/Battery

Sexual assaults are the result of violent, nonconsensual sexual actions against the victim. Common manifestations include the presence of sperm or blood, contusions, local evidence of forceful vaginal penetration, orthopedic injuries, abdominal trauma, and lacerations. The emergency care of the victim of sexual assault is focused on identifying and treating all injuries; appropriate testing and preventive treatment for all possible STDs, HIV, and hepatitis; prescribing preventive antibiotic therapy; and administering interventions aimed at preventing posttraumatic stress disorder (PTSD). Although assault victims are often reluctant to provide a detailed account of the assault, emergency providers are responsible for meticulous and comprehensive documentation to protect the patient's rights. In addition, referrals to appropriate community resources for post-emergency care should be made prior to the patient's discharge from the acute care facility. The patient should also be referred to a GYN for follow-up evaluation for potential infections or complications.

Trauma

The pelvic organs may be affected by blunt trauma, penetrating trauma, and injury due to trauma of adjacent structures such as pelvic fractures. Wounds may be due to automobile accidents, sports injuries, attacks by another person, gunshot wounds, or self-inflicted trauma. Penetrating wounds of the urethra can interrupt urine flow, while penetrating wounds of the vagina and uterus can compromise the abdominal cavity, leading to systemic effects. Blunt trauma to the lower abdomen can cause intrauterine bleeding and kidney contusions, which can compromise fluid volume status. In addition, all patients presenting with a history of trauma and complaints of groin pain should be assessed for the presence of pelvic fractures.

Common diagnostic studies include CBC, electrolytes, coagulation studies, type and screen, radiography, ultrasonography, CT scanning, urinalysis, and possible paracentesis to assess for penetration of the abdomen. Treatment is specific to the specific injuries and commonly includes fluid resuscitation, possible transfusion, Foley catheter insertion, and orthopedic, surgical, and GYN referrals as necessary. Possible surgical interventions include stabilization of pelvic fractures, possible hysterectomy due to severe blunt or penetrating trauma, or removal of ischemic ovaries.

Depending on the extent of the injuries, the patient may be assessed by the Revised Trauma Score, which is a risk prediction assessment tool used to assess the probability of survival in trauma patients. The patient's initial data set obtained upon arrival in the ER is used to calculate the risk. Parameters include the Glasgow Coma Scale score, the systolic BP, and the respiratory rate. Possible scores range from 0 to 7.8, and a score greater than 5.0 is associated with 80 percent or greater chance of survival. Emergency care of the patient with GYN trauma is based on the ABCDE protocol with attention to the possibility of "hidden" injuries that are not readily apparent.

Obstetrical

Abruptio Placenta

Abruptio placenta refers to the premature separation of the placenta from the uterine wall and is the most significant cause of hemorrhage in the third trimester. Descriptive terms for the condition include the identification of the degree of separation (either partial or complete), or the location of the separation (either marginal or central). Clinically, Class 0 indicates only the identification of a blood clot in the expelled placenta, while the manifestations in Classes 1, 2, and 3 progress from mild vaginal bleeding to hemorrhage, from mild uterine pain to tetanic or continuous contractions, from normal vital signs to maternal shock, from absent fetal distress to fetal demise, and from normal clotting to fibrinogen deficiency and hemorrhage. The exact cause is not known. However, there are several common risk factors, including maternal hypertension, which occurs in 40 percent of the cases of abruptio placenta; smoking; trauma in the form of car accidents, falls, or assaults; cocaine or alcohol abuse; maternal age greater than thirty-five or less than twenty years old; and previous history of abruptio placenta.

Depending on the patient's presenting manifestations, diagnostic studies include CBC, coagulation tests, type and screen, Kleihauer-Betke test in Rh-negative mothers to identify fetal-to-maternal transfer of blood, a nonstress test, fetal monitoring, and the possible use of ultrasonography; however, ultrasounds have a low sensitivity for identifying the separation of the placenta. The emergency care of the patient starts with fetal monitoring, initiation of IV access for fluid resuscitation with crystalloids and colloids,

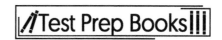

assessment and correction of any coagulopathy, administration of RhoGAM as needed, consideration of steroids for fetal lung maturity in preterm newborns, and preparation for delivery of the newborn.

Ectopic Pregnancy

Sites of Implantation of Ectopic Pregnancies

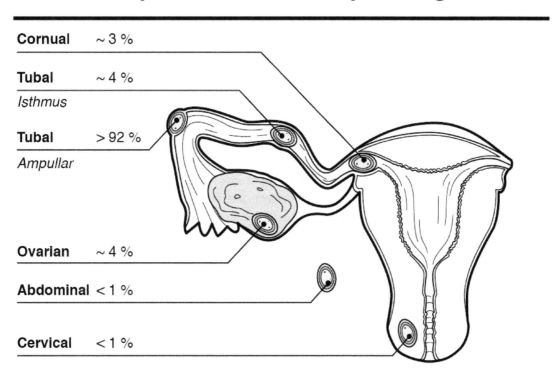

An ectopic pregnancy results from the abnormal implantation of the fertilized ovum at an alternative anatomical site—most commonly the fallopian tube—that is physiologically incapable of sustaining the pregnancy. An undetected or untreated ectopic pregnancy is a life-threatening emergency. The majority of patients do not have any identifiable risk factors; however, the most common defect is an alteration in the structure of the fallopian tubes that impedes the movement of the fertilized ovum to the appropriate site in the uterus.

Common causes of damage to the fallopian tubes include PID, a history of previous ectopic pregnancies, smoking (because it decreases the motility of the fallopian tube), the use of intrauterine devices (IUDs), and assisted reproduction, which doubles the risk for this disorder. Although the three classic symptoms are pain, amenorrhea, and vaginal bleeding, only 40 to 50 percent of patients with an ectopic pregnancy present with all three manifestations. Additional manifestations will be dependent on the implantation site, most commonly the fallopian tube, or rarely, the abdomen, and the "age" of the pregnancy, and may include signs of early pregnancy or abnormal signs such as dizziness, weakness, flu symptoms, and in the extreme, cardiac arrest.

To decrease the morbidity associated with undiagnosed ectopic pregnancies, all women of childbearing age who present with pain, vaginal bleeding, and amenorrhea must be screened for pregnancy. Testing of the urine and serum for beta human chorionic gonadotropin (βhCG) will be positive before the first missed menstrual period, and transvaginal ultrasonography is the recommended imaging modality. Laparoscopy is the treatment of choice for patients who are experiencing pain or hemodynamic instability. Intramuscular methotrexate, which impedes DNA synthesis and prevents cellular replication, is the recommended expectant treatment for ectopic pregnancy. The protocol requires an initial assessment of βhCG, liver and kidney function, blood type, Rh status, and bone marrow function. Methotrexate is administered in a single dose, and its effectiveness is measured by evidence of decreasing βhCG levels. Emergency treatment of an ectopic pregnancy is focused on identification of the location and characteristics of the abnormal pregnancy and the patient's systemic manifestations, which may include hemorrhage and cardiac arrest.

Emergent Delivery

An emergent delivery occurs when a pregnant patient presents with signs of imminent delivery as manifested by complete effacement and dilation of the cervix; strong, effective uterine contractions; and possible visualization of the presenting part at the vaginal orifice. The Emergency Medical Treatment and Labor Act (EMTALA) dictates that all patients who present to the ER must be treated; however, in the case of an imminent delivery, the provider must decide whether delivery in the ER or transfer to the obstetrical department is the most appropriate course for the individual patient. An emergent delivery will trigger the department protocol that includes notification of all personnel required to care for the mother and newborn after the delivery.

Maternal and fetal vital signs, fetal monitoring, IV access, and baseline lab studies will be initiated. Trained personnel will facilitate the delivery, resuscitate and warm the newborn, assess the newborn's Apgar score at 1 and 5 minutes after delivery, monitor the delivery of the placenta, and maintain surveillance of uterine involution. Prompt transfer of the mother and baby to the postpartum unit and newborn nursery, respectively, is required. In addition to common obstetrical and fetal complications, an emergent delivery due to the rapid descent of the fetus may also include vaginal and/or perineal lacerations. Emergency care of this patient is based on the presenting manifestations and the agency-specific protocol for emergent deliveries.

Newborn Apgar Assessment			
	Score of 0	Score of 1	Score of 2
Appearance (skin color)	Blue or pale	Pink body but blue extremities	Pink; no cyanosis
Pulse	Absent	< 100 bpm	> 100 bpm
Grimace (irritability reflex)	No response	Feebly cries or grimaces when stimulated	Cries or pulls away when stimulated
Activity (muscle tone)	None	Some flexion in the limbs	Flexed limbs that resist extension
Respiration	Absent	Gasping, weak, or irregular	Strong cry

Hemorrhage

Postpartum hemorrhage is commonly defined as the loss of more than 500 milliliters following a vaginal delivery or 1000 milliliters after a Caesarean section (C-section) in a pregnancy that has progressed for at least twenty weeks. Less substantial losses can result in alterations in fluid volume status in patients with comorbidities such as anemia, cardiac disease, dehydration, or preeclampsia, which means that

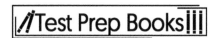

postpartum hemorrhage is the loss of any amount of blood that results in altered hemodynamic status. There are multiple contributing factors; however, the most common precipitating pathophysiology for hemorrhage is uterine atony. These factors are related to tone, tissue, trauma, or thrombosis. Alterations in tone may be due to uterine atony resulting from distention of the uterine muscles in prolonged labor or with a large-for-gestational-age (LGA) newborn. Tissue alterations include retained placental tissue or placenta accreta. Trauma may result from manipulation of the fetus during delivery, history of previous C-section, prolonged labor, and internal version and extraction of a second twin. Alterations in coagulation may be due to preexisting coagulopathies.

The diagnosis depends on the presenting manifestations of postpartum vaginal bleeding and deteriorating hemodynamic status. Commonly, the emergency care of postpartum hemorrhage includes notification of obstetrical, anesthesia, and surgical suite providers; type and cross match for six units of packed red blood cells (PRBCs); assignment of data recording to one provider; aggressive fluid management, including appropriate blood products; assessment of the placenta for missing fragments of tissue; baseline lab studies, including CBC, coagulation studies, renal function tests, and electrolytes; and oxygen by mask. The goal of treatment is to reverse the coagulopathy, resolve the underlying defect, and maintain close surveillance of the contractility of the uterus, or surgical intervention in the event of massive hemorrhage.

Hyperemesis Gravidarum

Hyperemesis gravidarum is an acute form of nausea and vomiting that is associated with fluid volume depletion, resulting in ketosis and up to a 5 percent weight loss. This extreme form of "morning sickness" may also be manifested by fatigue, weakness, dizziness, sleep disturbance, and mood changes. Diagnostic studies include urinalysis to assess acid-base balance and to rule out UTI, liver function studies to rule out hepatitis, CBC, and thyroid function studies. Obstetrical ultrasonography is done to assess the condition of the pregnancy and to confirm the number of fetuses.

The condition typically begins before eight weeks of gestation and rarely persists beyond twenty to twenty-two weeks of gestation. The symptomatic treatment includes close assessment of the fluid volume status and vital signs, antiemetics, and IV fluid replacement. In the event of severe nutritional deficits, acid-base dysfunction, or electrolyte imbalance, hospitalization may be required. The emergency care of the patient with hyperemesis gravidarum is focused on correction of fluid volume deficit, resolution of ketosis and electrolyte imbalances, and relief from nausea and vomiting.

Neonatal Resuscitation

In the United States, 50 percent of all newborn deaths occur in the first 24 hours after delivery. The two most common causes of newborn distress are perinatal asphyxia and extreme prematurity. Neither of these conditions is 100 percent predictable; therefore, all emergency departments must have skilled personnel and all appropriate resources to care for these patients. Additional complications that must be recognized include the presence of pneumothorax, esophageal atresia, multiple gestation, and/or congenital anomalies. Emergency providers must be knowledgeable about the events of the newborn's transition from intrauterine to extrauterine life with respect to respiratory and cardiovascular adaptation. Respiratory adaptation requires the absorption or removal of the amniotic fluid from the airways and alveoli.

In the full-term newborn, there are physiological fetal and maternal resorption mechanisms, which together with the stresses of delivery, decrease the amount of fluid that remains at birth; however, these mechanisms are less effective in preterm newborns. Cardiovascular adaptation involves the redirection of blood flow through the heart and the pulmonary vasculature with normal closure of the ductus arteriosus and the foramen ovale in the heart as a result of changes in the systemic and pulmonary vascular resistance.

The emergency resuscitation of the newborn begins with thermoregulation, which focuses initially on prevention of heat loss, prior to the application of additional heat. The goal is to achieve an initial axillary temperature of 36.5 °C (97.7 °F). Airway management initially involves clearance of amniotic fluid from the airway. It is recommended that only bulb syringes are used because catheters may stimulate a vagal response, resulting in apnea, bradycardia, and hypotension. Drying and clearing of secretions often provide sufficient stimulation to induce spontaneous respirations; however, rubbing the back or tapping the feet may be necessary.

Supplemental oxygen therapy will be initiated depending on heart rate, color, and oxygen saturation. The pulse oximetry goal for full-term newborns is 92 to 96 percent and 88 to 92 percent for premature newborns. If there is sustained bradycardia (less than sixty beats per minute) and cyanosis, mechanical ventilation is required. Additional emergency measures will be ineffective unless a patent airway and an effective ventilatory pattern are present. IV or ET tube administration of epinephrine to stimulate cardiac function, intravenous infusion of 0.9 percent normal sodium chloride for volume expansion and reversal of metabolic acidosis, and cardiac compresses consistent with the PALS protocol will be instituted as necessary.

Placenta Previa

Placenta previa is defined as the abnormal placement of the placenta with either complete coverage of the internal cervical os (complete) by the placenta, or location of the placenta within two centimeters of the internal cervical os (marginal). The condition generally presents with painless vaginal bleeding during the third trimester of pregnancy and is associated with the possibility of hemorrhage at the onset of labor, due to cervical dilation and the relative inability of the lower uterine segment to effectively contract the vessels of the exposed maternal implantation site. Risk factors for this condition include maternal age greater than thirty-five years, infertility treatments, increased number of previous pregnancies, multiple births, previous C-sections, previous abortions, previous placenta previa, and smoking or cocaine use.

Once the condition is identified, the patient can be safely observed as long as the maternal and fetal monitoring parameters remain stable. Betamethasone therapy is indicated for the maturation of the fetal lungs if the pregnancy duration is less than thirty-four weeks. At the first sign of bleeding, immediate surgery is necessary. The care of the patient who presents with hemorrhage without prior identification of the placenta previa will trigger the agency protocol for obstetrical emergencies, which will include the transvaginal ultrasound confirmation of the condition and preparations for emergency surgery, including coagulation studies and type and cross match for six units of blood. Depending on the cause of the placenta previa, surgical removal of the uterus may be the only alternative surgical approach.

Postpartum Infection

There are several infectious conditions that may occur after a vaginal or Caesarean birth or during breastfeeding. There is rarely sufficient postpartum observation of the new mother to identify the onset of infection, usually from the second to the tenth postpartum day, which is manifested by a

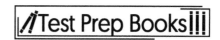

temperature greater than 38 °C (100.4 °F). Common infectious conditions include endometritis, postsurgical wound infections, perineal cellulitis, urinary tract infections, mastitis, and inflammation of the pelvic veins. The manifestations are specific to the anatomical site of the infection, while the causative agents are most often commonly occurring pathogens in the vagina and abdomen. Research indicates that the occurrence of severe sepsis is associated with preexisting conditions, including chronic liver disease, chronic kidney disease, congestive heart failure, and lupus.

Routine diagnostic studies include CBC; electrolytes; coagulation studies; blood, cervical, and wound cultures; and urinalysis. Ultrasonography is used to identify abscess formation, while CT and MRI scans are used to identify septic pelvic thrombosis or other systemic infection such as appendicitis. Antimicrobial treatment is specific to site of the infection. Emergency care of the patient with a postpartum infection is focused on aggressive fluid replacement to support hydration and hemodynamic status, identification of the source of the infection, and administration of the appropriate antimicrobial agent. Patients who present with thrombosed pelvic veins may also require anticoagulant therapy that will necessitate in-hospital care. All patients with systemic manifestations will be considered for admission, and all patients who present with infection will require follow-up care with an obstetrician.

Preeclampsia, Eclampsia, HELLP Syndrome

Preeclampsia is characterized by the onset of hypertension and proteinuria after twenty weeks of gestation and may persist for four to six weeks postpartum. The cause is unknown; however, there is evidence of alterations in the endothelium of the vasculature accompanied by vasospasm. Risk factors include nulliparity, maternal age over forty years old, family history, chronic renal disease, obesity, hypertension, and diabetes. Early manifestations include visual disturbances, altered mental state, dyspnea, facial edema, and possible upper right quadrant pain. Severe manifestations include hypertension on bedrest, increasing liver enzymes with increased pain, progressive renal dysfunction, pulmonary edema, and thrombocytopenia. Routine labs, fetal nonstress testing, and corticosteroids for lung maturation are done prior to delivery, which is the only known cure.

Eclampsia is the life-threatening complication of severe preeclampsia that is manifested by the onset of seizure activity and/or the development of coma and is associated with hypertension, proteinuria, intrauterine fetal growth delay, and diminished amniotic fluid. There are no specific diagnostic tests, and while the specific etiology is unknown, there are indications that the condition results from the interchange of maternal and fetal tissue or allografts. Magnesium sulfate is recommended for short-term use for 24 to 48 hours to stabilize the patient for delivery, which is the only curative measure.

HELLP syndrome is also associated with significant maternal and fetal mortality, resulting from liver rupture and strokes due to cerebral edema or hemorrhage. The syndrome is characterized by hemolysis of RBCs, elevated liver enzymes, and low platelet levels (HELLP). Some authorities consider HELLP syndrome to be a severe form of preeclampsia, while others view it as a separate entity. The coagulation defects and liver dysfunction are the result of microvascular changes in the endothelium in the presence of hypertension; however, the cause is unknown. Risk factors are similar to risk factors for preeclampsia. Manifestations include elevated liver enzymes, coagulation defects including thrombocytopenia and hemolytic anemia, and right upper quadrant pain, and there are classification systems that assess the condition according to the extent of hepatic dysfunction. The treatment involves stabilization of the patient and prompt delivery with attention to correction of the coagulation defects and liver dysfunction. The emergency care of all of these life-threatening conditions is focused on treating hypertension, safe delivery of the fetus, and prevention of associated complications.

Preterm Labor

Most neonatal deaths in the United States are due to preterm labor, which is defined as the onset of uterine contractions that are of adequate strength and frequency to result in effacement and dilation of the cervix between twenty and thirty-seven weeks' gestation. Although the exact etiology is unclear, the most significant predictor for preterm labor is a positive history for preterm labor. Additional risk factors include abruptio placenta, cervical incompetence due to prior surgery, uterine fibroids, cervical infections, fetal distress, and placental defects due to systemic conditions that include diabetes, hypertension, smoking, and alcohol and drug abuse.

The routine testing for a patient with a history of second-trimester pregnancy loss includes coagulation studies, cultures for chlamydia and gonorrhea, glucose tolerance assessment, and immune antibody studies. Two additional parameters—the cervical length as measured by transvaginal ultrasonography and the fetal fibronectin level (fFN)—are used to assess the risk for preterm labor in a patient with inconclusive manifestations. Preterm labor is treated with tocolytic agents and progesterone. The primary purpose of tocolytic therapy is to delay delivery for up to 48 hours to optimize the effect of betamethasone therapy on fetal lung maturation, thereby decreasing the incidence of respiratory distress syndrome in the newborn.

Tocolytic therapy with magnesium sulfate is recommended for preterm labor from twenty-four to thirty-three weeks of gestation. Common side effects of magnesium sulfate are headache, lethargy, blurred vision, and facial flushing. Toxic manifestations include respiratory depression and cardiac arrest. Progesterone is believed to prevent preterm labor by direct effect on the uterus after the placenta is fully formed, and it may also be used to delay delivery. The emergency care of the patient with preterm labor is focused on confirming the presence of true labor, assessing fetal health, and administering tocolytic agents and progesterone, which help inhibit the labor process.

Threatened Spontaneous Abortion

Abortion is defined as any form of early pregnancy loss; however, the term **miscarriage** appears more commonly in lay literature. Up to 80 percent of spontaneous abortions occur in the first trimester and may be categorized as threatened, inevitable, incomplete, complete, or missed. In addition, abortions are labeled as sporadic or recurrent. Chromosomal anomalies of the fetus are generally accepted as the most common cause of early abortions. In addition, several maternal risk factors have been identified that may be associated with first- or second-trimester pregnancy losses. Advanced maternal age and a history of type 1 diabetes, renal disease, severe hypertension, thyroid dysfunction, anatomical defects of the uterus, illicit drug use, smoking, alcohol abuse, and non-ASA NSAID use have all been associated with an increased risk of an initial or recurrent early pregnancy loss.

The diagnosis of a threatened spontaneous abortion will be based on the patient's history and physical, lab studies, and ultrasonography. The first priority is to confirm the presence of the pregnancy; therefore, lab studies will include the assessment of βhCG (human chorionic gonadotropin) in addition to CBC with differential, blood and Rh typing, hemoglobin and hematocrit, and coagulation studies. Transabdominal and transvaginal ultrasonography are the recommended imaging modalities. Treatment is dependent on the stage of the pregnancy, the presenting manifestations, and in some cases, the patient's preference for the treatment approach. A threatened abortion of a first-trimester pregnancy will be treated with expectant management, which includes close observation of maternal hemodynamic status and blood loss. If the abortion continues to an incomplete abortion, surgical or pharmacologically-induced evacuation of the products of conception will be considered. Emergency

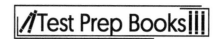

treatment is focused on the prevention and/or treatment of hemorrhage and the prevention of infection.

Trauma

Trauma care of pregnant women requires attention to the needs of two patients—mother and fetus—and the injury and complication risks are dependent on the gestational age of the fetus. Motor vehicle accidents, which include seat belt injuries in addition to blunt trauma, and domestic partner violence are the most common causes of trauma in pregnant women, and it is also noted that substance abuse is commonly related to these injuries. Research suggests that, collectively, accidental and violent trauma are responsible for more maternal injuries and death than all other complications of pregnancy. Patient complaints of pain must be differentiated as to an obstetrical or non-obstetrical etiology. There is an inherent risk of the onset of preterm labor and abruptio placenta with all maternal trauma.

The emergency care of the pregnant patient is focused on the assessment of maternal hemodynamic status and fetal wellbeing. Lab studies aimed at the identification and assessment of traumatic injuries may include CBC, electrolytes, glucose, blood typing and cross match, Rh typing, pregnancy testing, coagulation studies, urinalysis for presence of infection and/or RBCs, Kleihauer-Betke testing, toxicology screening, D-dimer testing for identification of placental abruption, and testing for a base deficit that may indicate intra-abdominal injury. In addition to the attention to special concerns related to the pregnancy, the trauma protocol will be initiated according to agency protocol. The emergency care of a pregnant trauma victim is focused on assessment of both patients, identification and emergency treatment of all injuries, preparations for emergency delivery of the fetus as necessary, prevention and/or treatment of hemorrhage, and appropriate fluid volume support. Emergency providers will also report the occurrence of domestic or criminal violence as mandated by applicable HIPAA and state laws.

Practice Questions

1. The nurse is caring for a patient with cirrhosis who arrives in the emergency room complaining of increasing abdominal distention. The nurse assesses the presence of ascites. Which of the following statements correctly describes the pathogenesis of ascites?
    a. Epinephrine and norepinephrine levels are decreased.
    b. Plasma albumin levels are decreased.
    c. Portal hypotension is the initial defect.
    d. Plasma oncotic levels are increased.

2. The nurse is caring for a patient with endoscopic evidence of esophageal varices. Which of the following statements correctly identifies the interventions associated with primary prevention of hemorrhage for this condition?
    a. Sclerotherapy ablation of the esophageal arteries
    b. Vasopressors to maintain the hepatic venous pressure gradient above 20 mmHG
    c. Transjugular intrahepatic portosystemic shunt implantation
    d. Endoscopic band ligation

3. The nurse is caring for a nineteen-year-old woman who presents in the emergency department with manifestations of acute hepatitis. She tells the nurse that she thinks she might be pregnant and asks the nurse how this disease could affect her baby. The nurse understands that which of the following genotypes is associated with the most significant risk for perinatal transmission of the hepatitis virus?
    a. HAeAb negative
    b. HBeAg positive
    c. HCeAg negative
    d. HDeAb positive

4. The nurse is caring for a thirty-eight-year-old male who presents with marked left-sided scrotal swelling and distention of the abdomen. The nurse understands that which of the following is an UNEXPECTED finding in this patient?
    a. Diarrhea
    b. Tachycardia
    c. Rebound tenderness
    d. BUN 27

5. The nurse is providing discharge teaching for a patient recently diagnosed with Crohn's disease. Which of the following patient statements indicates the need for additional instruction?
    a. "I understand that once I get through this surgery, my disease will be cured."
    b. "I know that I have a risk for the development of arthritis."
    c. "I know that vitamin B-12 is important for me."
    d. "I will tell my doc if my pain localizes to the right lower quadrant of my abdomen."

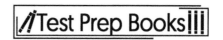

6. The nurse in the emergency department is caring for a patient who is being evaluated for a small-bowel obstruction. The nurse understands that which of the following assessment findings is consistent with this condition?

    a. pH 7.32, pCO_2 38, HCO_3 20 mmol/L

    b. Serum osmolality 285 mOsm/kg

    c. Serum sodium 128 mmol/L

    d. Lower abdominal distention

7. The nurse is preparing a discharge plan for a patient with risk factors for acute pancreatitis. Which of the following information should be included in this plan?

    a. Endoscopic retrograde cholangiopancreatography (ERCP) imaging is required to confirm the diagnosis.

    b. Ultrasonography is the most useful imaging study when significant abdominal distention is present.

    c. Current research confirms the efficacy of rectal administration of indomethacin to reduce the incidence of pancreatitis due to the ERCP procedure.

    d. There is no scientific rationale to explain why some individuals with chronic ETOH abuse develop acute pancreatitis, while others do not develop pancreatitis.

8. The nurse is caring for a patient with manifestations of peptic ulcer disease. Which of the following statements is correct?

    a. Stomach pain begins 20 to 30 minutes after eating.

    b. The condition is associated with an increased risk of malignancy.

    c. Endoscopy is used to establish hemostasis.

    d. Chronic NSAID use is the most common etiology.

9. The nurse is caring for a patient in the emergency department who has manifestations of diverticulitis. The patient asks the nurse to explain the difference between diverticulosis and diverticulitis. Which of the following statements is correct?

    a. Diverticulosis rarely occurs in adults.

    b. Diverticulitis is associated with chronic NSAID use.

    c. The initial treatment for diverticulitis is surgery to remove the affected bowel segment.

    d. The patient's age at onset of diverticulosis is associated with the risk of diverticulitis.

10. The nurse in the emergency department is caring for a patient with low-flow priapism. The patient also has a history of sickle cell disease, and the nurse understands that this disease is a significant risk factor for priapism. Which of the following statements identifies the pathology of this relationship?

    a. Sickle cell disease results in decreased free hemoglobin, which leads to vasodilation in the penis.

    b. Hemolyzed red cells decrease nitric oxide stores, resulting in vasodilation and priapism.

    c. Sickle cell is an autoimmune defect associated with altered arterial pressure in the penis.

    d. Prophylactic use of sildenafil effectively reduces the recurrence of priapism in this population.

11. The nurse is preparing a discharge plan for a patient who has chronic urinary retention and will be performing self-catheterization at home. Which of the following statements indicates the need for additional teaching?

    a. "My doctor told me that I can use my catheters more than once."

    b. "If I have chills and fever, it may mean that I am not emptying my bladder."

    c. "The acid in coffee will help to maintain the acidity of my urine, which decreases infection."

    d. "I should have about 700 milliliters to 1000 milliliters of urine output every day."

12. The nurse in the emergency department is caring for a fourteen-year-old boy with testicular torsion. The prehospital provider reported a TWIST score of 5; however, at the time of the patient's arrival in the ER, the urologist established a TWIST score of 6. The nurse understands that which of the following is the recommended treatment plan for this patient?

a. The patient most probably has an alternative condition causing his symptoms.
b. The patient will need an immediate ultrasound to confirm the diagnosis.
c. The patient requires immediate surgical intervention.
d. The treatment recommendations are the same for scores of 5 and 6.

13. The nurse is caring for a patient with a history of STDs who presents with right upper quadrant pain. The nurse understands that this pain may be associated with Fitz-Hugh–Curtis syndrome. Which of the following statements is consistent with the pathophysiology associated with this disorder?

a. This inflammatory process of Glisson's capsule results in adhesions.
b. It is an abnormal autoimmune response to the antimicrobial treatment of PID.
c. It is an infection of the liver that manifests in the tertiary stage of syphilis.
d. The syndrome is most often associated with severe pelvic pain.

14. The nurse is reviewing the history of a patient who is being evaluated for ovarian cancer. Which of the following risk factors is UNRELATED to the incidence of ovarian cancer?

a. Infertility treatment
b. Hyperthyroidism
c. Tubal ligation
d. Tamoxifen use

15. The nurse is providing emergency care for a patient who is the victim of a sexual assault by an unknown person. Which of the following statements regarding the reporting of sexual assault by health care providers is correct?

a. HIPAA requires mandatory reporting of all suspected sexual assaults by health care providers.
b. All of the individual states have mandatory reporting statutes for all suspected sexual assaults by health care providers.
c. HIPAA requires reporting of suspected sexual assault only if the assault occurs outside of a domestic relationship; in other words, the victim is not in a relationship with the abuser.
d. HIPAA defers to individual state laws when the abuse occurs outside of a domestic relationship.

16. The nurse is caring for a patient with a suspected ectopic pregnancy. The patient asks the nurse to explain how her smoking history is related to this condition. Which of the following statements correctly identifies the relationship between smoking and the development of an ectopic pregnancy?

a. Smoking decreases the oxygen saturation of the fetal circulation, which compromises the process of implantation.
b. Smoking alters progesterone levels, which interferes with the transfer of the fertilized ovum to the uterus.
c. Smoking alters the endometrial lining, making it an inhospitable environment for the fertilized ovum, thereby preventing implantation.
d. Smoking damages the cilia in the fallopian tube, which decreases motility and alters the movement of the fertilized ovum.

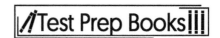

17. The nurse is caring for a patient who is thirty-six weeks pregnant with manifestations of abruptio placenta. Which of the following statements is consistent with the use of the Kleihauer-Betke test?
    a. The test is a highly sensitive indicator of the onset of preterm in pregnant patients with trauma.
    b. The test measures the amount of fetal blood in the maternal bloodstream, which guides RhoGAM dosing.
    c. The test is only used in the assessment of Rh-negative patients who present with abruptio placenta during a second pregnancy.
    d. Based on the amount of fetal blood that is transferred to the maternal circulation, the test is predictive of the degree of separation of the placenta.

18. The nurse is caring for a patient after an emergency delivery in the ER. The newborn had an Apgar score of 8 at 1 minute and a score of 9 at 5 minutes after delivery. Which of the following statements is consistent with these scores?
    a. The scores are normal.
    b. The deficit is most likely due to decreased muscle tone.
    c. The newborn will require only short-term mechanical ventilatory support.
    d. The newborn is at risk for cardiac anomalies.

19. The nurses in the emergency department are reviewing the treatment protocol for the emergency resuscitation of the newborn. Which of the following statements correctly identifies the rationale for the use of intravenous 0.9 percent sodium chloride (normal saline) as the initial treatment of metabolic acidosis?
    a. Normal saline can be administered intraosseously and is, therefore, more readily available.
    b. Sodium bicarbonate ($NaHCO_3$) causes adverse fluid shifts due to its low osmolarity.
    c. Normal saline does not generate additional CO_2, which can be harmful to cardiac and cerebral function.
    d. Sodium bicarbonate is not as effective as normal saline for the treatment of hyperkalemia resulting from prolonged resuscitation of the newborn.

20. The nurse is caring for a patient who has a complete placenta previa and is twenty-two weeks pregnant. She asks the nurse to explain the action of betamethasone. Which of the following statements is consistent with the action of this medication?
    a. The medication reduces newborn infections if the membranes rupture prematurely due to the placenta previa.
    b. Prolonged gestation is more effective than treatment with betamethasone for lung maturation.
    c. The therapy eliminates the occurrence of respiratory distress syndrome in the newborn.
    d. Betamethasone is a tocolytic agent that can be used long-term to stop preterm labor.

21. The nurse is caring for a patient with suspected HELLP syndrome. The patient asks the nurse to explain the complications associated with this diagnosis. Which of the following statements correctly identifies the complications of this syndrome?
    a. The syndrome creates a state of hypercoagulation that can result in infarction of the hepatic vasculature.
    b. Liver dysfunction is reversible with correction of the coagulation defects.
    c. Cerebrovascular effects are rare.
    d. The "complete" form of HELLP is manifested by red cell hemolysis, elevated liver enzyme levels, and low platelet levels.

Answer Explanations

1. B: Hypoalbuminemia is an essential element in the development of ascites. Decreased oncotic pressure resulting from deficient plasma proteins allows the movement of fluid from the vasculature into the extracellular fluid where it accumulates as ascites. Cirrhosis can result in increased levels of nitric oxide, which leads to vasodilation. The renal response to this abnormal condition is sodium retention and the secretion of increased epinephrine and norepinephrine due to stimulation of the sympathetic nervous system. Therefore, Choice *A* is incorrect. The development of ascites is a complication of portal hypertension, not hypotension. Portal hypertension is defined as the blockage of blood flow through the vasculature of the liver due to fibrotic changes resulting from cirrhosis or hepatitis; therefore, Choice *C* is incorrect. Plasma oncotic levels are decreased, rather than increased, because the diseased liver is not able to synthesize albumin; therefore, Choice *D* is incorrect.

2. D: Endoscopic band ligation should be implemented for all varices that are 5 millimeters or more in diameter or are associated with red wales, because these characteristics are associated with a greater risk for hemorrhage. Band ligation decreases this potential but may be associated with stricture formation and obstruction of the esophageal lumen. This procedure may need to be repeated as the liver failure progresses. Therefore, Choice *D* is correct. Sclerotherapy of the esophageal veins is considered as a form of secondary prevention by many because beta-blocker therapy is readily available, well tolerated, and equally effective as compared to sclerotherapy. In the event of hemorrhage due to ruptured esophageal varices, sclerotherapy can be used to decrease the blood loss; therefore, Choice *A* is incorrect. The recommended use of nonselective beta-blockers as primary prevention is intended to decrease the hepatic venous pressure gradient (HVPG) to less than or equal to 12 mmHg. An increase of this measurement would result in enlargement and possible rupture of the varices; therefore, Choice *B* is incorrect. The transjugular intrahepatic portosystemic shunt (TIPS) connects the portal and systemic circulations to decrease portal hypertension. The TIPS is appropriate to the care of the patient with active hemorrhage of esophageal varices and is not currently recommended as primary prevention of hemorrhage; therefore, Choice *C* is incorrect.

3. B: The greatest risk for perinatal virus transmission occurs with the antigen-positive hepatitis B virus. Hepatitis A virus spreads most commonly by the fecal-oral route, and perinatal transmission has not been established; therefore, Choice *A* is incorrect. Hepatitis C is rarely transmitted to the fetus, and the antigen-negative genotype would be less likely than the antigen-positive genotype to affect the fetus; therefore, Choice *C* is incorrect. Perinatal transmission of the hepatitis D virus is rare, and release of the hepatitis D virions requires coinfection with the hepatitis B virus; therefore, Choice *D* is incorrect.

4. A: The patient's manifestations are consistent with an incarcerated or strangulated hernia that is progressing to a small-bowel obstruction as evidenced by the abdominal distention. This complication is associated with decreased peristalsis and eventual absence of bowel activity, which means that diarrhea would be an uncommon manifestation. Tachycardia and a BUN of 27 are related to fluid volume losses resulting from the accumulation of fluid proximal to the obstruction in the small bowel; therefore, Choices *B* and *D* are incorrect. Rebound tenderness is also an expected finding in a bowel obstruction due to the trapped gas and fluid proximal to the obstruction; therefore, Choice *C* is incorrect.

5. A: Crohn's disease is recurrent. Surgery may be necessary to excise a segment of the intestine that has been damaged by the transmural effects of the disease process; however, progression to additional areas is common because Crohn's disease can affect the entire length of the GI tract. This is in contrast to ulcerative colitis, which may be cured by a total colectomy because the disease can only affect the

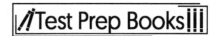

colon. Therefore, Choice *A* reflects the need for additional teaching and is the correct answer. Crohn's disease is an autoimmune-mediated disease and is associated with an increased risk for other immune diseases such as arthritis; therefore, Choice *B* does not reflect the need for additional teaching. Crohn's disease commonly affects the terminal ileum, which is the site of vitamin B-12 absorption. Deficiency of this vitamin can result in decreased red cell production and anemia; therefore, Choice *C* does not reflect the need for additional teaching. Crohn's disease is often complicated by fistulae formation between bowel segments, which results in localized pain in the right lower quadrant of the abdomen. Early recognition and treatment are necessary to prevent systemic effects including sepsis; therefore, Choice *D* does not reflect the need for additional teaching.

6. C: Small-bowel obstruction is associated with severe fluid and electrolyte losses. The normal serum sodium level is 135 to 145 mEq/L; therefore, Choice *C* is indicative of deficient serum sodium and severe alterations in fluid balance. Small-bowel obstruction is manifested by metabolic alkalosis due to the loss of acids with vomiting. Choice *A* is consistent with metabolic acidosis, not alkalosis, and is therefore incorrect. As noted, small-bowel obstruction is associated with fluid volume deficits; however, the reported serum osmolality of 285 mOsm/kg is within the normal range for serum osmolality (275–295 mOsm/kg); therefore, Choice *B* is incorrect. Abdominal distention in large-bowel obstruction most commonly occurs in the lower abdomen, while abdominal distention in the small bowel most commonly occurs in the epigastric or upper abdominal area; therefore, Choice *D* is incorrect.

7. D: Chronic alcohol abuse and biliary tract dysfunction are the most frequent causes of acute pancreatitis; however, there are no identified criteria that explain why some individuals will experience pancreatitis while others do not. Acute pancreatitis is most often diagnosed by the presenting history and physical examination. ECRP is only indicated in patients with acute pancreatitis and concomitant biliary disease; therefore, Choice *A* is incorrect. Ultrasonography is generally less useful than CT imaging for pancreatitis, and its efficacy is significantly decreased in the presence of abdominal distention, which distorts the images; therefore, Choice *B* is incorrect. Although rectal indomethacin is used commonly to treat acute pancreatitis resulting from ERCP imaging, controversy remains regarding the efficacy of the therapy; therefore, Choice *C* is incorrect.

8. C: Endoscopy is used to diagnose the condition and to cauterize hemorrhagic sites. The treatment algorithm for peptic ulcer disease recommends surgical intervention if two endoscopic attempts at hemostasis are unsuccessful. The pain related to peptic ulcer disease does not begin until the ingested food has reached the duodenum; therefore, the pain does not begin for 2 to 3 hours after a meal, while the onset of pain with gastric ulcers is 20 to 30 minutes after a meal. Choice *A* is incorrect. Gastric ulcers are associated with an increased incidence of malignancy, not peptic ulcers; therefore, Choice *B* is incorrect. NSAID use is a commonly-associated cause of peptic ulcer disease. However, even excluding patients who use NSAIDs, more than 60 percent of the cases of peptic ulcer disease are related to *H. pylori* infection; therefore, Choice *D* is incorrect.

9. D: There is evidence that patients who are diagnosed with diverticulosis before the age of fifty have a greater risk for episodes of diverticulitis, which may be due to an unidentified difference in the infective process, living longer, or delays in seeking care for the initial episode. The presence of diverticulosis is age-dependent, affecting less than 5 percent of individuals less than forty years old and up to 65 percent of individuals over eighty years old; therefore, Choice *A* is incorrect. Diverticulitis is caused by infection of the diverticula due to impacted fecaliths and other cellular debris, which results in overgrowth of normal colonic bacteria with progression to an inflammatory process that is responsible for the clinical manifestations of the acute attack. Therefore, Choice *B* is incorrect. Initial episodes of diverticulitis are treated with bowel rest, antibiotics, and IV fluids. Emergency surgical intervention of an initial attack is required only for severe manifestations, and an elective colectomy is recommended after three episodes of diverticulitis; therefore, Choice *C* is incorrect.

10. B: Hemolysis is the underlying defect of sickle cell disease, due to the abnormally-shaped or sickled red blood cells, and hemolysis results in an increased concentration of free hemoglobin. Under normal circumstances, nitric oxide is responsible for triggering vasodilation and relaxation of the smooth muscle of the penis, resulting in tumescence. However, nitric oxide is scavenged by free hemoglobin, which means that the elevated levels of free hemoglobin due to hemolysis in sickle cell disease results in a deficit of nitric oxide and sustained venous outflow inhibition and failure of the tumescent process, causing priapism. Choice *B* is the correct answer. As noted, hemoglobin is released by hemolysis, which leads to *increased* free hemoglobin and continued venous outflow inhibition and sustained priapism; therefore, Choice *A* is incorrect. Sickle cell disease is an inherited autosomal genetic defect that affects the structure of the red blood cell. It is associated with specific genes and does not involve alterations in the immune response. Sickle cell disease affects vasodilation by the release of free hemoglobin. The disease does not directly affect vasodilation; therefore, Choice *C* is incorrect. There is little research evidence for the efficacy of the prophylactic use of medications used to treat erectile dysfunction, and their use is not commonly recommended; therefore, Choice *D* is incorrect.

11. C: While it is recommended that patients maintain an acidic pH in the urine to limit the growth of *E. coli,* coffee is to be avoided because caffeine intake is associated with increased feelings of the need to void and urgency. Therefore, Choice *C* indicates the need for additional instruction and is the correct answer. The physician will prescribe the correct catheter for the individual patient, and usually clean technique and the reuse of the catheter is appropriate. The providers must be convinced that the patient and/or caregiver understand the procedure and the identification of complications that require medical intervention; therefore, Choice *A* is incorrect. The onset of chills and fever may indicate an infection of the bladder or kidney due to incomplete emptying of the bladder and should be immediately reported to the health care provider. Therefore, Choice *B* is incorrect. Urine output will depend on the patient's intake and diet; however, an average output of 30 mL/h is acceptable in most instances; therefore, Choice *D* is incorrect.

12. C: The TWIST score was devised by urologists for use in establishing the diagnosis and treatment protocol for testicular torsion. The points assigned to the individual assessments include testis swelling (2 points), hard testis (2 points), absent cremasteric reflex (1 point), nausea/vomiting (1 point), and high-riding testis (1 point). The scoring system has also been validated for use by prehospital providers. In the presence of scrotal pain, a TWIST score of 0 is an indication that there is an alternative cause for the patient's manifestations. A TWIST score between 1 and 5 requires immediate ultrasonography to confirm the diagnosis. Immediate surgical intervention, without any delay to obtain ultrasonography, is the recommended intervention for a TWIST score of 6; therefore, Choice *C* is correct. The possibility of an alternative condition is associated with a TWIST score of 0; therefore, Choice *A* is incorrect. Ultrasonography is only recommended for patients with a TWIST score of 5 or less; therefore, Choice *B* is incorrect. Ultrasonography to confirm the diagnosis is recommended for a TWIST score of 5. However, immediate surgery is required for a TWIST score of 6; therefore, the scores have different implications, and Choice *D* is incorrect.

13. A: Fitz-Hugh–Curtis perihepatitis presents with characteristic "violin string" adhesions that are due to an inflammation of the surface of Glisson's capsule, which is a layer of connective tissue that surrounds the liver and encloses the hepatic artery, the portal vein, and the bile ducts within the liver. The condition is most often secondary to pelvic inflammatory disease caused by chlamydia or gonorrhea. Therefore, Choice *A* is correct. The hepatitis is the result of the infection by the pathogen

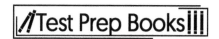

that causes PID; it is not an autoimmune response. The pathogen is thought to migrate to the abdomen and liver from the fallopian tubes, causing the inflammatory process that results in right upper quadrant pain and altered liver function; therefore, Choice *B* is incorrect. The inflammatory process is most often caused by chlamydia or gonorrhea and is not associated with the late stages of syphilis infection; therefore, Choice *C* is incorrect. The patient may report little or no pelvic pain with this syndrome; therefore, Choice *D* is incorrect.

14. B: Risk factors for ovarian cancer include hypothyroidism, a history of infertility treatment, tubal ligation, or the use of tamoxifen; therefore, Choice *B* is the correct answer, and Choices *A*, *C,* and *D* are incorrect.

15. D: HIPAA requires mandatory reporting of suspected domestic abuse; however, HIPAA regulations do not address suspected criminal assault. In that instance, the reporting statutes in the individual states apply to health care providers. In addition, there is no universal reporting mandate among states, which means that health care providers must understand their responsibilities, provide meticulous documentation, and follow agency protocol for the care of patients in this special population. Therefore, Choice *D* is the correct answer, and Choices *A*, *B,* and *C* are incorrect.

16. D: An ectopic pregnancy results from the abnormal implantation of the fertilized ovum at a site other than the uterus. The fallopian tube is the implantation site in 94 percent of ectopic pregnancies, which means that there is some impedance to the normal eight- to ten-day passage of the fertilized ovum from the fallopian tube to the uterus. The fallopian tube is lined by hair-like extensions, or cilia, which provide the motility that propels the ovum from the point of fertilization to the appropriate implantation site in the uterus. There is clear research evidence that one of the effects of smoking is the blunting or destruction of the cilia, which decreases the efficiency of this process, thereby contributing to the likelihood of faulty implantation. The process of implantation and initial development of the placenta is a hypoxic environment in the initial weeks of the first trimester due to "plugging" alterations in the vasculature of the endometrium that prevent maternal hemorrhage. Hypoxia from smoking is associated with fetal intrauterine growth delay later in the pregnancy. However, it does not directly affect implantation; therefore, Choice *A* is incorrect. Smoking affects the lining of the fallopian tube but has no identified effect on progesterone levels; therefore, Choice *B* is incorrect. Smoking directly affects the lining of the fallopian tubes. However, there is no evidence of any similar effect on the endometrium; therefore, Choice *C* is incorrect.

17. B: In the event of major trauma, there is an increased incidence of fetal-to-maternal hemorrhage, which can alter the amount of Rho(D) immune globulin (RhoGAM) that is required to protect the fetus. The Kleihauer-Betke test can be used to quantify the concentration of fetal hemoglobin in the maternal blood, which then is used to calculate the appropriate dose of Rho(D) immune globulin (RhoGAM) in Rh-negative mothers; therefore, Choice *B* is correct. Although some authors recommend the use of the test in all patients as an indicator of preterm labor, the research indicates that this test is not specific for, or sensitive to, the occurrence of preterm labor and is not a reliable indicator for preterm labor; therefore, Choice *A* is incorrect. The transfer of fetal hemoglobin to the maternal circulation must be addressed with the first pregnancy to avoid the formation of anti-D antibodies; therefore, Choice *C* is incorrect. The test can only measure the concentration of fetal hemoglobin in the maternal circulation. It is not sensitive or specific to the degree of the precipitating trauma; therefore, Choice *D* is incorrect.

18. A: Apgar scores of 8 and 9 are normal scores for a healthy newborn with acrocyanosis, which is a benign condition manifested by peripheral cyanosis of the hands and feet that usually resolves within the first few hours after birth. Decreased muscle tone or flexion is most often associated with other deficits that would result in a lower Apgar score; therefore, Choice *B* is incorrect. If the newborn required ventilatory support, there would also be deficits of muscle tone and heart rate, resulting in lower Apgar scores; therefore, Choice *C* is incorrect. The Apgar score is not predictive of specific anomalies, and the indicated scores are considered as normal; therefore, Choice *D* is incorrect.

19. C: Normal saline is preferred for the treatment of metabolic acidosis in the event of a brief episode of cardiopulmonary resuscitation because sodium bicarbonate (bicarb) generates additional carbon dioxide, which is potentially harmful to the heart and brain. Normal saline can be administered intraosseously. However, that has no bearing on the use of normal saline versus bicarb for the treatment of metabolic acidosis; therefore, Choice *A* is incorrect. Bicarb exhibits hyperosmolarity; therefore, Choice *B* is incorrect. Bicarb is effective in the treatment of hyperkalemia, but its use is not recommended except in the case of prolonged resuscitation and must be administered only after effective ventilation and circulation have been restored; therefore, Choice *D* is incorrect.

20. B: Betamethasone therapy can improve the maturity of the fetal lungs by increasing the amount of available surfactant, which allows adaptation of the respiratory system immediately after birth. However, prolonged gestation, which permits additional time for the lungs to mature naturally is more effective than administration of additional corticosteroids; therefore, Choice *B* is correct. Research indicates that the administration of steroids such as betamethasone in the presence of the premature rupture of membranes (PROM) increases the incidence of infection; therefore, Choice *A* is incorrect. Successful treatment with betamethasone may reduce the incidence of respiratory distress syndrome in the newborn. However, there is no evidence that the risk is eliminated by betamethasone; therefore, Choice *C* is incorrect. Betamethasone is only used to mature the fetal lungs by increasing the amount of surfactant that is available to facilitate the expansion of the newborn lungs. It is not a tocolytic agent (an agent that decreases uterine contractions in preterm labor), and in addition, tocolytic agents cannot be used for longer than 48 hours; therefore, Choice *D* is incorrect.

21. D: The Tennessee Classification System designates complete HELLP syndrome as having a platelet count of less than 10^{11}/L, AST greater than or equal to 70 units/L, and LDH greater than 600 units/L, which account for the alterations in liver function. Additional manifestations include red cell hemolysis, elevated liver enzymes, and coagulation defects. The syndrome is associated with abnormal blood clotting that commonly creates a hematoma in the liver tissue, not in the liver vasculature; therefore, Choice *A* is incorrect. The liver function is related to the degree of severity of the syndrome; however, the liver damage may or may not improve in a liver that has been previously damaged by systemic disease, prior trauma, or infection. Irreversible damage to the liver, including rupture of hematomas and liver capsule destroying a significant part of the liver, are commonly associated with this condition; therefore, Choice *B* is incorrect. Cerebral edema and hemorrhagic stroke are among the most common complications of the HELLP syndrome due to altered coagulopathy; therefore, Choice *C* is incorrect.

Psychosocial and Medical Emergencies

Psychosocial

Psychosocial emergencies consist of situations that cause extreme mental distress and the presence of psychological or societal harm to an individual or a group.

Abuse and Neglect

Abuse and neglect can take many forms and affect people of various demographics. Children, women, and the elderly tend to be the vulnerable victim populations. Abuse and neglect cases can often put the victim in the emergency room, so nurses and other medical personnel should be aware that they likely will come across these unfortunate situations, and intervention may be necessary. It is important to know how to spot abuse and neglect cases for legal and ethical reasons.

In children, abuse and neglect can come from a biological or adoptive parent, guardian, close adult in the child's life, or stranger. Younger children are the most vulnerable individuals in this demographic. This is because they may not be able to speak, defend themselves, or understand that they are being abused, or they may be fearful of reporting a caregiver.

Child abuse can be emotional (such as refusal to provide affection or emotional comfort, criticizing the child in a cruel or unusual manner, or administering humiliation or shame tactics) and may be hard to detect or penalize legally. Physical abuse of a child involves intentional acts of physical violence that could result in injury. Sexual abuse of a child includes sexual acts or interactions by an adult; even if the child provides consent, it is considered abuse, due to the emotional and mental immaturity of the child. In the United States, legal age of consent varies by state. Signs of abuse in children can include physical indicators, such as cuts, bruises, genital pain or bleeding, and persistent yeast infections. There can also be behavioral indicators, such as slow development, aggression, anxiety, suicidal tendencies, fearful natures, antisocial or awkward behavioral habits, statements describing inappropriate physical or sexual interactions, visibly unusual relationships or interactions with a parent or caregiver, and a lack of desire (or even refusal) to go home.

Child neglect refers to a parent, guardian, or other caretaker's inaction to provide basic care such as food, water, education, medical and dental treatments, safe supervision, and clean and safe living accommodations. Signs of neglect in children can include chronic illness, malnutrition, lack of personal hygiene, above-average school absenteeism, anxiety and depression, and substance abuse.

A single sign may not mean that abuse or neglect is present, but it should be taken seriously by asking further questions and potentially seeking resources, such as social support agencies and legal counsel, to prevent further abuse. Most states require that knowledge of potential abuse or neglect be reported to legal and child protective services. The process of reporting varies by state, and practitioners should familiarize themselves with abuse and neglect reporting practices of the state in which their nursing services will be provided.

Domestic violence between adult partners, also known as **intimate partner violence and abuse**, is also a common form of abuse that can require emergency department visits. While this type of abuse can be experienced by partners of either gender or orientation, it is most commonly inflicted by male partners on female victims. Physical indicators of abuse from a partner include marks such as bruises, black eyes, genital or anal damage, scratches, and welts. Behavioral indicators include a fearful nature, low self-esteem, isolation, anxiety, depression, constant excuses for the abusing partner's dangerous actions, and suicidal tendencies. Again, the presence of one sign may not indicate that abuse is occurring, but it can be a call to action to provide resources for the victim's safety.

Elder abuse and neglect may occur by family members or other caregivers. Elderly people are vulnerable, as they may be physically weak or have other physical and mental limitations, handicaps, or disabilities. Signs of abuse in elders are similar to those seen in children but can also include the occurrence of adult-minded activities that happen without the elder's consent, such as mishandled financial transactions or health care fraud. Physical indicators of abuse in the elderly include bruises, broken bones, and signs of physical restraint. Behavioral indicators include poor relationships with caregivers, anxiety, depression, and a fearful nature. Indicators of neglect in the elderly include missed or improper medication administration, signs of poor hygiene, genital or anal rashes, and malnutrition.

Unfortunately, many signs of elder abuse and neglect are similar to signs of dementia, a natural reaction to ailing health, and other behaviors commonly exhibited by this age demographic. Therefore, due diligence by nurses and medical personnel is necessary. All states have elder abuse prevention laws, though procedures for reporting may vary by state, so it is important to know the process for the state in which nursing services will be administered.

Aggressive/Violent Behavior

Nurses sometimes must contend with aggressive and violent behavior from patients in the emergency department. An aggressive or violent patient can be characterized by the exhibition of any nonverbal behaviors or verbal communication that intend to cause conflict, harm, pain, or injury. An aggressive or violent patient may invade personal space, make verbal threats or obscene gestures, mimic or follow through with physical threats, speak unnecessarily loudly or in a hostile manner, or be generally abusive in some other verbal or physical way. The causes motivating these behaviors are variable. Patients may show aggressive or violent behavior due to a psychiatric or physiological issue, such as drug abuse, delusions, head injuries, and infections of the brain. However, aggressive or violent behavior can also be a result of the patient's personal background and history, such as family upbringing, socioeconomic status, and current personal stressors.

Nurses should assess each patient for potential aggressive or violent behavior. This can include looking for known risk factors on intake forms (i.e., medical and psychological history, documented history of violence or substance abuse, history of detention or imprisonment, or personal stressors such as unemployment). This can also include assessing the patient directly and taking note of appearance, mental and physical state, pupil size, level of perspiration, mood, tone of speaking, and any comments made by the patient that could indicate current feelings of hostility or anger.

Nurses should be knowledgeable of their health care setting's policies and local laws as they relate to managing or sedating aggressive or violent patients. To protect the safety of medical personnel, the patient, and other patients in the vicinity, if a patient becomes visibly aggressive or violent, physical restraint may need to be provided by a dynamic team from the facility. In some cases, it may be necessary to administer antipsychotic medication or sedation.

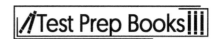

Anxiety and Panic

Anxiety and panic attacks are characterized by extreme, sudden, and often unpredictable feelings of paralyzing fear, nervousness, and discomfort. These situations are often debilitating for the individual experiencing them, with some reporting symptoms such as chest pain, the inability to breathe, and feeling a sense of impending death. Other common symptoms include overwhelming dizziness, nausea, sweating, trembling, accelerated heart rate, and feelings of "checking out" from reality. For a true medical diagnosis, four or more of these symptoms must be present. Typically, these episodes can last anywhere from 10 minutes to over an hour. Individuals who experience an anxiety or panic attack for the first time may be unfamiliar with the event, and it can warrant a trip to the emergency department. Consequently, it is important for nurses to know how to address these situations to help the patient to receive proper, adequate, and cost-efficient treatment in the future. It is important to show support and compassion toward the patient's feelings, even if the patient's fears seem irrational.

For recurrent anxiety and panic attacks, medication and/or psychotherapy is often needed to support the patient's quality of life. Selective serotonin reuptake inhibitors (SSRIs) are often prescribed to help manage anxiety symptoms. Brand names include Prozac®, Zoloft®, Paxil®, and Lexapro®.

Bipolar Disorder

Bipolar disorder is characterized by extremes in mood, energy, and function. The individual tends to experience manic periods, marked by highly energetic, almost frenzied behaviors and excitable moods, as well as depressive periods, marked by lethargy, sadness, and isolation. Clinically, manic periods must last at least a week and depressive periods at least two weeks for an individual to be diagnosed with bipolar disorder. Bipolar is a brain disorder that may be caused by physiological distinctions in the brain or genetics. It is often treated with mood-stabilizing medications in conjunction with psychotherapy. Common medications to manage symptoms of bipolar disorder include lithium and brand names such as Depakote®.

Due to the nature of the disorder, the extremes experienced by an individual with bipolar disorder can result in a trip to the emergency department. Individuals experiencing a manic period are at risk of engaging in impulsive behaviors such as drug abuse, violence, unsafe sexual encounters, and following through with suicidal thoughts. Individuals experiencing a depressive period are also at risk of having suicidal thoughts or tendencies due to a marked increase in feelings of hopelessness. Individuals with bipolar disorder can also experience periods of psychosis and have delusions or hallucinations. Nurses should be prepared to show sympathy and compassion while still being firm and direct with the patient. Patient behavior will likely be unpredictable, especially if he or she is in a manic phase. Nurses may need to use these interactions to deduce the risk factors a patient has for bipolar disorder so they can deliver effective treatment.

Depression

Depression is characterized by feelings of lethargy; hopelessness; an inability to derive pleasure from once pleasurable activities; problems with sleep, eating, and substances; and/or sexual dysfunction that lasts longer than two weeks. It can be caused by genetics, an imbalance of neurochemicals, or situational contexts. Depression often presents differently in men, women, children, and older adults. Men tend to exhibit increased anger and irritability, while women tend to feel sad, worthless, and guilty. Women tend to internalize symptoms and experience depression at a higher rate and frequency than men due to unique societal issues, hormonal changes, and other factors. Children present symptoms of depression through isolation, anxiety, or acting out. Older adults are more prone to hide symptoms of depression, attribute the feelings to another health problem, or be taken less seriously than other age demographics. It should be noted that these are generalizations and not hard rules.

Depression is usually managed through psychotherapy and sometimes medication. Common medications to treat depression include SSRIs, similar to those used to treat anxiety. Depression can also be treated with serotonin and norepinephrine reuptake inhibitors, such as the brand names Cymbalta® and Effexor®. When these options don't work, tricyclic antidepressants may be prescribed. These drugs tend to have more intense side effects, so they are usually not prescribed unless other options have been exhausted. Even with medication, some periods of depression can become so intense and unmanageable that they place the individual in a crisis or suicidal mode. In this context, emergency services are usually needed. It is important to show the depressed patient reassurance, comfort, and support, including directly asking the patient what would help comfort and support him or her during this time. Noting verbal and nonverbal communication will help determine if the patient is at risk for suicide and how severe that risk might be.

Homicidal Ideation

Homicidal ideation is characterized by recurrent thoughts of homicide and is an immediate cause for concern or emergency intervention. Homicidal ideation can consist of fleeting, ambiguous thoughts of homicide or long-term, detailed plans that are made with the intention of following through to completion. It often stems from another psychological disorder in which delusions or hallucinations may be present, such as bipolar disorder or schizophrenia. Other risk factors include a tendency toward violence or hostile behavior, victimization, and head injury; however, it is important to note that individuals who experience homicidal ideation can often be normal, otherwise healthy people who may be triggered by distress (e.g., betrayal). Consequently, it can be hard to detect and manage unless the individual makes direct comments about his or her homicidal thoughts or documents it in some other way (e.g., comments on social media, drawings, or journaling).

Psychosis

Psychosis is a broad term encompassing any mental condition in which the individual experiences thoughts or exhibits behaviors that indicate a detachment from reality. Psychosis can be its own diagnosis or a part of another mental health issue. It is often associated with schizophrenia, a cognitive disorder characterized by episodic hallucinations and delusions. Acute or short-term episodes of psychosis may be seen in patients diagnosed with bipolar disorder; episodes can also stem from drug abuse, especially in patients who have used methamphetamines, cocaine, or LSD.

Psychosis can be characterized by abnormal or awkward social behavior, indecipherable verbal communication or writing, catatonia, visual or auditory hallucinations, and/or extreme paranoia. Individuals experiencing psychotic episodes are often brought to the emergency department by concerned friends, family, or legal professionals, as they may pose a threat to themselves or others while detached from reality. It is important to rule out any concerns or influences of a physiological nature (such as head trauma or a brain tumor) before diagnosing the patient as having a psychotic episode. The patient should be approached gently and asked about the delusions in a neutral manner (without openly denying or accepting the patient's storyline), and all effort should be made to not excessively stimulate or frighten the patient.

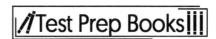

Situational Crises

A situational crisis refers to specific, often sudden and acute contexts that are not the norm in an individual's life, but are currently the source of extreme duress. Often, the situational crisis is something that is overwhelming to the point where the individual is unable to healthily cope. Events that can result in a situational crisis include major life changes such as sudden unemployment, divorce, death of a loved one, an unexpected but severe medical diagnosis, and an unanticipated relocation. It is important to note that, in these cases, the individual does not have a chronic mental illness but is experiencing a short-term episode that can result in panic attacks, depression, homicidal ideation, or suicidal tendencies (often for the first time in the individual's history).

If an individual comes to the emergency department when experiencing a situational crisis, he or she may be extremely agitated, angry, or anxious and present physical indicators of distress such as muscle pain, nausea, crying, and shortness of breath. Medical personnel should try to obtain as much information as possible about the patient's medical and mental health history and the events leading up to the clinical visit. They should appropriately assess the risk for violent or aggressive behavior, self-harm potential or the potential to harm others, risk for substance abuse, and impulsivity in behavior.

Suicidal Ideation

Suicidal ideation refers to having thought of suicide. It is often a component of another mental health diagnosis in an individual, such as depression. It can range from a spectrum of fleeting suicidal thoughts without a plan of action (also referred to as **passive suicidal ideation**) to suicidal thoughts with a plan of action (also referred to as **active suicidal ideation**). Suicidal ideation, like homicidal ideation, is an immediate cause for concern and emergency intervention. Risk factors for suicidal ideation include family history, above-average number of negative life experiences, chronically high levels of stress, inability to cope with or manage stressors, mental illness, guns in the home, domestic violence, and imprisonment. Men are more likely to experience suicidal ideation than women. Medical personnel should note patient symptoms associated with depression, comments made about death or dying, history of or visible marks from past suicide attempts, marks from self-harm, mood swings, extreme anxiety, and intense negative emotions. Suicide attempts that are not fatal can result in severe consequences, such as brain damage or falling into a long-term coma.

Medical

Medical emergencies include any instance of poor physical health, injury, or sickness that could result in long-term complications or fatality if not immediately mitigated.

Allergic Reactions and Anaphylaxis

An allergic reaction occurs when an individual's body responds negatively to a substance it has come in contact with, either through touch, consumption, or inhalation. The substance that causes an allergic reaction in an individual is referred to as an **allergen,** and the reaction occurs as a result of the individual's immune system treating the allergen as a threat. Since immune systems between individuals vary widely, the presence and severity of an allergic reaction—even to the same allergen—varies also. A potential allergen (e.g., a plant pollen or a peanut) may cause no response in one individual, cause a mild uncomfortable response in a second individual, and be life-threatening to a third individual.

Usually, allergic reactions happen relatively soon (immediately to within a few hours) after exposure to an allergen. Repeated exposure can eventually result in hypersensitivity to the allergen and produce more intense allergic reactions. Family history typically influences the presence and severity of allergies. Symptoms of a mild allergic reaction include rashes, itching, congestion, watery eyes, and other cold-like symptoms. Many mild allergic reactions can be treated by eliminating the presence of the allergen or taking anti-allergy medications.

More severe allergic reactions can include symptoms such as physical pain in the chest or stomach, diarrhea, skin swelling or redness, fainting, and trouble breathing deeply. The most severe allergic reactions occur almost instantly and can intensify to result in anaphylaxis, which is a medical emergency requiring immediate attention. Anaphylaxis comprises severe swelling of the tongue or throat (which can result in suffocation), vomiting, dizziness, or rashes. If anaphylaxis goes untreated, it can result in death. The most common treatment of anaphylaxis is an epinephrine injection, and many individuals who know they have a severe allergy carry an epinephrine injection pen (EpiPen®) with them.

Common allergens include nuts, shellfish, some fruits, eggs, dairy, gluten, a variety of pollen types, latex, animal dander and hair, and insect or reptilian venom. Some of these allergens, like food allergens, can be present from birth onward; others will develop later in life. Allergens such as bee venom or snake venom may remain unknown unless there is an attack.

Blood Dyscrasias

Blood dyscrasias broadly refer to disorders of the blood.

Hemophilia

Hemophilia is a hereditary blood disorder in which an individual's blood lacks proteins (specifically, clotting factors VIII or IX) that aid in clotting, resulting in wounds bleeding for a longer period of time. Hemophiliacs are not usually in danger if they have a small or superficial cut, but the risk of excessive bleeding with deeper cuts or internal wounds is especially critical. This can result in hemorrhage or damage to the internal organs. In addition to excessive bleeding in response to relatively normal situations such as minor surgery, symptoms of hemophilia include abnormal and frequent bruising, abnormal and frequent nosebleeds, joint pain, and blood in the urine or stool. Hemophiliac episodes that constitute a medical emergency include extreme swelling of large joints, prolonged headaches, chronic vomiting, neck pain, vision problems, major injuries, and lethargy. Hemophilia and associated emergencies are usually treated by manually replacing the insufficient clotting protein via drip or injection directly into the hemophiliac's vein.

Von Willebrand Disease

Von Willebrand disease is another type of genetic coagulopathy that affects how an individual's platelets stick to form a clot. This disease can range from very mild in nature to severe, as designated by the individual's bleeding tendency. Those on the mild end of the spectrum may show no symptoms or minor symptoms such as occasional bruising. Severe cases are rare but can result in heavy internal bleeding and hemorrhage. The majority of cases are treated proactively with intranasal and intravenous (IV) hormone therapies, typically administered before surgeries, childbirth, menstruation, or other instances where bleeding may be a concern.

Thrombocytopenia

Thrombocytopenia is a disease that causes individuals to have platelet counts significantly below normal healthy levels, usually without symptoms. But some individuals may experience increased nosebleeds,

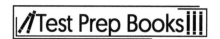

bleeding wounds, or bruising, and women may experience longer menstruation periods. Another obvious indicator of thrombocytopenia is the presence of visible blood-filled sacs in the mouth. This disease can be genetic but can also result from dehydration, malnutrition, the use of certain medications, liver failure, sepsis, Lyme disease, or snake bites. Treatment will vary among individuals by cause and may include steroid therapy.

Some diseases require the formation of clots to be slowed or decreased. For example, patients who have congenital heart disease or a lifestyle disease that requires any kind of heart surgery or who are at high risk of heart attack or stroke are often required to take anticoagulants. Anticoagulants thin the blood to decrease or prevent the formation of clots, which can obstruct other blood vessels and lead to a heart attack or travel to the brain and cause a stroke. The most common anticoagulants include the medications warfarin and heparin. These medications work by blocking the body's ability to adhere platelets together or by limiting the ability to produce clotting factors. The medications can be delivered orally (a slower release) or intravenously (more rapid results); the attending physician will usually decide what is best on an individual basis.

Anemia

Anemia is a nonhereditary blood disorder in which an individual's blood has a low number of red blood cells. Mild forms of anemia may have no symptoms or manageable symptoms such as tiredness. Severe forms of anemia can result in extreme fatigue, shortness of breath, or unconsciousness. Anemia can be caused by low iron levels as a result of poor diet, heavy menstrual cycles in women, or stomach and intestinal cancers. In these instances, low iron levels can typically be remedied with iron supplementation or dietary changes. Sometimes, iron-deficiency anemia will need to be treated with blood transfusions; however, this is quite rare. A type of anemia called pernicious anemia is caused by vitamin B-12 deficiencies. Other forms of anemia are caused by chronic diseases, especially diseases related to the kidney, disorders within the bone marrow (aplastic anemia), or autoimmune disorders (autoimmune hemolytic anemia). These situations usually require stronger medication, synthetic hormones, blood transfusions, and sometimes transplants to rectify the low red blood cell count.

Leukemia

Leukemia refers to any form of cancer of the blood cells. Different forms of leukemia are categorized by the blood cell type they affect and the rate at which they spread. Leukemia can affect lymphocytes, a type of white blood cell associated with the body's immune system, or myelocytes, a type of young blood cell found in the bone marrow. Leukemia can be categorized as acute, meaning that young blood cells are affected and likely will not mature to carry out their intended function. This form of leukemia tends to progress quickly. Leukemia can also be categorized as chronic, meaning that older blood cells are affected; however, these cells may still be able to carry out their intended function to some extent.

This form of leukemia tends to progress more slowly. The four most common types of leukemia take these two factors into consideration. They are acute lymphocytic leukemia (most common in young children), acute myeloid leukemia (affecting children and adults), chronic lymphocytic leukemia (most common in adults aged fifty-five years or older), and chronic myeloid leukemia (mostly found in adults). Symptoms of leukemia include unexplained bruising, weight loss, bleeding, and fevers. Most patients have to undergo chemotherapy; some may have to have bone marrow transplants. The immune system of most leukemia patients is compromised, so the risk of infection and complications from infections is high. Prognosis varies widely by individual diagnosis.

Sickle Cell Crisis

Sickle cell crisis is a complication of sickle cell disease, a type of genetic blood disorder that affects the functioning of hemoglobin throughout the lifespan. Normally functioning hemoglobin is physically flexible, therefore allowing the red blood cell to easily travel throughout arteries to deliver oxygen to tissues. In a person with sickle cell disease, the hemoglobin can become inflexible and distort the entire shape of the red blood cell into a crescent shape. This makes it difficult for the red blood cell to travel through smaller arteries.

A sickled red blood cell can get stuck in arteries, ultimately blocking oxygen from reaching tissues. When this occurs, it is referred to as a **sickle cell crisis**. It brings sudden and debilitating pain that can occur anywhere in the body, but tends to more commonly affect the limbs, torso, and chest. Most people cannot predict when they will experience a sickle cell crisis, but common triggers include stress, dehydration, sickness, and high altitudes. Most sickle cells end up bursting within ten to twenty days after being formed, and these episodes are generally managed with pain relievers and heat therapy. Sometimes IV fluids, a blood transfusion, or spleen surgery is needed; severe sickle cell crisis episodes can lead to organ damage.

Disseminated Intravascular Coagulation (DIC)

DIC is a nonhereditary disorder in which normal clotting and fibrinolysis processes become disrupted. The body fails to recognize when an adequate number of clots have been formed to stop a bleeding wound in or on the body and continues to create new clots without breaking them down. These extra clots can clog arteries and block blood supply to vital organs. They can also travel to the brain and cause strokes. It is also possible for the body to absorb the clots or to run out of resources (such as platelets or clotting factors) with which to create new clots. This can result in heavy (and sometimes spontaneous) internal bleeding—a risk that comes in addition to the risks presented by extra clots. People with DIC also run the risk of losing healthy red blood cells, as the presence of so many clots can cause red blood cells to rupture if the two come into contact with one another.

DIC may affect up to 1 percent of a hospitalized population. It does not occur spontaneously; it always follows the presence of another serious disease, injury, or systemic inflammation. It is most commonly seen in patients who have leukemia, pancreatitis, fungal or bacterial blood infections, or liver disease, or in patients who are suffering from burns or pregnancy complications or have recently had surgery. Symptoms include heavy bleeding from multiple wounds, blood clots, bruises, and sudden drops in blood pressure. Testing for DIC includes conducting a blood count with blood smear (to show platelet counts and state of the patient's red blood cells), partial prothrombin time test (which measures how long it takes for the patient's blood to clot), and a prothrombin time test (which measures how long it takes for the patient's plasma to clot). Fibrinogen counts may be tested; high counts can serve as another indicator of DIC. This test is not always a reliable indicator, as most patients' levels will be higher than normal due to the presence of disease or injury.

The presence of DIC usually makes the underlying disease riskier and the chances of death from the disease higher due to the occurrence of simultaneous clotting and heavy bleeding, which can be uncontrollable. The severity of DIC varies widely, as do treatment options. Generally, treatment remains focused primarily on treating the underlying disease or condition. Sometimes, blood transfusions are given to correct imbalanced platelet and clotting factor levels; this varies on a case-by-case basis. While thrombosis is often treated with heparin, patients with DIC are only given this anticoagulant if their risk of bleeding is low. Overall prognosis is usually poor once a DIC diagnosis has been made, as it can be

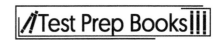

difficult to treat a system that is simultaneously producing extra clots and hemorrhaging. Up to half of all patients who have been diagnosed with DIC do not survive.

Electrolyte/Fluid Imbalance

Electrolytes are minerals that, when dissolved, break down into ions. They can be acids, bases, or salts. In the body, different electrolytes are responsible for specific cellular functions. These functions make up larger, critical system-wide processes, such as hydration, homeostasis, pH balance, and muscle contraction. Electrolytes typically enter the body through food and drink consumption, but in severe cases of imbalance, they may be medically-administered. They are found in the fluids of the body, such as blood.

Key electrolytes found in the body include the following:

Sodium and Chloride

Sodium (Na^+) is mainly responsible for managing hydration, blood pressure, and blood volume in the body. It is found in blood, plasma, and lymph. It is important to note that sodium is primarily found outside of cells and is accessed by a number of different systems and organs to tightly regulate water and blood levels. For example, in cases of severe dehydration, the circulatory and endocrine systems will transmit signals to the kidneys to retain sodium and, consequently, water.

Sodium also affects muscle and nerve function. It is a positively-charged ion and contributes to membrane potential—an electrochemical balance between sodium and potassium (another electrolyte) that is responsible for up to 40 percent of resting energy expenditure in a healthy adult. This balance strongly influences the function of nerve impulses and the ability of muscles to contract. Healthy heart function and contraction is dependent on membrane potential.

Sodium is available in large quantities in the standard diets of developed countries, especially in processed foods, as it is found in table salt. Consequently, sodium deficiencies (hyponatremia) are possible, but rare, in the average person. Hyponatremia can result in endocrine or nervous system disorders where sodium regulation is affected. It can also result in excessive sweating, vomiting, or diarrhea, such as in endurance sporting events, improper use of diuretics, or gastrointestinal illness. Hyponatremia may be treated with an IV sodium solution. Too much sodium (hypernatremia) is usually a result of dehydration. Hypernatremia may be treated by introducing water quantities appropriate for suspending the sodium level that is tested in the patient's blood and urine.

Chloride (Cl^-) is a negatively-charged ion found outside of the cells that works closely with sodium. It shares many of the same physiologic responsibilities as sodium. Any imbalances (hypochloremia and hyperchloremia) are rare but may affect overall pH levels of the body. Chloride imbalances usually occur in response to an imbalance in other electrolytes, so treating a chloride imbalance directly is uncommon.

Potassium

Potassium (K^+) is mainly responsible for regulating muscular function and is especially important in cardiac and digestive functions. In women, it is believed to promote bone density. It works in tandem with sodium to create membrane potential. Potassium is a positively-charged ion and is usually found inside cells. It plays a role in maintaining homeostasis between the intracellular and extracellular environments.

Potassium is found in all animal protein and animal dairy products and in most fruits and vegetables. Low potassium levels (hypokalemia) may be caused by dehydration due to excessive vomiting, urination, or diarrhea. In severe or acute cases, hypokalemia may be a result of renal dysfunction and may cause lethargy, muscle cramps, or heart dysrhythmia. It may be treated by stopping the cause of potassium loss (e.g., diuretics), followed by oral or IV potassium replenishment.

High potassium levels (hyperkalemia) can quickly become fatal. Hyperkalemia is often the result of a serious condition, such as sudden kidney or adrenal failure, and may cause nausea, vomiting, chest pain, and muscle dysfunction.

It is treated based on its severity, with treatment options ranging from diuretic use to IV insulin or glucose. IV calcium may be administered if potentially dangerous heart arrhythmias are present.

1.

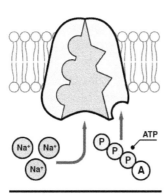

The sodium-potassium pump binds three sodium ions and a molecule of ATP.

2.

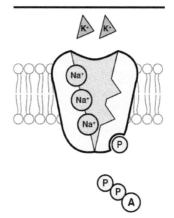

The splitting of ATP provides energy to change the shape of the channel. The sodium ions are driven through the channel.

3.

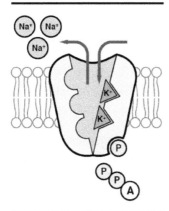

The sodium ions are released to the outside of the membrane, and the new shape of the channel allows two potassium ions to bind

4.

Release of the phosphate allows the channel to revert to its original form, releasing the potassium ions on the inside of the membrane

Calcium and Phosphorus

Calcium (Ca^{2+}) is plentiful in the body, with most calcium stored throughout the skeletal system. However, if there is not enough calcium in the blood (usually available through proper diet), the body will take calcium from the bones. This can become detrimental over time. If enough calcium becomes present in the blood, the body will return extra calcium stores to the bones. Besides contributing to the skeletal structure, this electrolyte is important in nerve signaling, muscle function, and blood coagulation. It is found in dairy products, leafy greens, and fatty fishes. Many other consumables, such as fruit juices and cereals, are often fortified with calcium.

Low calcium levels (hypocalcemia) can be caused by poor diet, thyroid or kidney disorders, and some medications. Symptoms can include lethargy, poor memory, inability to concentrate, muscle cramps, and general stiffness and achiness in the body. Supplementation can rapidly restore blood calcium levels. In cases where symptoms are present, IV calcium administration in conjunction with an oral or IV vitamin D supplement may be utilized.

High calcium levels (hypercalcemia) is usually caused by thyroid dysfunction but can also be the result of diet, limited mobility (such as in paralyzed individuals), some cancers, or the use of some diuretics. Symptoms can include thirst, excess urination, gastrointestinal issues, and unexplained pain in the abdominal area or bones. Severe or untreated hypercalcemia can result in kidney stones, kidney failure, confusion, depression, lethargy, irregular heartbeat, or bone problems.

There is an intricate balance between calcium levels and the levels of phosphorus, another electrolyte. Phosphorus, like calcium, is stored in the bones and found in many of the same foods as calcium. These electrolytes work together to maintain bone integrity. When too much calcium exists in the blood, the bones release more phosphorus to balance the two levels. When there is too much phosphorus in the blood, the bones release calcium. Therefore, the presence or absence of one directly impacts the presence or absence of the other. Indicators of hypocalcemia and hypercalcemia usually also indicate low levels of phosphorus (hypophosphatemia) and high levels of phosphorus (hyperphosphatemia), respectively.

Magnesium

Magnesium (Mg^{2+}) is another electrolyte that is usually plentiful in the body. It is responsible for an array of life-sustaining functions, including hundreds of biochemical reactions such as oxidative phosphorylation and glycolysis. It is also an important factor in DNA and RNA synthesis, bone development, nerve signaling, and muscle function. Magnesium is stored inside cells or within the structure of the bones. It can be consumed through leafy greens, nuts, seeds, beans, unrefined grains, and most foods that contain fiber. Some water sources may also contain high levels of magnesium.

Low levels of magnesium (hypomagnesemia) are primarily caused by chronic alcohol or drug abuse and some prescription medications and can also occur in patients with gastrointestinal diseases (such as celiac or Crohn's). Symptoms of hypomagnesemia include nausea, vomiting, depression, personality and mood disorders, and muscle dysfunction. Chronically depleted patients may have an increased risk of cardiovascular and metabolic disorders.

High levels of magnesium (hypermagnesemia) are rare and usually result in conjunction with kidney disorders when medications are used improperly. Symptoms include low blood pressure that may result in heart failure. Hypermagnesemia is usually treated by removing any magnesium sources (such as salts or laxatives) and may also require the IV administration of calcium gluconate.

Magnesium imbalance can lead to calcium or potassium imbalance over time, as these electrolytes work together in achieve homeostasis in the body.

Hydration is critical to fluid presence in the body, as water is a critical component of blood, plasma, and lymph. When fluid levels are too high or too low, electrolytes cannot move freely or carry out their intended functions. Therefore, treating an electrolyte imbalance almost always involves managing a

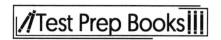

fluid imbalance as well. Typically, as fluid levels rise, electrolyte levels decrease. As fluid levels decrease, electrolyte levels rise. Common tests to determine electrolyte fluid imbalances include basic and comprehensive metabolic panels, which test levels of sodium, potassium, chloride, and any other electrolyte in question.

Endocrine Conditions

The endocrine system is responsible for hormone production and messaging. These hormones are produced by glands through the brain and body. They regulate a vast number of mental, emotional, and physiological functions, such as mood, growth, metabolism, sleep, sexual function, and reproduction. Consequently, some pathological conditions can have system-wide repercussions.

Adrenal Conditions

Located on top of each kidney, the adrenal glands are responsible for producing a number of hormones. These include sex hormones, such as DHEA and androstenedione; corticosteroids, such as cortisol; and mineralocorticoids, such as aldosterone. These hormones influence sexual function, metabolism, electrolyte balance, blood volume, blood pressure, immunity, and stress management. Dysfunctional conditions of the adrenal glands include the following:

Cushing's Syndrome

This disease results from an excess of glucocorticoid, which is responsible for producing steroids that manage inflammation and other stresses in the body. One example of a glucocorticoid is cortisol. Symptoms of Cushing's syndrome include excessive weight gain that cannot be managed, excessive growth of body hair, high blood pressure, and decreased elasticity in the skin. This disease is typically treated with medication that controls hormone production. In severe cases, adrenal surgery may be required.

Addison's Disease

This disease may be referred to as **adrenal insufficiency**. It results when the adrenal glands produce insufficient amounts of glucocorticoids and mineralocorticoids. Mineralocorticoids are another group of steroids influencing electrolyte and fluid balance. This can be the result of an underlying autoimmune disorder or systemic infection. Symptoms include fatigue and skin discoloration. Addison's disease is usually treated with steroid injections but may become a medical crisis if the patient goes into shock, a stupor, or a coma. This can occur if the patient does not realize he or she has the disease, as some of the primary symptoms can be quite generic.

Conn's Syndrome

This disease is characterized by excess aldosterone production. Symptoms include hypertension, muscle cramping, weakness, dehydration, and excessive thirst. It is usually treated by surgically removing any tumors on the adrenal glands, and the patient may be asked to minimize table salt consumption. If Conn's syndrome goes untreated, it can result in serious cardiovascular and kidney disease.

Adrenal Tumors

The presence of malignant or benign tumors on the adrenal glands may affect hormone production, which can cause one of the above disorders to develop.

Glucose-Related Conditions

The endocrine system handles processes related to the metabolism of glucose.

Disorders relating to glucose include the following:

Diabetes Mellitus

This is a condition that affects how the body responds to the presence of glucose. Glucose is needed for cellular functions, and all consumable calories eventually are converted to glucose in the body. A hormone produced by the pancreas, called **insulin,** is needed to break down food and drink into glucose molecules. In patients with type 1 diabetes, the pancreas fails to produce insulin, leading to high levels of glucose in the bloodstream. This can lead to organ damage, organ failure, or nerve damage. Patients with type 1 diabetes receive daily insulin injections or have a pump that continuously monitors their blood insulin levels and releases insulin as needed. These patients need to be careful to not administer excess insulin, as this will cause their blood sugar to become too low. Low blood sugar can lead to fainting and exhaustion and may require hospitalization.

In patients with type 2 diabetes, the pancreas produces insulin, but the body is unable to use it effectively. Patients with type 2 diabetes typically need to manage their condition through lifestyle changes, such as losing weight and eating fewer carbohydrate-rich and sugary foods. There are also some medications that help the body use the insulin that is present in the bloodstream. Gestational diabetes is a form of diabetes that some women develop during the second to third trimester of pregnancy, when their systems temporarily become resistant to insulin. High blood sugar in a pregnant woman can affect fetal growth and influence the baby's risk of becoming obese. Pregnant women with gestational diabetes are encouraged to exercise daily, avoid excessive weight gain, and carefully monitor their diet. Gestational diabetes is similar to type 2 diabetes in the way symptoms present and in treatment options.

Diabetic Ketoacidosis

This is an acute complication that primarily occurs in patients with type 1 diabetes who lack adequate insulin. When the body does not have enough insulin in the blood to break down macronutrients into glucose, it defaults to breaking down fatty acids into ketones for energy. This typically does not cause major issues in a person who does not have diabetes, as eventual insulin production and uptake will balance the level of ketones in the blood. In a patient with diabetes who cannot produce enough insulin, the body will continue to release fatty acids into the bloodstream. Eventually, this will result in too many ketones in the blood and will shift the body's pH level to an excessively acidic one. This is a crisis situation, and the patient may eventually go into a coma if left untreated. Symptoms include dehydration, nausea, sweet-smelling breath, confusion, and fatigue. Treatment includes oral or IV electrolyte and insulin administration. Diabetic ketoacidosis can occur with type 2 diabetes but occurs more frequently with type 1 diabetes. Often, a ketoacidosis event is the first indicator that a person may have diabetes.

Glycogenoses

Glycogenoses refer to a number of hereditary disorders in which the body is unable to convert stored glycogen to glucose when glucose is needed by the body. This inability is the result of the absence of an enzyme, although the specific enzyme that is missing can vary from patient to patient. Symptoms include failure to thrive (in infants), growth and development issues, kidney stones, confusion, and general weakness. More severe cases can result in chronic gout, seizures, coma, intestinal sores, and kidney failure. These disorders are usually treated by timing carbohydrate consumption so that blood sugar levels remain stable throughout the day.

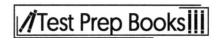

Metabolic Syndrome/Syndrome X

Metabolic syndrome, or *Syndrome X,* refers to the presence of comorbid cardiovascular and insulin-related conditions. Patients diagnosed with metabolic syndrome must have three or more of the following conditions: hypertension, elevated fasting blood glucose levels, low HDL cholesterol, high triglycerides, and excess belly fat. This syndrome is believed to result from insulin resistance, causing high blood glucose, insulin, and lipid levels. Patients with metabolic syndrome tend to be overweight or obese and at an increased risk of organ failure, heart attacks, and strokes. They often suffer from another underlying condition, such as diabetes or polycystic ovary syndrome, that leads to metabolic syndrome. Metabolic syndrome is often treated with prescription medications that lower cholesterol and blood pressure, but diet and exercise changes are strongly recommended. Weight loss is a key component in managing metabolic syndrome.

Thyroid Conditions

Located at the front of the throat, the thyroid is one of the most influential glands in the endocrine system. The hormones it produces are involved in a multitude of functions throughout the body, including an assortment of metabolic, muscle, and digestive functions. Thyroid hormones also play a key role in neurological processes. When thyroid conditions develop, they can cause systemic effects. Testing for thyroid conditions goes beyond simply testing thyroid hormone levels. It can also include a physical exam, blood tests to determine how much thyroid-stimulating hormone (TSH) is being produced by the pituitary gland, tests to determine blood antibody levels, ultrasounds to check for tumors, and uptake tests to determine the rate at which the thyroid uses iodine.

Hyperthyroidism

When patients are diagnosed with hyperthyroidism, they may also be referred to as having an **overactive thyroid**, which results in the overproduction of T4 and/or T3 hormones. Symptoms include feelings of anxiety, trouble focusing, feeling overheated, gastrointestinal problems such as diarrhea, insomnia, elevated heart rate, and unexplained weight loss. Hyperthyroidism is commonly caused by Grave's disease, an autoimmune disorder. The extent to which symptoms of Grave's disease manifest can be broad, depending on the severity of the disease. Family history, stress, smoking, and pregnancy can increase the risk of developing Grave's disease. Women under the age of forty are most likely to be diagnosed.

Medical treatment options can include methimazole and propylthiouracil, two common antithyroid medications. Prescription corticosteroids may also be used. In nonpregnant patients, radioactive iodine may be used. This is a long-term, repeat-dose solution that can sometimes result in hypothyroidism, which can be easier to treat. In serious cases, some or all of the thyroid may be removed, although this also usually results in hypothyroidism. It is also recommended that most patients with Grave's disease modify their lifestyle to limit stress, eat a healthy diet, and exercise regularly.

Hypothyroidism

When patients are diagnosed with hypothyroidism, they may also be referred to as having an underactive thyroid, which results in the underproduction of T4 and/or T3 hormones. Symptoms include depression, excessive fatigue, chills, dry skin, lowered heart rate, gastrointestinal problems such as constipation, and unexplained weight gain. Hypothyroidism is commonly caused by Hashimoto's disease, another autoimmune disease that affects thyroid function. This disease is usually treated with synthetic thyroid hormone replacement therapy, which involves taking a daily dose of the T4 hormone. T3 supplementation is rare, as it is derived from T4. Hypothyroidism can also be caused by the presence of too much iodine. The thyroid uses iodine to make T4 and T3 hormones. If there is too much iodine in the blood, the pituitary gland releases less TSH. The low levels of TSH can later result in the thyroid not producing enough T4 and/or T3 hormones. In some cases of hypothyroidism, surgery is required.

Goiter

A goiter refers to any enlargement in the thyroid gland. Goiters can occur in healthy thyroids or in thyroids producing abnormal levels of hormones. Their presence can indicate a lack of iodine, an autoimmune disease, an injury, or cancer.

Thyroid Cancer

Thyroid cancer is rare but can result in goiters and thyroid dysfunction. Thyroid cancer is more common in people who have nodes or goiters already present on the thyroid, which later turn malignant. The disease is also more prevalent in people who have been exposed to radiation. Thyroid cancer is usually treated through surgery, and thyroid hormone replacement therapy is a part of follow-up treatment.

Fever

Normal body temperature averages around 98.6 degrees Fahrenheit. A fever is an increase in body temperature. It is often the first indicator that the body is fighting an infection or injury, as most bacteria and viruses cannot survive high temperatures. Mild fevers can be treated with over-the-counter pain and fever relievers, such as ibuprofen or acetaminophen. Increased risks for more serious fevers include hospitalization, surgery, travel to high-risk countries, a suppressed immune system, drug abuse, and some medications. These are risk factors due to the increase in exposure to viruses and bacteria that can cause a fever. Usually, individual risk factors will be assessed as a part of the intake process (where personal, demographic, medical, and insurance history are usually retrieved) when the patient is admitted.

Infants, Toddlers, and Children

Fevers in infant and young children are managed differently than fevers in adults. In infants under two months of age, fevers can indicate a systemic infection or hereditary disease. Fevers in this age group can result in irritability, colic, vomiting, and refusal to feed; consequently, this can result in a failure to thrive. Skin changes, such as rashes, may also present in many feverish newborns. Older infants often show similar symptoms. In older infants and toddlers, it is important to know their vaccination schedule and any medications given. Vital signs should be recorded. Any important details from birth, such as delivery method and documented concerns, will be factored into the diagnostic process. Administering tests for herpes simplex viruses, urinary tract infections, **Streptococcus** bacteria, and blood abnormalities are often the first diagnostic steps.

Fevers are a common reason for emergency department visits. High fevers can cause rashes, neck pain, hallucinations, extreme lethargy, abdominal pain, and headaches. In young children, febrile seizures can occur if the fever reaches higher than 100.4 degrees Fahrenheit. These types of seizures usually do not cause long-term harm but can be traumatic for caregivers. In children, especially very young children, even moderate fevers may be a cause for concern. They can be the initial indicators of the following serious diseases:

Familial Mediterranean Fever

This is a hereditary fever disease that results in recurrent fever events with pain and swelling in the abdomen, chest, and joints. It is most commonly seen in people of Mediterranean and Middle Eastern origins and usually presents before the age of ten. This condition is not contagious. Fever events can last up to four days but may change in frequency and duration over time. However, some events can be

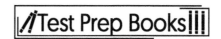

debilitating to the point of long-term damage, especially if this syndrome is misdiagnosed. This disease can often be misdiagnosed as appendicitis, arthritis, an infection, or a strained joint or muscle. It cannot be cured but can be managed well with colchicine. By adulthood, the episodes that most patients experience are far less severe and frequent.

Hyperimmunoglobulin D Syndrome

This is a rare, hereditary fever disease that results from high immunoglobulin type D proteins. It is characterized by recurrent, painful fevers that occur alongside skin rashes, swollen lymph nodes, and gastrointestinal distress. Fevers begin soon after birth, and episodes can last up to two weeks. The fever is not contagious, but symptoms are similar to that of the flu, so it is often misdiagnosed. While the fever tends to decrease in severity and frequency as the patient ages, there are no cures or episode prevention options. This disease is most commonly seen in people of French and Dutch origin but can be present in anyone.

Measles

This is a highly contagious viral disease, characterized by high fever (up to 104 degrees Fahrenheit) and flu-like symptoms. Its most commonly recognized characteristic—a full-body, red rash—occurs a few days after the onset of fever. Though most people in the United States are vaccinated, a recent surge in parents choosing to not vaccinate or delay vaccinations in their children has affected the benefits of herd immunity in some areas. Most children cannot receive their first dose of the measles vaccination until one year of age, so infants can be highly vulnerable in cases of measles outbreaks. An unvaccinated person has a 90 percent chance of contracting measles if he or she comes into contact with the virus. The disease can take up to ten days to present symptoms. An antibody treatment is available for unvaccinated people who have been exposed to measles. It may lessen the severity of the outbreak or prevent an outbreak from occurring. Otherwise, the fever and rash gradually subside over one to two weeks, although more serious complications—such as blindness and meningitis—may occur. The person should remain at home for at least twenty-one days after symptoms appear.

Neonatal-Onset Multisystem Inflammatory Disease

This is a rare, hereditary fever disease that presents at birth or almost immediately after. In addition to fever, classic symptoms include rash, chronic meningitis, and impaired hearing and vision. As the patient grows, joint abnormalities may present and result in stunted growth. There are no long-term treatment options, although anti-inflammatory and steroidal drugs may be given in the short term to manage symptoms. Prognosis and overall quality of life are poor.

Varicella

This is a highly contagious viral disease, more commonly known as **chicken pox**. It is characterized by high fever (up to 102 degrees Fahrenheit), fatigue, and an itchy rash. The rash begins as raised pink papules that turn into blisters. The blisters eventually burst and scab. A person with varicella is contagious from two to three days before the rash appears, until all scabs have healed. In high-risk patients, such as newborns, infants, the immunocompromised, or pregnant women who have not been vaccinated, complications may result, including sepsis, meningitis, Reye's syndrome, and toxic shock syndrome. Finally, people who have chicken pox as children are susceptible to shingles as adults. In the United States, the first dose of the varicella vaccination is typically administered around twelve to eighteen months of age.

Adults

In adults, a temperature over 100.4 degrees Fahrenheit is considered high. A fever over 103 degrees Fahrenheit is cause for immediate medical attention, as it can be associated with seizures, comas, breathing problems, confusion, bodily pain, swelling, and inflammation. A high fever with other telltale symptoms may indicate a serious condition. A high fever with brown phlegm is indicative of pneumonia. A high fever with abdominal pain can be indicative of appendicitis. A high fever with neck or head pain, nausea, vision distortion, or light sensitivity is indicative of brain inflammation or infection. Populations particularly vulnerable to fevers include older adults (over sixty-five years of age), pregnant women, and immunocompromised adults.

Immunocompromised Patients

An immunocompromised person refers to any individual who has a less than optimally functioning immune system. This could be the result of a genetic disorder, a viral or cancerous disease, medication, injury, surgery, age, or nutrition. An immunocompromised person is more susceptible to infection and illness than someone whose immune system is functioning optimally.

HIV/AIDS

The human immunodeficiency virus (HIV) is a sphere-shaped virus that is a fraction of the size of a red blood cell. There are primarily two types of HIV: HIV-1 and HIV-2. HIV-2 is not highly transmissible and is poorly understood. It has mainly affected people in West Africa. HIV-1 is more severe and more highly transmissible. It is the dominant strain among global HIV cases, and when literature and media refer to HIV, this is usually the type that is being referred to.

HIV is highly contagious. It is found in human bodily fluids and can be transmitted through infected breast milk, blood, mucus, and sexual fluids. The most common forms of transmission are through anal or vaginal sex, but transmission can also occur through contaminated syringe use, blood transfusions, or any other method where membranes are compromised. Once in the body, HIV attacks and destroys CD4/T cells. These cells are responsible for attacking foreign bodies (e.g., bacteria, infections, other viruses). As the body's CD4/T-cell count diminishes, the patient is left immunocompromised.

The HIV-1 type can be broken further into four groups: M, N, O, and P. M is the most commonly seen group globally. Within group M, there are ten different subtypes of HIV. These are noted as A, B, C, D, E, F, G, H, J, and K. Subtype B is prevalent in the Western world, and most research has been conducted on this subtype. This research has led to the manufacturing of antiretroviral (ARV) drugs. Antiretroviral therapy (ART) has been a major breakthrough in the management of HIV and in the quality of life for patients with HIV. In conjunction with medical care, many patients with HIV are able to have completely normal, healthy, active lives. It is important to treat HIV as early as possible. The better a patient's HIV is managed, the lower his or her viral load. Viral load refers to how much HIV is present in a patient's blood; when a viral load is low, transmission of the disease is far less likely to occur. With ART, many patients with HIV are viral-suppressed, and some even have an undetectable viral load. Viral load in other transmitting fluids, such as semen, cannot be detected but the virus is still present. Therefore, transmission is still possible, and all precautions should be taken.

Globally, most HIV patients have subtype C, but subtypes are mixing as travel and migration become more widespread. Most subtypes can be treated with ART, though these drugs were researched and manufactured to treat subtype B. However, ART is not always physically available or financially accessible in countries that need it most.

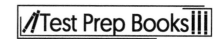

Without early intervention or adequate managed care of HIV, the virus can deteriorate the host body's immune system to a point where it cannot be rehabilitated. This stage is marked by extremely low levels of CD4/T cells (less than two hundred cells per cubic millimeter of blood) and is referred to as **acquired immunodeficiency syndrome** (AIDS). When a patient's HIV diagnosis progresses to AIDS, he or she often succumbs to serious chronic diseases, such as cancer. Mild illnesses, such as a cold or flu, can also be fatal to someone with AIDS. Not everyone who is diagnosed with HIV will also be diagnosed with AIDS. Once diagnosed with AIDS, the patient has approximately one to three years to live unless he or she receives adequate treatment.

Patients Receiving Chemotherapy

Chemotherapy is a broad term referring to the use of drugs in cancer treatment. This type of therapy is intended to target and treat the entire body, especially in advanced stages of cancer where malignant cells may be widespread. However, it may also be used in earlier stages of cancer to eliminate many of the cancerous cells. This is done with the intention that the patient will go into remission and potentially not experience cancer again in the future. If this does not seem like a viable prognosis, chemotherapy can be used to control early stages of cancer from advancing. In advanced stages of cancer, chemotherapy can be used to manage pain and suffering from cancerous tumors, even if the patient's prognosis is poor.

The aggressiveness of chemotherapy (such as which drugs are used, dosing amount, and frequency) is contingent on many factors, such as the type and stage of cancer. Chemotherapy treatment plans also consider the patient's personal and medical history. Since this form of treatment is so aggressive, it is often effective in reducing or eliminating cancer cells. However, chemotherapy can also kill healthy cells in the process. The intensity of this side effect varies by person, but almost all patients experience some degree of immunocompromise. This is because chemotherapy almost always inadvertently targets bone marrow, where white blood cells are made. White blood cells, especially neutrophils, play an important role in fighting infection. When there are not enough white blood cells present in the patient's blood, he or she can become seriously ill from sickness or infection that would be mild in a healthy person.

Medical personnel usually monitor neutrophil counts during and between chemotherapy cycles to make sure these levels do not fall too low. Chemotherapy cycles can last up to six months, and patients are considered to have a compromised immune system for the entire time they are undergoing chemotherapy. Once a full cycle of chemotherapy ends, it takes approximately one month for the immune system to return to its normal state.

Patients undergoing chemotherapy should be especially mindful of personal hygiene habits such as handwashing and showering, as well as avoiding cuts, scrapes, insect bites, or other instances where the skin may break. They may also need help taking care of a pet and handling pet waste or other trash. Additionally, it is important to practice extra caution when handling foods, such as cooking meats well, avoiding unpasteurized foods, washing produce with produce cleaner, cooking many foods that typically could be eaten raw, and avoiding certain moldy cheeses. They also need to be more careful of their surroundings in public places; since these areas tend to be dirtier and more populated, there is an increased risk of contracting infections. Medical personnel and those visiting the patient should be aware of these practices as well.

Renal Failure

Renal failure is also known as **kidney failure**. The kidneys are a pair of organs located in the posterior portion of the abdomen. They filter the blood for waste that later leaves the body in urine. The kidneys are also influenced by antidiuretic hormone, which signals when the kidneys should retain water. Consequently, the kidneys play an important role in electrolyte balance and hydration.

Renal failure is usually a gradual process; often, it is the last stage of chronic, progressive renal disease. However, renal failure can also be sudden. This is referred to as **acute kidney injury** and usually results from sudden trauma to the kidneys. Acute kidney injury is often caused by drug overdose, lengthy surgeries, heart attack, or crush syndrome. Chronic kidney disease is often the result of poorly managed diabetes over time, poorly managed high blood pressure over time, or overusing over-the-counter pain and fever reducers. Acute kidney injury is typically treatable, although patients live with an increased risk of kidney failure for the rest of their lives. Patients may also experience permanently decreased kidney function. However, many patients do go on to enjoy a normal quality of life after an acute kidney injury.

Renal failure that results from chronic kidney disease is not treatable, but managed based on the progression of disease. Stage 1 kidney disease shows few symptoms. Stage 5 kidney disease requires dialysis and may result in the need for a kidney transplant. During the progression of these five stages, lifestyle changes are usually incorporated alongside medical interventions to manage symptoms and hinder disease progression. These changes usually include dietary modifications, such as decreasing red meat and sugar intake, along with smoking cessation and increasing exercise frequency and duration. These changes decrease the strain on the body's cardiovascular system, and therefore ease the process of blood filtration for the kidneys.

Renal failure results in the body's inability to filter waste and balance fluids and electrolytes. Symptoms include nausea, swelling of the extremities and abdomen, cramping, decreased urine output, blood or excess protein in the urine, excess waste products in the blood, acidic blood pH levels, and elevated or low electrolyte levels. Testing includes checking blood creatinine and urea levels and may also include comprehensive metabolic panels.

Sepsis and Septic Shock

Sepsis is a serious condition in which the body has an out-of-control response to a wound, infection, or illness. It can progress through three stages of severity, with septic shock being the most life-threatening stage. It always accompanies the presence of an underlying condition, including pneumonia, kidney infections, and blood infections. The frequency of cases has been rising in the United States; this increase is attributed to aging populations, antibiotic resistance, increased chronic illness rates, and increased reporting of sepsis cases.

Sepsis refers to the first stage. It is characterized by a high fever, extreme pain, sleepiness, an accelerated heart rate, and/or rapid breathing. If other serious physiological symptoms are also present, such as low platelet count, low urine output, or mental confusion, the patient diagnosis shifts to severe sepsis—the second stage. If the patient also has low blood pressure that doesn't respond to treatment, the diagnosis is septic shock.

It is important to administer treatment as soon as possible to keep a sepsis diagnosis from progressing through these three stages. The first line of intervention usually includes antibiotics and IV fluid administration. In more severe cases, surgery to remove affected tissues may be necessary to prevent septic shock. Once a patient goes into septic shock, he or she may experience organ failure. Half of all septic shock cases are fatal. Prognosis after treatment for mild and severe sepsis varies. With early and adequate treatment, most people who experience mild sepsis return to their normal quality of life.

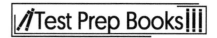

However, immunocompromised patients or patients who have other health problems may quickly progress to severe sepsis status or go into septic shock. They may require surgical amputation if gangrene sets in or if all the tissues in an extremity die, experience irreparable organ damage, or suffer from other long-term complications. Even in the event of a full recovery, most of these patients remain with an increased risk of another sepsis episode in the future.

Practice Questions

1. Which of the following are vulnerable populations at high risk of being abuse and neglect victims?
   a. Dogs, fish, and gerbils
   b. Immigrants, women, and minority races
   c. Children, women, and the elderly
   d. Children, pets, and immigrants

2. Mary is a seven-year-old in second grade. She has been absent from school nine days in one month. When Mary's teacher asks her why she has been absent or contacts her parents to ask about the absences, they all simply say she was sick and don't provide any additional information. Mary looks extremely frightened when asked about her absences. She regularly comes to school in large, baggy clothing that smells unpleasantly, and her hair always looks dirty. She falls asleep often in class, and one day her teacher saw her crying as she prepared to leave for home. Mary's teacher is probably concerned that Mary is dealing with which of the following issues?
   a. She is suffering from a hormonal imbalance or disorder.
   b. She is too emotional.
   c. She is hungry.
   d. She is being abused or neglected by a caregiver.

3. Which of the following options correctly names the type of common medication used to treat anxiety and depression?
   a. Antipsychotics
   b. Selective serotonin reuptake inhibitors (SSRIs)
   c. Norepinephrine reuptake inhibitors
   d. Homeopathic options

4. Psychosis is a common side effect of which of the following?
   I. Schizophrenia
   II. Methamphetamine, cocaine, or LSD use
   III. Bipolar Disorder
   IV. HIV antiviral medications

   a. Choices II and IV
   b. Choices I and II
   c. Choices I, II, and III
   d. All of the above

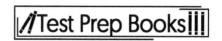

5. Jack and Jill are two nursing students who are on rotation in their county's emergency department. One afternoon, a woman comes into the waiting area and collapses on the floor. She says she cannot breathe and rambles about feeling blindsided. She begins thrashing on the floor and starts to sob. Upon reviewing her intake forms, Jack and Jill notice that the woman's health insurance shows she is employed, and she has not had any notable medical or mental health issues. However, she keeps mentioning that her partner has left her. Jack says, "I think she must have an undiagnosed anxiety disorder; we should look into medication options." Jill disagrees with him, saying that this seems more like which of the following?

    a. A situational crisis

    b. A case of cocaine abuse

    c. A case of intimate partner violence

    d. A nonemergency situation that they should send to the scheduling department

6. Which of the following statements is correct?

    a. Self-destructive ideation is characterized by thoughts of harming oneself, while global destruction ideation is characterized by thoughts of harming others.

    b. Suicidal ideation is characterized by thoughts of harming oneself, while homicidal ideation is characterized by thoughts of harming others.

    c. Internal ideation is characterized by thoughts of harming oneself, while external ideation is characterized by thoughts of harming others.

    d. Intrinsic ideation is characterized by thoughts of harming oneself, while extrinsic ideation is characterized by thoughts of harming others.

7. Middle school student Johnny stores an epinephrine injection pen in his locker, lunch bag, and pencil case. Johnny likely suffers from which of the following?

    a. Homicidal ideation

    b. Narcolepsy

    c. Depression

    d. A severe allergy

8. Which of the following is a commonly used anticoagulant that works by blocking the body's ability to adhere platelets together?

    a. Paxil

    b. Coumadin

    c. Heparin

    d. Thromblok

9. Which of the following is a commonly used anticoagulant that works by limiting the body's ability to produce clotting factors?

    a. Paxil

    b. Warfarin

    c. Heparin

    d. Thromblok

10. Which form of leukemia is most common in young children?

    a. Acute lymphocytic leukemia

    b. Acute myeloid leukemia

    c. Chronic lymphocytic leukemia

    d. Chronic myeloid leukemia

11. Which form of leukemia is most common in adults aged 55 years or older?
    a. Acute lymphocytic leukemia
    b. Acute myeloid leukemia
    c. Chronic lymphocytic leukemia
    d. Chronic myeloid leukemia

12. Billie is a 20-year-old college student who faints in the campus recreation center weight room while exercising. She is rushed to health services where she regains consciousness, but the medical personnel order blood and urine tests. Billie's blood tests show iron levels of about 10 grams of hemoglobin per deciliter. Her urine is darker and a bit bloody. Billie shares that she has had very heavy and long menstrual cycles lately. Billie is suffering from which of the following?
    a. Iron-deficiency anemia
    b. Anabolic steroid use
    c. Polycystic ovary syndrome
    d. An eating disorder

13. Which of the following statements is true?
    a. As fluid levels decrease, electrolyte levels increase.
    b. As fluid levels increase, electrolyte levels increase.
    c. As fluid levels osmose, electrolyte levels diffuse.
    d. As fluid levels homogenize, electrolyte levels dissipate.

14. What are two sex hormones produced by the adrenal glands that play an important role in reproductive processes?
    a. Cortisol and follicle-stimulating hormone
    b. DHEA and androstenedione
    c. Aldosterone and sodium
    d. Ovary hormone and vas deferens hormone

15. Maya eats a nutrient-rich, balanced diet and exercises vigorously for 30 minutes each day. However, she has gained almost 25 pounds over the course of four months. She has also started growing patches of facial hair. She visits her primary care physician seeking insight as to why these issues are suddenly occurring. He takes her blood pressure as they are talking and finds it to be 130/85. Maya's physician refers her to an endocrinologist, believing she is showing signs of which of the following?
    a. Bulimia nervosa
    b. Gestational diabetes
    c. Chronic kidney disease
    d. Cushing's syndrome

16. Which of the following statements about diabetes is correct?
    a. Type 2 diabetes mellitus is diagnosed based on the pancreas's inability to produce insulin.
    b. Gestational diabetes mellitus is diagnosed based on the mother's inability to produce glucose.
    c. Type 3 diabetes mellitus is diagnosed based on the pancreas's inability to produce insulin.
    d. Type 1 diabetes mellitus is diagnosed based on the pancreas's inability to produce insulin.

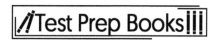

17. Patients with type 2 diabetes can manage their symptoms with which of the following?
    a. An insulin pump and finger prick testing strips
    b. Steroid injections and stevia sugar substitutes
    c. A regular yoga practice
    d. Lifestyle changes and metformin

18. Which of the following statements about thyroid conditions is correct?
    a. T4 deficiency is an example of a hyperthyroidism disease, while T3 deficiency is an example of a hypothyroidism disease.
    b. Grave's disease is an example of a hyperthyroidism disease, while Hashimoto's disease is an example of a hypothyroidism disease.
    c. Goiter is an example of a hyperthyroidism disease, while gout is an example of a hypothyroidism disease.
    d. Cancer is an example of a hyperthyroidism disease, while gestational diabetes is an example of a hypothyroidism disease.

19. Characterized by high fevers and a full body rash, which of the following types of cases has been on the rise in the United States recently, due to more people choosing to delay or avoid childhood immunizations?
    a. Measles
    b. Varicella
    c. Chicken pox
    d. Familial Mediterranean fever

20. Pregnant women, infants, patients with cancer, and patients with HIV are all considered which of the following?
    a. Handicapped
    b. Immunocompromised
    c. A burden on the health care system
    d. At high risk of experiencing disseminated intravascular coagulation

21. Which of the following statements is correct?
    a. The sodium-potassium pump is responsible for membrane potential.
    b. The calcium-phosphorus balance is responsible for membrane potential.
    c. The sodium chloride molecule is responsible for hormone production.
    d. The magnesium channel is responsible for regular waste excretion.

22. Diabetic ketoacidosis is an acute complication that occurs primarily in patients who have which of the following?
    a. Type 1 diabetes
    b. Type 2 diabetes
    c. Gestational diabetes
    d. A primarily ketogenic diet

23. Immunocompromised patients should do which of the following?
    I. Always practice extraordinary personal hygiene and handwashing habits
    II. Avoid eating moldy cheeses, such as blue cheese
    III. Only drink bottled water
    IV. Ask for help with caring for pets and taking out trash

   a. Choices I and IV
   b. Choices I, II, and III
   c. Choices I, II, and IV
   d. All of the above

24. Stage 5 of chronic kidney disease usually requires which of the following to manage the condition?
   a. Steroid and antidiuretic hormone injections
   b. Dialysis or a kidney transplant
   c. A full-time home health aide
   d. Hospice services

25. A patient with HIV who has CD4/T-cell levels of less than two hundred cells per cubic millimeter of blood is diagnosed with which of the following?
   a. Leukemia
   b. Remission
   c. AIDS
   d. Subtype C

Answer Explanations

1. C: Children, women, and the elderly are vulnerable populations due to tendencies to be physically weaker than their attackers, possibly disabled, unable to communicate, or dependent in some other way.

2. D: All the signs that Mary is showing, such as poor hygiene, absenteeism, withdrawn behaviors, and crying before going home are red flags for abuse and neglect.

3. B: Selective serotonin reuptake inhibitors (SSRIs) are a class of drugs that can treat both anxiety and depression symptoms. Therefore, brand names of this drug, such as Prozac®, Zoloft®, and Lexapro®, may be prescribed to individuals who are suffering from anxiety, depression, or a combination of both.

4. C: Schizophrenia and bipolar disorder are mental disorders in which hallucinations and delusion (key components of psychosis) are common. These characteristics can also result from mind-altering drugs, specifically methamphetamines, cocaine, and LSD. Antiviral medications used to treat HIV do not normally cause psychosis.

5. A: The patient is having many symptoms of panic, such as struggling to breathe, having difficulty controlling her emotions, and acting agitated. However, she mentions that her partner just left, and there are no other indicators of previous physical or mental health problems in her history. This is a good clue that the patient's partner's leaving is a very stressful event for her and a situational crisis that is likely causing these acute, short-term behaviors. Jack and Jill can help this patient by providing comfort, support, and counseling to help her reach a place where they can calmly discuss treatment options needed, if any.

6. B: Suicidal ideation is characterized by recurrent thoughts of suicide, ranging from passive ideation to active ideation. Homicidal ideation is characterized by thoughts or plans to kill another person or a group of people.

7. D: Severe allergies can be life-threatening and lead to anaphylaxis. An epinephrine injection pen is the first line of defense if a person comes into contact with an allergen to which he or she has a serious or life-threatening reaction.

8. B: Coumadin® is a brand name for the drug warfarin, which can be administered orally or intravenously. It works by decreasing platelet adherence to prevent clot formation. Paxil® is used to treat anxiety and depression and Thromblok is fictitious.

9. C: Heparin can be administered orally or intravenously. It is often given before surgery. It works by decreasing the presence of clotting factors in the blood. Paxil® is used to treat anxiety and depression and Thromblok is fictitious.

10. A: Acute forms of leukemia affect young cells and tend to affect younger people. Acute leukemia of the lymphocytes is the most common form of leukemia seen in children.

11. C: Chronic forms of leukemia affect older cells and tend to affect adults. Chronic leukemia of the lymphocytes is the most common form in older adults.

12. A: Iron deficiency anemia is characterized by iron levels lower than 12 g/dL in women, and Billie's tests showed she was below this level. She also shared that she has heavy, long menstrual periods, and it appears she is currently in her cycle. This heavy blood loss can deplete iron levels. Her fainting episode is also a symptom of anemia.

13. A: Since electrolytes need to be suspended in a certain amount of liquid to move optimally and carry out their intended function, fluid level in the body is important. As fluid levels increase beyond a state of fluid-electrolyte balance, electrolyte levels will decrease, since there is too much fluid present. If fluid levels are too low, such as in a state of dehydration, there will be too many electrolytes per unit of fluid, which also prevents the electrolytes from carrying out their intended function.

14. B: These hormones are produced by the adrenal glands and influence specific sexual and reproductive functions, such as building estrogen and testosterone.

15. D: Cushing's syndrome is characterized by unmanageable weight gain, hair growth, and high blood pressure. Due to excessive production of glucocorticoid by the adrenal glands, it is an endocrine system disorder that can be managed through medication.

16. D: Patients with type 1 diabetes cannot produce enough or any insulin and are required to manually administer it into their system. This answer option is the only one that has an appropriate, logical pairing; therefore, it is the correct statement.

17. D: Patients with type 2 diabetes cannot use the insulin their body produces to break down food into glucose. They can manage their symptoms with lifestyle changes, such as losing weight, diet, and exercise. They can also use the drug metformin, which helps regulate their blood glucose levels.

18. B: Grave's disease and Hashimoto's disease are both autoimmune disorders, but Grave's disease results in an overproduction of thyroid hormone, while Hashimoto's disease results in a deficiency of thyroid hormone. The other statements are not correct.

19. A: Many parents have been choosing to delay or not vaccinate their children, leading to a recent surge of measles cases in the country. The first sign of measles is a high fever, often reaching 104 degrees Fahrenheit. It is followed by a full-body rash. Measles is a highly contagious disease that can last up to a month in duration.

20. B: Pregnant women are considered immunocompromised due to the strain that the fetus places on the mother's health resources. Infants are considered immunocompromised, since their immune systems are not developed. Patients with cancer are considered immunocompromised, as their immune systems are stressed by fighting cancer cells, especially if undergoing chemotherapy. Patients with HIV are considered immunocompromised because they have a lifelong virus that directly targets their immune system.

21. A: The sodium-potassium pump is a cellular mechanism that maintains balance between sodium on the inside of a cell and potassium in the blood outside of the cell. Maintaining this balance creates membrane potential across the cell. The other pairings listed in the statements do not make logical sense.

22. A: Patients with type 1 diabetes are prone to diabetic ketoacidosis due to the absence of adequate insulin in their blood. This absence makes it more likely for the body to use fatty acids for energy rather than carbohydrates, and without insulin, this can lead to excessive ketones in the blood. Excessive ketones lead to an acidic blood environment.

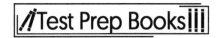

23. C: Immunocompromised patients need to minimize their contact with potentially infectious or illness-causing agents as much as possible, since even mild illnesses can be life-threatening to them. All the practices listed are recommended for patients who have a compromised immune system with the exception of only drinking bottled water. While clean water and clean drinking vessels should always be used, water does not need to necessarily be bottled.

24. B: Stage 5 chronic kidney disease is the last stage of progression for this condition. By this time, it is serious enough to require constant dialysis (a process that filters the blood for the kidneys) or a kidney transplant because the kidneys have failed.

25. C: AIDS, or acquired immunodeficiency syndrome, is the most severe stage of HIV due to the extremely low CD4/T-cell counts in the patient's body. This means the patient is extremely vulnerable to infectious diseases, and possibly death.

Maxillofacial, Ocular, Orthopedic, and Wound Emergencies

Maxillofacial

Abscesses

A maxillofacial abscess refers to any kind of localized, fluid-filled mass in a person's jaw or face. An abscess is normally easily visible, red or inflamed in appearance, and painful when touched. The mass often results from a wound in the area that fails to heal properly. Infections result in white blood cells, wound tissue, and other cellular debris mixing into pus, and pooling into the area.

Common maxillofacial abscesses include dental abscesses, which occur around teeth and within the gum line, and peritonsillar abscesses, which occur around the tissues of the throat. Dental abscesses most commonly occur when dental procedures do not heal correctly, or as a result of untreated gum disease or cavities. Peritonsillar abscesses are less common, but can result in untreated or improperly treated cases of tonsillitis and strep throat. When treated early, maxillofacial abscesses can be removed through drainage procedures; mild cases may be treated with antibiotics. However, if they go untreated, maxillofacial abscesses can rupture and become life-threatening. The bacteria in the abscess can travel to the brain, spinal cord, or blood. This can result in infections of the nervous system or sepsis.

Dental Conditions

In addition to maxillofacial abscesses, a number of dental conditions are treated as emergencies. Trauma to the facial region that results in broken or avulsed teeth, a broken or dislocated mandible or upper or lower jaw, or broken or fractured facial bones around the nose or chin often requires emergency care.

In patients with broken or avulsed teeth, uncontrollable bleeding from the tooth socket may be an issue. Individual wound care should be administered for each affected tooth. Avulsed permanent teeth should be reinserted into their point of origin; avulsed baby teeth should not be replanted, but the patient should be thoroughly examined for any potential injuries to the respective permanent tooth.

In patients with broken or dislocated jaws or other facial bones near the nose, the airway may become compromised. This often occurs in cases where the resting position of the tongue after maxillofacial trauma moves and covers the throat. In these instances, adequate airway management is vital so that respiration stays intact.

Epistaxis

Epistaxis refers to nasal bleeding. This event can frighten patients, which often brings them to emergency services. However, most events are not true emergency cases. Epistaxis events are most like to occur when blood vessels in the nasal region rupture. This can result from dry or irritated nasal membranes, other underlying diseases (such as hypertension or genetic blood disorders), nasal infections, or localized trauma. Since the network of blood vessels in the nasal region is extensive and delicate, trauma can result from something as mundane as excessive nose-blowing. Most cases of epistaxis are acute and stop on their own. Treatment involves applying pressure to the nose, and

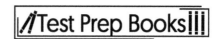

occasionally administering medications that promote vasoconstriction. Antibiotics can help reduce epistaxis events in patients who are prone to them.

A few cases can become life-threatening. This includes posterior nasal trauma where blood is able to occlude the nasopharyngeal airway, and in some cases in immunocompromised patients. If the patient's airway becomes blocked, suction techniques may be necessary to manage the airway. Immunocompromised patients are vulnerable to excessive bleeding and blood loss, so these symptoms will need to be addressed.

Facial Nerve Disorders

Facial nerve disorders often present as excessive (such as twitching) or weakened (such as paralysis) activity in the facial region. This can affect movement associated with the eyes or mouth, as well as sensory input perceived by the eyes, nose, mouth, tongue, or ears. Some disorders are acute and temporary, but are frightening for the patient upon onset. Facial nerve disorders can be genetic and chronic, or can result from an event that affected the nerves in the face.

Bell's palsy is a facial nerve disorder with an acute onset. It results from trauma to the facial nerve, often as a result from swelling due to a virus, physical injury, respiratory infection, or other chronic inflammatory disorder. This causes communication disruption between the brain and various muscles of the face. Bell's palsy is characterized by weakness or paralysis on one side of the face (although in cases of severe trauma, it may be seen on both sides). The patient's eyelid and mouth on the affected side tend to excessively droop, and they will often be unable to control drooling, swallowing, or crying on that side. Taste and hearing may also be affected. The condition typically lasts anywhere from two to fourteen days, with full recovery occurring within six months. Bell's palsy is treated with steroid injections, facial massage, and physical therapy. Rarely, some degree of nerve damage remains even after primary symptoms have passed.

Trigeminal neuralgia results from pressure on a cranial nerve, which is responsible for sensory perception relating to the face. It is common in patients with multiple sclerosis, history of stroke, or brain tumors. In afflicted patients, routine daily habits that affect the face (such as tooth brushing) can feel severe, manifesting as sharp shooting pain, excessive pressure, or unrelenting tenderness. It normally affects the area around the mouth. Painful episodes can occur spontaneously and last anywhere from a few seconds to several months. Short-term treatments usually involve administering anticonvulsants or muscle relaxers to the patient; long-term solutions may include vascular or radiation surgeries around the nerve.

Other instances of facial nerve disorders can occur from surgeries in the area, such as major oral surgeries.

Foreign Bodies

Foreign bodies in the maxillofacial region are often the result of, or quickly progress to, an emergency situation. A foreign body in this context includes any object that is not normally in the area, so it may include otherwise natural biological entities (such as blood or mucus present in the airway, or bone pieces that protrude into surrounding tissues). Foreign bodies in the maxillofacial region are especially common with blunt force or other contact trauma cases, such as in motor vehicle injuries where a patient's face may come in contact with glass, metal, gravel, dirt, plastics, or other environmental agents. Microscopic or deep pieces may go undetected in the initial assessment of the patient, but imaging studies can help with this process.

In maxillofacial puncture wounds, such as gunshot wounds, a large foreign body may be more visible. However, any impact with skeletal structures can cause the bone to fragment and travel into surrounding tissues.

Finally, any form of trauma can lead to excessive bleeding around or into the nasopharyngeal cavity. This can result in the patient's airway becoming compromised and should be managed immediately. Lack of adequate respiration will quickly progress to additional complications for the patient. Undetected foreign bodies can lead to painful and long-term patient discomfort, infection, abscesses, deformities, and/or unsightly scar tissue. They can also lead to more severe outcomes, such as sepsis or death.

Removing foreign bodies of any size requires precise surgical technique, as many fragmented pieces have rough edges that can easily rupture nearby blood vessels. These procedures will almost always require large interdisciplinary groups of medical professionals.

Infections

Infections are always a potential threat to the human body; the risk increases significantly during emergency situations since there are more opportunities for various bacteria and viruses to enter a system that is already under duress. Post-surgical wounds are also susceptible to infections that require emergency treatment, and pre-existing moderate infections can progress to infections that require urgent care.

Ludwig's angina refers to an oral infection that results in rapid swelling of the tissues under the tongue. It can occur after surgical dental procedures or in the presence of a tooth abscess. If not immediately treated, the swelling can push the tongue over the throat and block this airway. It also can result in facial paralysis, chest pain, or sepsis. Clearing the airway, draining any excess fluids, and then managing the bacteria through antibiotics (with regular follow-ups) is the common treatment protocol.

Otitis refers to ear infections. Ear infections can affect any part of the ear and are fairly common. They can be divided into categories: otitis externa refers to infections of the outer ear, and otitis media refers to infections behind the eardrum. Otitis externa is common in swimmers or other individuals who are prone to having fluid in their ears. Otitis media is common in very young children whose ear canals and immune systems are still developing. Recurring ear infections in either category can lead to hearing loss. Severe cases of otitis media can lead to membrane rupture in the middle ear, which can cause temporary hearing loss, speech development delays, and emotional anxieties. Additionally, untreated otitis media can lead to mastoiditis—inflammation of a space within the skull. Complications of mastoiditis include brain abscesses, hearing and balance problems, and meningitis. Luckily, it is relatively rare in developed countries.

Sinusitis refers to infections of the membrane lining of the air passages around the nasal cavity. This is a fairly common condition that often presents after another respiratory illness, such as a cold, which causes the sinuses to become filled with mucus and fluid. If these fluids remain stagnant, they are susceptible to breeding bacteria in the space. Sinusitis events can last anywhere from one to two weeks, and may require the use of antibiotics if the event is determined to be bacterial in origin. Untreated, however, bacteria and viruses in the sinus cavities can travel to the brain and cause serious repercussions.

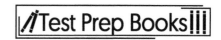

Acute Vestibular Dysfunction

Acute vestibular dysfunction refers to any disorder or infection affecting the inner ear and/or the vestibular nerve, therefore disrupting normal vision capabilities and balance.

Labyrinthitis refers to inflammation of the vestibular nerve, rendering it incapable of communicating effectively with the brain. Patients with labyrinthitis often experience dizziness, nausea, vomiting, falling, ringing in the ears, and vision problems. These secondary problems can lead to emergency situations, such as experiencing a dangerous fall. For an accurate diagnosis, labyrinthitis normally requires a full physical examination, hearing tests, image scans, and brain wave tests. This condition should be treated early, and it can take up to two months for complete recovery.

Meniere's disease is believed to be caused by high pressure from fluid buildup, usually in a single ear. A number of conditions are believed to exacerbate Meniere's disease, including trauma of the head or ear, alcohol abuse, extreme stress, immune system disorders, family history, or a history of migraines. The onset of the disease begins with a strong sensation of inner ear pressure, hearing loss, and dizziness.

Most vestibular dysfunctions are treated with antihistamines, nausea medications, and/or steroid prescriptions in conjunction with behavior modifications, such as moving slowly, practicing exercises that focus on balance, avoiding screens, and avoiding bright lights.

Ruptured Tympanic Membrane

The tympanic membrane, more commonly referred to as the inner eardrum, is located right behind the middle ear. Small holes or tears can commonly result from events such as untreated ear infections, fluid buildup, loud noises, or trauma (such as from inserting a foreign object inside the ear canal). Rupture involves short-lived but sharp ear pain, liquid drainage into the ear canal or to the outer ear, and ringing in the affected ear. Often, ruptured tympanic membranes can heal on their own or with the assistance of simple prescription medications; this can take a few weeks. During this time, temporary hearing loss or decreased hearing capability in the patient is a possibility. Ruptured tympanic membranes are common in pediatric patients.

Improper healing can result in the need for scheduled surgery to repair the membrane, or the area can become infected and emergency surgery may be required. Additionally, the cause of the ruptured tympanic membrane can indicate a need for urgent care. For example, if the foreign object that caused the rupture is still inside the ear, it will need to be medically removed. Dizziness, inability to walk properly, migraines, neck pain, or heavy bleeding from the ear are symptoms that also warrant emergency care. In these instances, preventing and treating infection, minimizing blood loss, patching the membrane, or performing surgery on large tears are likely courses of action. If the patient is experiencing recurring dizziness or nausea, additional surgeries of the inner and middle ear may be required. Rare but life-threatening complications of ruptured tympanic membranes can include brain infections.

Temporomandibular Joint (TMJ) Dislocation

The TMJ is found just below the ear and joins the jawbones with the rest of skull. It allows the mouth to open and close, and for the lower jaw to move across various planes of space. Dislocation of this joint can occur from blunt force trauma to the area, arthritis, or muscular or ligament imbalances around the joint. People with chronic issues in this area, known as temporomandibular joint disorder (TMD), are more likely to experience dislocation. TMD is characterized by facial pain, headaches, audible clicking of the mouth when moving the lower jaw (such as when eating), muscle spasms near the joint, or feeling the jaw lock at times.

The TMJ is a ball-and-socket joint that can dislocate (slip out of place). This normally results in the patient's inability to close the jaw. In addition to being awkward and physically uncomfortable, it can also be quite painful until the joint is reset. TMJ dislocation is considered an emergency situation. Treatment measures can be mild, such as utilizing local anesthesia in the mouth, resetting the TMJ, and providing physical therapy exercises that treat any laxity and tenderness in the ligaments that support the joint. However, chronic dislocation of the jaw (common in people that have laxity in the stabilizing ligament or arthritis) may require surgical intervention to shorten the ligament, or to place elastics around the joint in order to limit mobility. People with history of TMJ dislocation are likely to experience recurring events.

Trauma

Maxillofacial trauma can refer to a number of damaging events involving facial, nasal, temporal, ocular, and oral bones, muscles, and soft tissues. These injuries can be categorized into three broad categories: soft tissue injuries, bone injuries, and special area injuries (involving nerves). Due to the wide spectrum of potential injuries, as well as the depth of sensory functions associated with the maxillofacial region (since the primary sight, taste, hearing, and smell structures are located here), maxillofacial trauma can be complex and life-altering. Additionally, trauma in this region can threaten the primary airways. Initial assessment of a traumatic maxillofacial event should include airway management and spinal assessment. Disfigurement is also a risk, and it can lead in to psychological consequences for the patient. Recovery is often a long process.

Maxillofacial trauma is most commonly caused by motor vehicle accidents, but can also result from assault, recreational accidents, drug abuse, or side effects from neurological disorders (such as a brain tumor that makes a patient more prone to falling). After stabilizing the patient, the patient should be checked for the following:

- Visible skin bruising or swelling, lacerations, or bleeding

- Foreign bodies embedded in the skin, ears, or eyes

- Injury to the inner eyelids, pupil dilation, and eye movements

- Nasal fractures and swelling at the nasal bridge

- Inner ear or tympanic membrane ruptures

- Jaw mobility, Le Fort 1 (when teeth are able to move) fractures, Le Fort 2 (when bones in the nose are able to move) fractures, ability to open and shut the mouth, and avulsed teeth

- Le Fort 3 fractures, when multiple or all facial bones are fractured and may be able to move; a patient's face will often appear flat if they have Le Fort 3 fractures

- Sensory input abilities (if the patient can hear, smell, taste, see, and feel sensations associated with the cranial nerves)

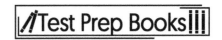

Additionally, continuous monitoring of vital signs can help detect early warning signs of infection, hemorrhage, shock, cardiac events, or sepsis.

Ocular

Abrasions

Ocular abrasions, commonly called corneal abrasions, refer to any scratch made on the surface of the eye. These cases normally heal easily, but can be uncomfortable during the healing process. Ocular abrasions are usually caused by routine activities, such as wearing contact lenses, applying eye makeup, or roughhousing with a child or pet. Traumatic events, such as motor vehicle crashes or explosions, can cause foreign bodies to enter the eye. This can lead to deeper abrasions, which can cause issues like scarring and vision loss. Foreign bodies can also enter the eye from improperly handled or improperly disinfected contact lenses.

Ocular abrasions are most commonly treated with antibiotics and pain medication. Infection is always a concern during the healing process, but antibiotic use for minor emergency cases is not recommended. An ocular abrasion can become an ulcer if fungal or bacterial infections take hold of the area; early detection is key. Infection is characterized by red and itchy eyes, blurred vision, light sensitivity, eye pain, the sensation of something being in the affected eye, and abnormal fluid discharge. Most emergency cases will be discharged for in-home self-care, such as resting the eyes, applying medications, and wearing sunglasses for at least 48 hours.

Burns

Ocular burns almost always require emergency care. They are categorized as chemical burns (resulting from corrosive chemical agents) or ultraviolet burns (resulting from heat or ultraviolet rays).

Chemical ocular burns can be caused by alkaline substances, which are able to quickly penetrate layers of superficial eye tissue. Alkaline substances can destroy collagen and other fatty tissues in the eye; inflammation occurs as a result and causes further functional impairment. Acidic substances do not penetrate or break down fatty tissues, but can cause significant surface level damage to the eye. Chemical ocular burns are most commonly found in incidences of motor vehicle explosions (due to the presence of gasoline and car batteries), or in laboratory settings where hazardous chemicals are present. However, alkali and acids, which are often associated with ocular burns, are routinely found in household items such as cleaners, disinfectants, and laundry detergent pods.

Thermal, ultraviolet, and radiation ocular burns can occur in a number of ways; fire exposure, inadequate sun or tanning bed protection, ultraviolet ray reflection at high altitudes, steam exposure, and cooking accidents are common causes. Often, these can be prevented with the use of safety goggles or safe handling practices.

Ocular burns are categorized on a four-tier severity scale, known as the Roper-Hall scale. Grade 1 burns have positive prognoses, while Grade 4 burns normally result in opaque, necrotic tissues with negative prognoses (including full vision loss).

Foreign Bodies

Foreign bodies in the ocular area refer to any object that is not normally present in a healthy, fully functioning eye. In this context, foreign bodies can refer to external objects including, but not limited to: dirt; bugs; debris consisting of a variety of metal, wooden, composite, or plastic materials; grass; or smoke. However, it can also include organic materials near the eye (such as a loose eyelash) that happen to fall under the eyelid or onto the cornea.

Symptoms of a foreign body in the ocular region include pain, burn, blurry or double vision, feelings of pain and scratchiness, bleeding or bruising of the eyeball, and headaches. In mild cases, removing the foreign body (usually through gentle, repetitive flushing of the eyes) eliminates symptoms. Urgent cases normally result when a foreign body has not been completely removed, resulting in corneal scratching, infection, scarring, and/or vision loss. Emergency cases involving foreign bodies can result from traumatic events, such as motor vehicle crashes, construction mishaps, or laboratory explosions, where the propulsion of small pieces can cause puncture wounds in the eyeball. Covering the affected eye until it can be anesthetized and treated will prevent eyeball movement; this prevents a foreign body from potentially becoming further lodged into the tissues.

Glaucoma

A diagnosis of glaucoma indicates that the patient may have any one of several eye diseases that cause excessive pressure, or other damage, to the optic nerve. The optic nerve is located deep to the eyeball, and relays sensory input from the retina to the brain. A healthy optic nerve is crucial for accurate visual perception.

Glaucoma can present in multiple forms. Open angle glaucoma is the most common form and results from gradual fluid buildup in the eyeball. This leads to increased intraocular pressure and compromises the optic nerve. The optic nerve is also vulnerable in individuals who have high blood pressure or poorly managed diabetes. However, many people develop glaucoma even if they do not have increased intraocular pressure or other health risk factors. Some patients are predisposed; African-American and Mexican-American individuals tend to have disproportionately higher rates of glaucoma. For all individuals, the likelihood of developing glaucoma increases with age or with a family history of glaucoma.

Most cases of early stage glaucoma present no symptoms; in its early stages, glaucoma is usually detected during preventative care vision exams. Angle closure glaucoma is one form that rapidly progresses to an emergency situation. In this form, fluid ceases to drain from the eye completely. Fluid buildup is rapid and vision loss quickly occurs. Additionally, the patient may feel dizzy and nauseous. Without emergency intervention, this situation often leads to blindness.

Standard glaucoma care involves medicine—administered through eye drops—that reduces intraocular pressure. In cases where pressure that cannot be managed by topical medication, surgery to create new channels that help drain fluid (and therefore reduce buildup and pressure) may be required. Managing the risk of infection is crucial in the few weeks leading up to surgery and for up to several months after the surgery.

In cases of angle closure glaucoma, emergency intervention usually requires a type of laser surgery called laser trabeculoplasty. In this procedure, lasers burn spaces into existing draining channels to help

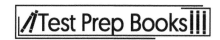

relieve fluid buildup immediately. Topical medication is required during short-term follow up care, and long-term surgical options may need to be reviewed to prevent another event.

Infections

Infections can occur in any of the ocular tissues in or around the eyeball, including in the eyelids and surrounding skin. These infections are commonly caused by bacteria, fungi, or viruses that enter through direct contact, contact with a foreign body (such as a contact lens or makeup brush), or improper wound healing.

Conjunctivitis, more commonly known as pink eye, is a broad term used to describe inflammation or swelling of the corneal surface and inner eyelids. Conjunctivitis causes the eye to appear bright red or pink and irritated. Thick discharge is also associated with conjunctivitis, especially upon waking. If caused by bacteria or viruses, conjunctivitis is highly contagious and spreads quickly through direct contact. Allergies or reactions to contact lenses or other eye products can also cause conjunctivitis; these cases are not contagious. Most will clear up on their own, but cases resulting from bacteria often require topical antibiotics.

Iritis refers to inflammation or swelling of the middle eye tissue, called the iris. The iris can readily be seen to an outside observer; it is the ringed tissue around a person's pupil that gives the person their eye color. Iritis is characterized by pain, red eyes, distorted vision, and headaches. In general, iritis should be seen immediately by a doctor or emergency care because vision distortion and light sensitivity are common symptoms that will not subside until the condition is treated. Treatment usually involves topical medication and resting the eye muscles (such as through the use of an eye patch or dark sunglasses); preventing further infection is key.

Blepharitis is a common result of bacterial infection in the eyelids. It causes red, inflamed tissue along the eyelid and eyelash hair follicles. This condition is often recurrent in patients that are susceptible to it, and can be associated with chronic conditions like rosacea. Treating the associated chronic condition can help reduce instances of blepharitis. Otherwise, treatment includes topical antibiotic use and regular cleaning and compressing of the eyelids.

Cytomegalovirus retinitis is a viral infection of the retina. It normally causes serious issues in immunocompromised patients; without treatment, it leads to blindness within six months. In immunocompromised patients, long-term treatment often is not effective due to the fact that the patient often cannot tolerate long antiviral dosing without the support of a healthy immune system.

Retinal Artery Occlusion

The retina, located behind the eyeball, is responsible for relaying images perceived by the lens of the eyeball to the optic nerve. Without a healthy, fully functional retina, the sense of vision would not occur. Like all tissues in the body, the tissues of the retina are supplied and detoxified through a network of arteries and veins. These can become blocked through blood clots or plaque, the way any other blood vessel can.

A retinal artery occlusion refers to a blockage in one of the arteries that brings oxygenated blood to the retina. Patients at higher risk of experiencing artery blockage—such as those with diabetes, hypertension, hyperlipidemia, arteriosclerosis, or general cardiovascular diseases—are more likely to experience retinal artery occlusion. Symptoms include total or partial vision loss. When total vision loss occurs, it is referred to as central retinal artery occlusion. This indicates that the primary artery that services the retina is experiencing the blockage. If partial vision loss occurs, it indicates that one of the branches stemming off of the primary artery is blocked. This is referred to as branch retinal artery occlusion. Vision loss can last anywhere from a brief second to indefinitely. Any indication of partial or total inclusion should immediately be examined; this is a serious risk factor for other blockages within the body, which can lead to a heart attack or stroke. Sometimes, retinal artery occlusion is an immediate precursor to a stroke.

The condition is treated with vasodilation or clot-eliminating medications. However, vision can remain impaired even with treatment.

Retinal Detachment

Retinal detachment occurs when the retina moves from its normal position behind the eye and is no longer attached to the superficial membrane covering the eyeball. This condition most commonly occurs due to trauma, infection, or inflammation; a history of cataracts, cataract surgery, or short-sightedness can also increase the chance of retinal detachment. Symptoms that indicate retinal detachment has occurred include an excessive number of opaque visual floaters (microscopic particles that are suspended in the vitreous humor of the eye but appear transparent when the retina is attached), central vision loss, excessive flashes of light in the patient's peripheral vision, and partial shadows in the line of vision. These symptoms indicate a medical emergency; without treatment, permanent vision loss is likely.

Retinal detachment can be categorized into three main types. Rhegmatogenous retinal detachment occurs as a result of a tear in the retinal tissue. The tear causes fluid to pass through, increasing the space between the retina and the membrane of the eyeball. Secondary retinal detachment occurs due to injury or inflammation, and occurs when a buildup of fluid presents without a visible tear in the retina. Sometimes, this can be caused by a cancerous growth. Tractional retinal detachment occurs when scar tissue or other fibrous tissue created as a result of a prior injury separates retinal cells.

All cases require surgery to re-attach the retina, but the success rate is high. Approximately 15 percent of cases may require additional surgeries, but approximately 90 percent of all surgical cases restore the patient's vision to his or her prior state, or close enough that it can be easily managed with standard eyewear.

Trauma

Ocular trauma often gets overlooked in emergency cases where more life-threatening conditions may be present. However, a number of traumatic events can cause serious damage to the eye that can have long-term effects on an individual's quality of life. Pediatric cases of ocular trauma can lead to cardiac events, so vital signs should be monitored diligently. Once stable, initial ocular examination should include a vision test, pupillary reaction, intraocular pressure monitoring, eye motility, fluid leaks, and angle recession (a factor in the development of glaucoma).

Hyphema refers to a painful pooling of blood at the front of the eye, behind the cornea. This results in blood covering the pupil and hindering vision. An increase in intraocular pressure usually coincides with hyphema, unless the instance of hyphema is a result of a hemophilic disorder. In healthy individuals, hyphema most commonly occurs as a result of a contact sport injury, but also results from general accident or falling contexts in which eye protection would not necessarily be present. Mild cases of hyphema can heal on their own, but emergency cases (such as those that present with an increase in

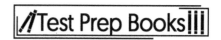

intraocular pressure) require immediate surgery to drain the pool of blood. This is primarily performed to decrease intraocular pressure or to prevent risk factors of glaucoma. Without treatment, these situations can lead to permanent vision loss.

Corneal laceration is an injury of the cornea. The cornea is a thin, clear membrane that creates the front, most superficial layer of the eye. A laceration of the cornea occurs when something punctures this membrane; it is usually the result of a flying foreign object making contact at high speed, or severe blunt force. It often occurs when people fail to wear adequate eye protection during risky activities, such as construction work or in a laboratory setting. This event is always considered an emergency, due to the high risk of vision loss if left untreated. Symptoms include severe pain, bleeding at the front of the eye, partial or full vision loss, and light sensitivity. Corneal laceration treatment requires the guidance of an ophthalmologist. One or more surgeries will be needed to repair the break in the cornea and any underlying tissues. Vision loss may still occur, and the patient will always remain at an increased risk for developing glaucoma or experiencing retinal detachment.

Globe rupture is another result of penetrating trauma; this refers to an event that affects all layers of the eyeball. Often, the wound is so severe that all fluid drains from the eye, giving it a deflated appearance. Globe ruptures can be caused by solid materials penetrating through the layers of the eye, but can also be caused by acidic chemical materials. Globe ruptures are difficult to remedy. Complete vision loss is expected, and often patients will need to permanently patch the eye socket or replace the affected eyeball with a prosthetic version.

Blowout fractures are a type of trauma affecting the orbital skull bones. These bones are crucial in protecting the eyeball, its surrounding tissues, and assisting with eye motility. When suffering from this type of fracture, patients may appear to have a deflated nasal and cheekbone region. When these bones are not intact, the eyeball is susceptible to additional trauma, such as corneal lacerations.

Ulcerations/Keratitis

Ocular ulcerations, sometimes referred to as keratitis, refer to situations where there is an open wound or active inflammation on the surface of the eye. They are often caused by organic infections and are common in contact lens wearers. Microscopic tears from small foreign bodies such as sand and dirt, dry eyes, improperly cleaned or worn contact lenses all create vectors in which bacteria, viruses, and fungi can invade and thrive. Symptoms of ulcers include redness, discharge, pain, blurred vision, and swollen and itchy eyelids. Large ulcers may be visible to the average observer; they will appear as a large, white dot near the iris. Severe infections require emergency care, including administration of topical or localized, intravenous antibiotics. Some cases may require a corneal transplant if the ulcer becomes too infected or is too large.

Another type of ulceration occurs in people with rheumatoid arthritis and other autoimmune disorders. Peripheral corneal keratitis results from the inflammatory response that occurs in patients with autoimmune disorders. This extreme response takes place in the eye when bacteria, viruses, or fungi enter and causes painful, blinding inflammation. Due to the body's inability to regulate this response, it responds to the extra inflammation by escalating the immune response further. This leads to deterioration and breakdown of the eye tissues.

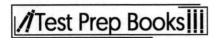

Orthopedic

Amputation

Amputation refers to the removal of a body part due to infection, trauma, or illness. It is often needed in cases where the region in question is no longer living and cannot be rescued, is ravaged by cancerous cells, or is susceptible to a life-threatening infection. The most common cause of amputation in the United States is due to poor circulation, which results in cell death and gangrene. If these areas are not removed, wide-spread infection in the blood (sepsis) can occur. However, removing cancerous bones, extra limbs or fingers, or deformed limbs and fingers also comprises a large number of amputations.

Amputation can also be spontaneous (such as the result of a traumatic accident where a limb is severed, construction injuries where fingers are cut, or falling injuries where a limb is crushed). Spontaneous amputations are at high risk for infection and hemorrhage. These incidents are most likely to be emergency situations, and emergency surgeons use the Mangled Extremity Severity scale to determine whether amputation is needed. This scale produces a score based on factors such as the patient's age, tissue necrosis, shock, and what caused the injury.

Surgical amputations are performed by sectioning off blood vessels that will be affected, and sawing through muscle and bone. The remaining edge of bone is smoothed, and the surrounding muscle and bone are neatly sutured around it. After this, the patient may choose to wear a prosthetic limb, or utilize a tool such as a cane or crutch to support their movements. Regardless, most patients suffer severe emotional and psychological distress as they adjust post-surgery. Adjusting to changed or limited mobility and a new appearance can reduce quality of life for many patients. A large majority experience sensory discomfort, such as itching, burning, or an unpleasant sensation of the limb still existing (phantom limb syndrome). This may reduce over time if the brain is able to adjust its neural signaling for the missing limb, or if the patient becomes comfortable with a prosthesis.

Most common amputations involve the legs, feet, arms, and hands; however, reproductive organs may also be amputated in late stage cancer cases. In some countries outside of the United States, amputations can be performed as acts of war, punishment, or cultural mutilation. These types of amputations can extend to the face and reproductive organs.

Compartment Syndrome

Compartment syndrome affects muscles and connective tissues. In this context, "compartment" refers to a grouping of individual muscle cells, muscle fibers, and groups of muscle fibers, encased in sheath-like structure of connective tissue known as fascia. Compartment syndrome occurs when a section of muscle is exposed to excessive fluid buildup, leading to increased pressure within the compartment. This causes the fibers to expand to a level beyond what the fascia can accommodate, resulting in the inability for adequate blood circulation to take place. As fluid and waste byproducts accumulate, the patient will experience excruciating pain and swelling. Compartment syndrome can take place in any part of the body. When it is not treated in the hand, forearm, and arm, it can progress to a condition referred to as Volkmann Contracture in which the muscle remains permanently contracted and causes permanent joint damage. This will often lead to a visible deformity of the arm. Volkmann Contracture can render the hand, arm, or forearm permanently useless in both moderate and severe cases.

Compartment syndrome can come on suddenly, such as in a traumatic event resulting the shattering of bone. This is referred to as acute compartment syndrome. It is considered an emergency situation

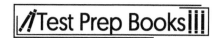

requiring immediate surgery to relieve the compartment and allow circulation to resume. Without this procedure, permanent nerve damage will occur within hours. Acute compartment syndrome is common after fractures, crushing injuries, the placement of a tight cast, and from abusing certain drugs that cause tissue swelling.

Chronic compartment syndrome normally results from heavy exertion that places a demand on muscle tissues that are unable to be healthfully managed. Individuals who participate in sports that require constant repetitive motions, such as swimming and running, are at a higher risk of developing chronic compartment syndrome. Failing to adequately rest between heavy workouts can also contribute to developing this condition. Chronic compartment syndrome is characterized by painful cramping, immobility and numbness in the affected compartment, and visible swelling or concentrated bulging in the area. Stopping activity immediately normally causes symptoms to subside within 30 minutes. However, if symptoms consistently present with particular activities, the individual may require surgery in that area to help the body deal with this load. Untreated, the individual is likely to ultimately experience a sports-related injury to the compartment. Chronic compartment syndrome is not well understood; it can affect people with excellent health and fitness, and most commonly affects younger people under the age of forty.

Compartments in the Leg

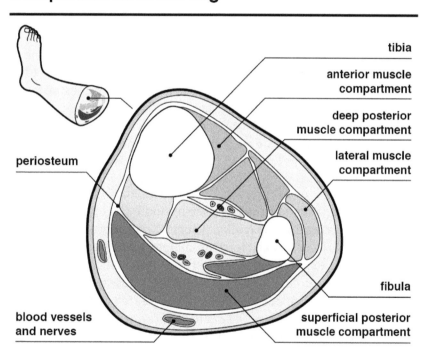

Contusions

Muscle contusions refer to bruising that occurs as a result of forceful trauma that injures the area's muscle fibers, connective tissue, and/or blood vessels. They range from Grade 1 (mild) contusions, which are normally able to quickly self-repair and have limited pain or long-term effects, to Grade 3 (severe). Grade 3 contusions are very painful, cause swelling and visible bruising, and may be accompanied by bone contusions or fractures. In all contusions, range of motion may be affected because of pain when moving actively or passively, as well as simply being unable to move the affected area very well.

Upon initial presentation, muscle contusions can be confused with delayed-onset muscle soreness (DOMS)—a condition that occurs when a muscle is overworked but presents physical symptoms (such as pain, stiffness, lactic acid buildup, and limited range of motion) 24 to 48 hours later. Muscle contusions often show with indicators of additional injuries, since the trauma experienced by the patient tends to be widespread. For example, victims of domestic violence or football players that are aggressively tackled will likely have other physical injuries to address in addition to any presenting contusions.

General treatment measures will include the RICE method—rest, ice, compression, and elevation—in addition to pain-relieving and anti-inflammatory medications, but serious contusions with large hematomas may require surgical draining of the pooled blood. Complications of contusions normally arise from improper or inadequate healing, with the most severe complications including compartment syndrome or myositis ossificans, where bone growth occurs within the damaged muscle fibers. These complications most commonly arise when rehabilitation treatments are performed too quickly or too aggressively, such as in an athlete who is trying to return to their sport sooner than what is optimal for the body.

Contusions that require urgent care tend to be those that affect pulmonary or cardiac tissues.

Costochondritis

Costochondritis refers to a condition where cartilage that holds the two halves of the ribcage to the breastbone becomes inflamed. When pressure is applied to the front of the chest, this area may feel tender and painful to the touch. Adult patients may also feel internalized chest pain and pressure, which may cause them to worry, as this sensation can feel similar to that experienced during a heart attack. Adult patients should be thoroughly assessed for any underlying cardiovascular conditions before receiving a diagnosis of costochondritis. True cases of costochondritis are often easily treated and do not progress to an emergency situation.

It is also more common in pediatric and young adult children, especially those in early adolescence, because the bodies of pediatric patients are still developing, more susceptible to infection, and because the inflammation sometimes occurs from recreational horseplay or sporting injuries. This condition is normally caused by bacterial, viral, or fungal infections, minor trauma, or overexertion of the chest and arm muscles. Most emergency situations will arise from infections that become severe and result in symptoms like an unmanageable increase in body temperature, nausea, swelling or fluid discharge near the chest, or an inability to breathe. Serious infections will be treated with intravenous antibiotics and/or steroids; some cases may require removal of affected cartilage. Adults experiencing any kind of chest pain or pressure may end up in emergency care.

Upon discharge, care involves avoiding strenuous activity until the cartilage heals. Additional oral medications may be required, as well.

Foreign Bodies

In the context of orthopedic emergencies, foreign bodies refer to any object lodged in the muscular or skeletal systems not usually present in a healthy, intact, fully functional system. Symptoms may include pain, pressure, redness, discharge, itchiness, and swelling at the site. Foreign bodies can be organic items, such as wood, thorns, or other body components (such as shattered bone pieces embedded in

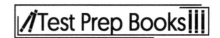

muscle), or they can be inorganic items, such as metal or glass. In patients who experience penetrating or abrasive trauma, foreign bodies are likely to enter the body's musculoskeletal system. Orthopedic foreign bodies can be especially worrisome if essential muscle or bone is compromised, as this commonly leads to long-term nerve dysfunction or regional paralysis. Bullet wounds, in particular, can cause tremendous impact not only to the area of impact, but also to the surrounding tissue, bone, and nerves. In general, large foreign bodies can become deeply embedded and affect nerve sensation and perception.

Foreign bodies in the extremities can be easily overlooked and lead to infection, which, in severe cases, can ultimately lead to amputation of the extremity. Diabetic patients are highly vulnerable to this situation. Many diabetic patients experience nerve disorders in their feet, and foreign bodies in this area can easily go undetected until severely infected. Granulomas, or areas of dense scar tissue, inflamed cells, pus, and/or other fluids can form around small foreign bodies left in the patient. Granulomas can form as a result of routine activities, such as getting a tattoo (where ink enters the skin cells) or receiving stitches to close a wound.

Once the patient's vital signs have been stabilized, immediate treatment involves the administration of a tetanus shot (unless the patient's medical history clearly shows having received the vaccination in the past five years). This vaccination prevents bacteria commonly present in dirt, dust, and soil from causing tetanus, a highly fatal condition that is characterized by widespread nervous system and muscular dysfunction. Some foreign bodies may not need to be removed if there appears to be no other physical risks. When foreign bodies do need to be removed from muscle or bone, it is a highly complex and risky surgical procedure.

Fractures/Dislocations

Fractures refer to a break in any of the bones in the human body. Symptoms of a bone fracture include pain, swelling, partial or total loss of mobility at the site, and visible deformity in the region. There are a number of different kinds of fractures that can occur. Closed fractures occur without any breakage in the skin. Open fractures occur when the broken portion of the bone pierces through the skin. Pathologic fractures occur when normally-tolerable levels of force are able to break a bone; this normally occurs in the case of bone diseases that cause the structure to weaken, such as osteoporosis or bone cancer cases.

Stress fractures occur from occurrences of force placed over the same area of bone repetitively, and are commonly seen in athletes. In general, fractures take place when a single forceful blow occurs. This blow can be direct, occurring directly at the place of fracture, or indirect, where the force occurs elsewhere but travels to another bone. Finally, the shape of the fracture can be categorized in different ways. Simple fractures refer to a single break line in the bone. Avulsion refers to a chunk of bone breaking away from the main structure. Comminuted refers to a bone with multiple simple breaks in it.

Dislocations refer to separations of bone at a joint and always occur as a result of spontaneous force applied to the joint. The sudden and forceful nature in which dislocations occur usually means that the entire area will require medical attention. For example, a dislocated shoulder would not only affect bones of the shoulder joint, but also may affect adjacent bones, connective tissues, and nerves. A dislocated joint is likely to remain fragile even after it has been treated and reset.

Spinal fractures and dislocations are especially serious due to the housing of the nervous system. While pediatric patients often experience bone fractures and joint dislocation, it usually takes a serious blow

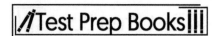

to cause these conditions. In elderly patients, a fall or bump can cause serious musculoskeletal injury from which recovery can take months. The incidence of hip fractures doubles every five years after the age of 60 in both sexes.

Types of Fractures

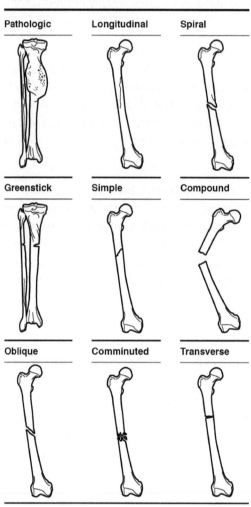

Inflammatory Conditions

Some musculoskeletal conditions result in chronic inflammation that can result in a loss of mobility. These conditions typically affect the spinal vertebrae, but some may affect the extremities or be widespread through the body. Inflammatory conditions are caused by aging, sedentary lifestyles, poor nutrition, genetic disposition, and autoimmune disorders. They are characterized by pain, swelling, and a lack of mobility around the joints of the neck, back, hips, hands, and feet. If inflammation occurs near nerve endings, the patient may experience sharp jolts of radiating pain.

Rheumatoid arthritis is an autoimmune disorder that causes cartilage between joints to become inflamed. This is often most noticeable and painful in the hands and fingers, but can also affect joints throughout the body. Rheumatoid arthritis is different than traditional arthritis (osteoarthritis), which results from the wear and breakdown of cartilage between joints over time or with overuse. Since it can

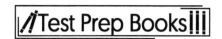

affect all areas served by the immune response, patients may also experience vision, heart, and skin problems. Due to the extreme swelling of the joints, limbs can become permanently deformed, and patients may be unable to perform basic functions like holding items. Rheumatoid arthritis is primarily treated with immunosuppressive drugs, but lifestyle changes, such as eliminating processed grains and sugars, can help alleviate symptoms as well.

Ankylosing spondylitis is a type of inflammatory arthritis that directly affects the vertebral column of the spine by causing discs to fuse. This compromises the structural integrity of the spine and results in kyphosis, a spinal curve that causes the patient to stoop over. Ankylosing spondylitis is characterized by slow onset lower back and hip pain and blurry vision. Severe cases can affect the ability of the ribcage to expand in order to allow full lung capacity, which can impair efficient and adequate respiration in patients. Inflammation of major cardiac arteries is also associated with ankylosing spondylitis. This condition is most commonly treated with immunosuppressant medications, tailored physical therapy, and non-steroidal anti-inflammatory drugs.

Sciatica, a compression of the large sciatic nerve that runs from the lower spine to the feet, often occurs as a result of musculoskeletal inflammation. It can also occur when lumbar or sacral vertebral discs slip from their space between the vertebrae; these spongy discs can cause inflammation of the nerve if they press against it. An inflamed or compressed sciatic nerve will cause tingling, pain, burning, and/or numbness down the leg. Severe sciatic cases can result in an inability to control bladder and bowel functions, or limited mobility.

Joint Effusion

Joint effusion refers to the symptom of a joint filling with fluid as result of trauma, infection, damage, or inflammation. Extreme, visible swelling is a common symptom; patients may also feel pain and uncomfortable warmth at the site of effusion. This condition commonly occurs in patients with both osteoarthritis and inflammatory arthritis types, as well as ankylosing spondylitis. It is also a symptom of gout, a type of arthritis that causes the deposition of uric acid crystals in one or more joints. Finally, joint effusion may occur in dislocated joints or joints that are surrounded by injured or inflamed tissues. Connective and muscle tissues that are unable to provide adequate circulation near the joint can cause fluid to accumulate in the region.

Depending on the level of severity, joint effusion can be treated in different ways. For mild cases, over-the-counter NSAIDs and pain-relieving drugs may be all that is needed to manage discomfort. Heat and ice treatment may also help. In severe cases, surgery to drain the fluid and repair any affected connective tissue that supports the joint may be required.

Low Back Pain

Low back pain is a common complaint of patients, and can be caused by a number of different factors, with just as many potential remedies. Some of the symptoms discussed in prior sections, such as arthritis, spinal disc herniation, and sciatica, are some of the more common causes. However, muscle injuries and imbalances, poor posture, pregnancy, labor and delivery injuries, being overweight, and stress are lifestyle factors that can contribute to low back pain as well. Low back pain can also present in many different forms, encompassing sensations from tense musculature to radiating, burning pain. It can come on suddenly, come intermittently based on rest or activities performed by the patient, or progressively increase in discomfort level.

Spinal stenosis is a condition where the spinal column narrows and compresses a region of the spine. It is a common occurrence of the natural aging process, and can result in numbness from the area of stenosis downward. It can also cause muscle and organ dysfunction, including an inability to control bladder and bowel functions. Common spinal stenosis symptoms include gradual onset, intermittent pain and numbness, and relief of symptoms upon lying down. Spinal stenosis in the low back is likely to produce sciatica and pain or localized leg weakness when walking. Lumbar spinal stenosis is aggravated by moving in the upright position (i.e. walking, running). This condition is treated with physical therapy, corticosteroid epidural injections, and prescription narcotics, muscle relaxers, or anti-depressants.

Degenerative disorders in the hips and lower spine can also cause general low back pain. In this context, degenerative disorders refer to any context where the vertebral column, sacral space, or pelvic region has broken down in some way. This typically causes bony spurs to form, or muscles in the area to overload, in order to compensate for the areas that have become structurally weakened.

Spinal tumors, whether malignant or benign, are also known to cause excess pain and pressure across the low back.

Any low back pain that presents with bowel or bladder dysfunction and lower body weakness should be considered an emergency. This is often indicative of cauda equina syndrome, a condition that causes dysfunction of a large mass of nerves responsible for sensations and bodily functions in the lumbar, sacral, and lower extremity regions. Cauda equina syndrome can present with a number of orthopedic conditions, including the ones listed in this section, as well as with a number of inflammatory conditions.

It is important to diagnose the exact cause of a patient's low back pain, as many different conditions cause similar symptoms. The use of imaging technologies can assist with this process. For patients that experience an acute low back injury, a visit to the emergency department to simply treat the pain often uncovers an underlying condition of which the patient was not initially aware.

Osteomyelitis

Osteomyelitis is an extremely rare and serious bone condition that results from a bacterial or fungal infection within a bone. It is characterized by pain in the region, fever, nausea, and limited mobility. Very young pediatric patients and elderly patients are most vulnerable to developing osteomyelitis. It is often a result of another infection (usually in the blood), metabolic syndrome, or trauma. Since very young children have bones that are still growing and spongy, infectious blood cells are easily able to transmit infection. Elderly patients are likely to have degenerated bones that can become infected by blood-borne pathogens, or to receive trauma through joint replacements that can introduce bacteria. Other risk factors include having a medical history of compromised immunity, such as in patients with HIV/AIDS or alcoholism. As the immune system responds to these areas of infection, it is likely to cause structural weakness and bone tissue death at the site of infection. Certain bones are more vulnerable to developing osteomyelitis, including the tibia, femur, and vertebrae.

Treatment measures include intravenous antibiotic administration, and sometimes amputation to remove compromised areas of bone or prevent severe cases of infection from spreading. Full treatment can take months to complete.

Strains/Sprains

Strains refer to injuries experienced by muscles and tendons—thick connective tissues that attach muscles to bone. Sprains refer to injuries experienced by ligaments—thick connective tissues that

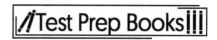

connect bones to one another. Strains and sprains show similar symptoms and require similar treatment methods. Both are characterized by pain, swelling, and limited mobility.

Strains occur when a muscle or tendon becomes overloaded or unstable. Acute strains occur spontaneously and are often accompanied by an audible popping, snapping, or tearing sound. Chronic strains occur from repetitive movements, and are common in athletes. They often occur suddenly. Sprains can occur in any instance where a ligament is forcefully stretched or loaded beyond its capabilities, such as in a joint dislocation. In both situations, low fitness and conditioning levels, hazardous environments, poor posture and biomechanics, and prior history of musculoskeletal injury make individuals more vulnerable to strains and sprains. Severe strains and sprains will require bracing, splinting, or surgery to repair or reattach affected tissues. In all cases of strains and sprains, tailored physical therapy can help rehabilitation. Often, it is a required prescription for full recovery.

Trauma

Orthopedic trauma refers to severe, often sudden and unexpected, injury to a component of the musculoskeletal system. This field covers conditions like fractures, tendon and ligament ruptures, bone and tissue transplants, bone and tissue reconstruction, correcting improperly healed fractures, treating bone infections, bone grafting, and general orthopedic surgeries. For most orthopedic trauma cases, care goes beyond emergency treatment. Intensive follow-up therapy, with the help of other medical specialists, may last for several months before traumatic cases are fully recovered. Many of the orthopedic injuries listed in this section, such as fractures, amputations, compartment syndrome, back pain, strains, and sprains can result directly from a traumatic event (such as assault, a motor vehicle accident, or bad falls). Some other common cases will be discussed in this section.

Achilles tendon ruptures occur just below the gastrocnemius, the main calf muscle. The Achilles tendon is a thick band of connective tissue that connects the gastrocnemius to the calcaneus (heel bone). It is most commonly seen in athletes that perform quick twists of the ankle to allow pushing off the balls of the feet, such as in football players, sprinters, and contemporary dancers. If too much force is loaded onto the tendon, it is prone to overstretching or snapping completely. When this occurs, an audible tear can be heard. The patient will have difficulty walking. Age, sex, steroid use, choice of recreational activities, lifestyle behaviors, and weight gain are all risk factors for Achilles tendon ruptures.

Surgical and non-surgical options are available to heal ruptured Achilles tendons, and both options are viable. Non-surgical options are less likely to develop infection, but take longer to heal. Non-surgical recovery is more likely to result in a relapse, most often due the patient's noncompliance to adequately rest the injury and keep the ankle joint immobile. By resting the tendon and immobilizing the lower leg, the connective tissue has the ability to reconstruct itself. However, most younger patients tend to opt for surgical reconstruction in order to heal faster. The surgical approach involves suturing the two sections of the tendon together. In addition to infection, this approach is vulnerable to nerve damage. Regardless of the recovery method, virtually all patients will need intensive strength- and mobility-focused physical therapy for approximately a year. During this time, pain and discomfort can continue. All patients have an increased susceptibility to re-injuring the Achilles tendon after it occurs once.

Blast injuries is an umbrella term referring to any physical trauma that affects multiple systems within the body (i.e., shrapnel from an explosion that penetrates the stomach and the lungs). However, blast injuries are categorized into primary, secondary, tertiary, and quaternary injuries based on the cause of injury and the damage sustained to the body. Primary injuries are caused by pressure waves, when an event causes a vibration so fast and forceful (supersonic) that the imbalance of pressure between the outside of the patient's body and the inside of the patient's body causes damage. This commonly occurs in loud explosions close to the body, such as in the case of combat militia near-improvised explosive devices. These explosions affect soft membranes and sac-shaped, fluid-filled organs of the body, such as the eardrums and the stomach. It can cause these structures to change in shape or rupture. In severe cases where the cause of vibration is especially close, blood cells and blood vessels can be affected.

Secondary injuries are caused by the impact of other external objects in the area when a pressure shift occurs, such as shrapnel from an explosive. Due the high velocity at which these pieces travel, they can cause severe puncture wounds if they make contact with people. Tertiary injuries refer to the physical movement of persons from blast forces. Quaternary injuries include any additional injuries that occur from a blast event, such as amputations. Blast injuries are most common in combat war zones.

All blast events have the potential to immediately kill. Sustained injuries are normally severe, and can include permanent damage of vital organs such as the brain, heart, and lungs. Any blast event that causes oxygen depletion is likely to result in multi-system bodily injury. Unfortunately, high numbers of victims are likely due to the nature of blast events, which cause geographically widespread hazards. This can tax emergency departments, as patients will slowly but steadily arrive. Even in patients that recover from bodily injuries, sensory dysfunction, such as loss of hearing and tactile abilities, are common. Finally, all victims of blast injuries are susceptible to experiencing mental health disorders, such as post-traumatic stress disorder, depression, and anxiety.

Wounds

Abrasions

Abrasions refer to wounds that result from the repetitive scraping or chafing of an area. They are rarely severe, as they normally occur at the most superficial layer of skin. Most mild skin abrasions, also categorized as first-degree abrasions, can be treated at home with a sterile bandage. Second-degree skin abrasions are often treatable at home as well, though they may involve more body fluids, affect deeper layers of skin, and require more detailed treatment in order to prevent infection. Treating a second-degree abrasion can include using antibiotic and antiseptic creams, removing debris, and bandaging the abrasion with sterile material. Second-degree skin abrasions that involve large amounts of debris or cover a large surface area on the body may require emergency care to ensure the wound is cleaned as diligently as needed to prevent infection. First- and second-degree abrasions can heal within two weeks, and often require half that time.

Third-degree skin abrasions are extremely painful for the patient, bloody, and are the most likely to necessitate emergency care. In these types of abrasions, the subcutaneous layer of skin under the dermis is often affected. This layer houses nerve endings, and its deep location can make it harder to remove all debris from the tissues, which can lead to infection, especially if additional fat or muscle is visible from the wound opening. Third-degree abrasions are most likely to occur from trauma that involves high impact and high velocity to the patient's skin, such as when a person falls over while driving a motorcycle and is dragged across asphalt. It is important to note the patient's medical history when treating urgent abrasion cases, to ensure that the patient has a tetanus shot.

The cornea is another area of the body that is vulnerable to abrasion injuries. These are covered in detail under the Ocular section.

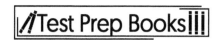

Avulsions

Avulsions are serious injuries when a part of or an entire structure is traumatically detached from the body. It can occur with any external structure of the body (such as skin, limbs, or ears), but can also affect bones, especially teeth. The skin is the most common structure to experience an avulsion; some severe third-degree abrasions can be considered avulsions depending on the contact with the subcutaneous layer and whether or not the injury proceeds to a depth beyond this layer. Some skin avulsions can be repaired through skin grafting, while others will require extensive reconstructive surgery; similarly, in amputation cases, some severed limbs will be able to be surgically reattached (though not all).

Spontaneous amputation, such as when a woodworker accidentally saws off a finger, is another cause of skin avulsion. Spontaneous amputations resulting in skin avulsions can often coincide with an avulsion fracture, which affects the bone. Avulsion fractures occur when bone fragments occur and disperse due to trauma. Common areas of avulsion fractures include dental traumas where a tooth is forcibly removed from its socket, the little toe of the foot (especially in dancers), and the tibia. Avulsions of the tibia are referred to as tibial tuberosity avulsions. They most commonly occur in young athletes who have powerful quadriceps femoris muscles that are overdeveloped in relation to the hamstrings muscles, their antagonistic counterpart. In running or jumping activities, the contraction of the quadriceps femoris can be strong to enough to fracture the tibia. When treating avulsion fractures, the limb can be reset through splinting or casting to allow the bone to heal; however, if the fractured part has traveled too far within the body, surgery will be necessary. Infection prevention is an important component of treating avulsion fractures, whether the recovery treatment is surgical or nonsurgical.

Foreign Bodies

Since wounds are open, functionally-impaired pathways into the human body, they are inherently susceptible to foreign bodies. In the context of this section, foreign bodies refer to organic or inorganic materials that become embedded in the soft tissues of the body. These materials are not normally present in the body. The type of foreign bodies that present in wounded areas depend on the type of injury that caused the wound, but commonly-seen materials include dirt, sand, rock, gravel, glass, wood, metal, plastic, and grass. Living organisms such as bacteria, fungi, and viruses may also enter open wounds either autonomously or upon one of these listed materials; this greatly increases the chance of wound infection.

Symptoms of a foreign body in a wound include pain, burning, discharge, or feeling like something is present, such as increased pressure in the area. Even microscopic foreign bodies can cause these sensations. Some foreign bodies cause no symptoms and may remain where they are, but bodies causing infections or preventing the wound from healing will require surgical removal. Granulomas refer to the development of inflamed, often infected, tissues around an embedded foreign body; they can even occur after medically-supervised injections. Granulomas look like thick bumps that raise on or under the skin. They are normally treated with topical or oral antibiotics, steroids, or laser surgery.

Infections

Infection refers to a foreign organism infiltrating tissues of another organism (referred to as the "host body") and triggering inflammation, tissue breakdown, or other pathology. Chronic disease or acute systemic illness can occur from infections. Most infections are caused by viruses, bacteria, or fungi; however, nematodes, amoebas, and other parasites can cause extremely volatile infections and illnesses. These organisms usually enter the body through the nose, mouth, eyes, genitals, or open wounds.

Human bodies react to the presence of a foreign organism with an immune system response that floods the area with white blood cells and increases general temperature and inflammation in the body in hopes of destroying the foreign organism. This can present as muscular aches and pains across the entire body, fever, fatigue, and pus at the site of the infection (especially if it is within or near an open wound). Most healthy individuals come into contact with multitudes of foreign organisms daily and do not fall ill. However, immunocompromised patients (such as young children, the elderly, HIV/AIDS patients, or cancer patients) can become fatally ill from foreign organisms that may not cause any symptoms in a healthy person.

In wounded patients or patients who have undergone surgery, infection is often a secondary health issue that results from a primary cause (such as trauma or the surgery itself). In cases of trauma or surgery, tissues are already injured and likely not functioning optimally, which makes it easier for a foreign organism to invade. Infections that cause long-term or serious problems are typically caused by viruses or bacteria. Viral infections cause systemic symptoms, while bacterial infections tend to produce localized symptoms near the area of foreign organism invasion. Some viral infections can be managed with anti-viral drugs that prevent the virus from infecting more cells or minimize associated symptoms. Once a human body has been infected with a virus, however, the virus cannot be completely eradicated from the human system.

Viruses remain dormant in the human body and are able to become active again when the body's immunity drops, such as during another illness or high periods of stress. Bacterial infections are most commonly treated with topical, oral, or intravenous antibiotics that inhibit the spread of infection by eliminating the foreign bacteria. In recent decades, antibiotics have been over-prescribed by physicians and improperly used by patients. Antibiotics have been prescribed for some conditions that will heal with time (such as ear infections), and patients often fail to finish the full dosing schedule, which can span up to ten days in length, because symptoms are often alleviated in the first few days of treatment. This causes bacteria to become resistant to antibiotic use, and for strengthened, antimicrobial resistant strains to proliferate. This has become a public health hazard, as a number of previously treatable bacteria have become resistant. Current microbiology research focuses on finding alternative treatments.

Injection Injuries

Injection injuries most commonly affect the wrists, hands, and fingers. They are considered to be the most dangerous injury affecting the hand and wrist. These injuries occur from a liquid material entering the body through a high-pressure gun, which inject at a pressure rate of up to 12,000 psi (where 100 psi is enough to cause a break in the skin). These guns shoot material at extreme pressure that cause the material to immediately penetrate the skin, blood vessels, and fascia. Skin avulsions, fracture avulsions, and burns are common byproducts of these injuries. Affected tissues are also highly vulnerable to rapid necrosis, leading to long-term nerve damage, disability, and deformity. The most common long-term dysfunctions that result from injection injuries are a loss of sensation in the affected region and extreme temperature sensitivity. Other complications include the invasion of the body's tissues by a noxious material, the forceful impact, and wound infection. These complications can have a systemic impact.

The severity of the injury will depend on the material inside the high-pressure gun, although all cases are considered emergency situations. Without rapid intervention, amputation of the affected area

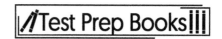

becomes likely. Injuries from guns holding paint or grease will always require emergency surgery, in addition to a tetanus shot, antibiotic use, and anticoagulant use. Paint injuries are likely to require amputation even with early response, due to the highly noxious nature of the material.

Lacerations

A laceration refers to a tissue injury that occurs due to a cut or a tear. It can be very deep, but normally presents as a single cut or break in the tissue. It usually occurs from a single blow with a sharp object. Emergency cases will be characterized by being large (deeper than a quarter of an inch, or spanning a long range on the surface of the skin), near extremities (as this is more likely to lead to an amputation), and heavy bleeding that does not stop after ten to fifteen minutes. Additionally, a laceration near or on soft tissues relating to sensory function, such as near the eyeball or eardrum, is often likely to be an emergency.

Like with any other open wound, lacerations are highly vulnerable to infection, and also commonly hold foreign bodies from any materials that came in contact with the tissue when the laceration occurred. Therefore, thorough cleaning of the site is crucial. While initial first-aid will involve cleaning the wound and covering it with a sterile bandage, almost all lacerations that extend beyond the superficial layers of skin will require emergency care, due to the fact that laceration injuries often need stitching to close the wound, or else they are susceptible to repetitively reopening. Additionally, deeper lacerations will impact the fat, muscle, and nerves underneath the superficial layers of skin. Stitching to connect separated connective tissues and muscle fibers may be required. In lacerations that are older than a day, the topmost layer of skin which is affected may remain open in order to monitor the healing of deeper stitches. This practice prevents internal infections from occurring underneath the skin.

Missile Injuries

Missile injuries can occur from anything that disperses an object at a high impact, but are most commonly referred to in the context of military combat. However, they are also associated with mechanical and construction equipment where gasoline or hydraulic mechanism are employed, such as lawnmowers. Missile objects may penetrate and exit the body, or remain embedded. The severity of the wound will depend on the velocity of impact, the object of impact, and the location of impact. Traveling missiles crush any tissue with which they come into contact, and they can affect surrounding tissue depending on the speed that the body was impacted and the type of missile used. For example, some bullets "spread" upon impact and cause increased tissue damage. In general, most missile injuries are quite traumatic to the body. Treatment that will include stabilizing and monitoring the patient is crucial, and the wound is often not completely closed for a week or so, in order to prevent deep infection or sepsis.

The stomach, intestines, spinal cord, chest, and head are critical areas to treat should they suffer from a missile wound. The stomach and intestines are susceptible to leaking their contents into the bloodstream, which can lead to sepsis. Wounds to the spinal cord can result in permanent paralysis. The chest houses vital organs like the heart and lungs; wounds to these organs can quickly result in brain damage or death if not treated in time. The head houses the brain and many sensory structures, such as the eyes and ears. Missile injuries to the head can cause long-term personality, concentration, and memory issues, even if the patient appears recovered otherwise.

Pressure Ulcers

Pressure ulcers occur due to repetitive, prolonged pressure on a part of the skin. They are more commonly referred to as bedsores and are more likely to occur on places of the body that rest against hard bone, such as the tailbone, or places that are constantly exposed to chafing or friction. Pressure ulcers are characterized by warm, tender spots on the skin, physical changes in the skin's appearance and touch, and swelling. They occur most often in patients who have limited mobility due to another condition and consequently remain in one position for long periods of time (such as in a bed or wheelchair).

If a pressure ulcer is spotted in its early stages, it can be managed by simply changing position. Early stage pressure ulcers are usually red and swollen. Later stage pressure ulcers will show signs of discharge and may be open wounds. These are prone to infection. Patients who show pressure ulcers should be asked about their living and caregiver arrangements, if applicable. While pressure ulcers can present quickly, they can also be indicative of neglectful caretaking or an unsafe living condition (such as a patient with limited sensory ability who lives alone). Complications from pressure ulcers include skin, bone, and joint infections that can permanently damage bone cells, cartilage, and soft tissue. Some unrelenting pressure ulcers may also be indicative of certain types of cancer. A pressure ulcer without these more severe complications will be treated through regular cleaning (with water, sterile saline solutions, or suctioning) and bandaging until it heals. Topical antibiotics may also be utilized.

Puncture Wounds

Puncture wounds refer to any instance where the skin is broken, stabbed, or pierced by a sharp foreign object and in which the entry point is often narrow and circular in shape. Puncture wounds may, however, be very deep. Emergency situations will include any puncture wounds near vital organs, such as in the torso, or near large arteries, such as in the neck or thigh. Puncture wounds that continue to bleed excessively, even after pressure has been applied, are also considered urgent situations. Initial treatment is to clean all debris from the wound, including removing any embedded objects. The patient should be assessed for any motor or sensory dysfunction, since deep puncture wounds can affect nerve endings or make contact with nearby bones.

It is important to ensure that bone has not been fractured or fragmented in any way. All puncture wound patients will likely need a tetanus shot, unless the patient's medical history indicates that one has been received in the past five years. Sterile bandaging is normally all that is required to cover the wound until it heals, while topical or oral antibiotics may also be administered to prevent infection. However, large puncture wounds that continue to bleed, even minimally, after receiving care may require stitches. The most common complication are infections, which may be characterized by swelling, redness, warmth, and pain in the area of the wound. In severe cases of the infection, the area around the wound may require amputation

The most common puncture wounds occur on the sole of the foot. These are called plantar puncture wounds and are most likely to occur due to a person stepping barefoot onto a nail. Other likely instances include puncture wounds from stabbing or gunfire assaults, animal bites, and recreational accidents. Gunfire wounds may have double the number of punctures, since they can have a point where the bullet enters the body, as well as a point where it exits.

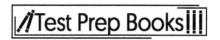

Trauma

Trauma wounds refer to severe, spontaneous injuries to the body, and can take the form of any of the wound types listed in this section. In order to be considered traumatic, the wound usually needs to affect both superficial layers of skin as well as underlying tissues, fat, and/or muscle. Traumatic wounds can be classified into three categories. The first category, acute wounds, are characterized by events of rips, tears, or other messy breaks in the skin. They can be difficult to neatly suture, and there may be a good deal of debris that requires removal. The deeper subcutaneous layer may be visible or affected, as well. The second category, cut wounds, always involve the subcutaneous layer. However, cut wounds may seem "neater" in appearance, though they can be fairly deep. Penetrating wounds are the third and most severe category. They are almost always emergency situations, as they are deep wounds often in conjunction with other acts of violence or grievous injury (such as domestic violence or a motor vehicle injury).

A degloving injury is an example of a traumatic wound. In these injuries, a large sheath of skin is torn away, similar to the motion that occurs when a glove is removed from a hand. Degloving injuries are most likely to happen to one's extremities, such as the hands or feet. Instances where these can happen include motor vehicle injuries and conveyor belt injuries, where a portion of the human body can become caught and dragged. Since traumatically removing such a large area of skin affects the underlying vascular system, musculoskeletal system, and blood vessels, critical conditions like ischemia, necrosis, and hemorrhage of the deeper tissues can happen rapidly. Sometimes these vessels can be surgically reattached and skin can be grafted, but amputation is often the end result. Even in cases of reattachment, the likelihood of infection is high.

Another example of traumatic wound injuries that has not been covered in this section are burns. Burns refer to damage of the skin and underlying structures due to contact with high heat or electricity. Burns can be classified into three tiers, with first-degree burns being the least severe, and third-degree burns always constituting as a traumatic wound. Third-degree burns damage skin as well as deep underlying structures. They can result in blistering, permanent scarring, and deformity that can make treatment and infection prevention difficult even after physiological recovery has been made.

All traumatic wounds are prone to infection, as foreign bodies, the depth of the wound, and the direct contact with open air as the wound heals may allow foreign organisms to invade the area. Traumatic wound repair is an extensive process that requires deep tissues to be repaired surgically and monitored for injury and infection before repairing the top layer. Then, the most superficial repair work has to be monitored for injury and infection as well. Additionally, all surgical repair work must be performed from an aesthetic viewpoint as well, to minimize any drastic scarring or physical deformity. These values are often important to patients and affect their overall quality of life after recovery.

Practice Questions

1. Maria has a root canal at her dentist's office. Which of the following is a concern Maria should be aware of as an emergency condition as she recovers from her procedure?
   a. Halitosis
   b. Dental abscess
   c. Plantar abscess
   d. The emergence of an impacted wisdom tooth

2. Jake, a 30-year-old male in good health, is visiting Denver, Colorado from his hometown in Miami, Florida. On his second day there, he begins showing signs of epistaxis. What are some actions he can take on his own to try to treat this condition?
   a. Pinch the bridge of his nose, and tilt his head back while maintaining a firm pressure
   b. Take some leftover antibiotics that he has with him from the last time he experienced this
   c. Immediately go to the emergency department
   d. Test his blood sugar and eat an apple to prevent diabetic shock

3. Which of the following is an ocular disorder that results from gradual fluid buildup in the eyeball, characterized by a slow increase in intraocular pressure?
   a. Open angle glaucoma
   b. Angle closure glaucoma
   c. Retinal detachment
   d. Ocular hypertension

4. Which of the following conditions is a risk factor for retinal artery occlusion?
   a. Vision acuity worse than 40/20
   b. A Cesarean section birth
   c. A history of hypertension
   d. A job that requires long hours of screen time daily

5. Joel is in a car accident where his left foot and lower leg are crushed upon impact. However, he remains conscious and waits for emergency services to arrive. He notices the outside of his calf is visibly swollen, and becoming noticeably more painful. By the time emergency services arrive, the pain is excruciating. What is Joel likely experiencing?
   a. Acute compartment syndrome affecting his lateral gastrocnemius
   b. Shock and hallucination from the trauma
   c. Deep vein thrombosis in his leg
   d. Sciatic nerve damage

6. Which of the following groups of symptoms are indicative of cauda equina syndrome, a condition that requires immediate treatment?
   a. An inability to stay awake, with excessive drooling from the mouth, occurring for at least ten minutes
   b. A loss of feeling along the cervical column and limited mobility along the shoulders and arms
   c. An inability to control bowel and bladder movements, and a sudden loss of strength in the lower body
   d. A history of horseback riding injury and a slipped sacroiliac joint

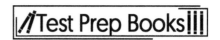

7. Where do most puncture wounds occur and from what cause?
    a. In the tips of the fingers, as a result of stapler, woodworking, and injection injuries
    b. In the stomach, as a result of gun violence
    c. Near the lumbar spine, as a result of epidural injections
    d. In the sole of the foot, as a result of stepping on nails

8. 100 psi is enough pressure to break the skin. Injection injuries occur from high-pressure guns that inject the skin at what pressure?
    a. Up to 12,000 psi
    b. Up to 14,000 psi
    c. Up to 15,000 psi
    d. Up to 22,000 psi

9. Marina was in a skiing accident where she broke both femurs. She is expected to make a full recovery, but recovery time is expected to be long. Marina, who is a very active person, is frustrated by her inability to move freely. She regularly feels irritable and sad. One day, she feels some pain near her tailbone. Her caregiver looks at it and finds that the area around her tailbone is red, inflamed, and swollen. What is Marina likely experiencing?
    a. Psychosomatic stress that is presenting itself on her body
    b. A pressure ulcer
    c. Referred fracture pain
    d. A broken tailbone

10. Which population of people are susceptible to blast injuries?
    a. Nomads
    b. The immunocompromised elderly
    c. Deep sea divers
    d. Military personnel

11. Which of the following conditions always requires emergency surgical treatment?
    a. Epistaxis
    b. Retinal detachment
    c. Iritis
    d. Sciatica

12. Elizabeth has rheumatoid arthritis. While she has to be mindful of her joints, which of the following is a condition of which she also needs to be aware?
    a. Plantar fasciitis
    b. Ocular ulceration
    c. Insomnia
    d. Developing new food allergies as she ages

13. Which of the following individuals is most at risk for chronic compartment syndrome?
    a. Eleanor, a 65-year-old woman who swims twice a week to maintain her fitness levels
    b. Susie, a 5-year-old child with diagnosed asthma
    c. Ray, a 36-year-old internationally renowned tennis player
    d. Micah, an 18-year-old graphic designer

14. Robbie was in a motorcycle accident that caused moderate road rash across his right arm. In addition, he experienced a severe cervical injury that was the primary focus of treatment when he was taken to the emergency department. His arm was cleaned, irrigated, disinfected, and bandaged. However, as he recovers, he notices two thick bumps under the surface of the skin on his forearm. They feel uncomfortable to touch. What do these bumps indicate?

    a. Robbie may have serious nerve damage in his wrist.
    b. Robbie may have skin cancer.
    c. Robbie is healing normally; the bumps will slough off soon.
    d. Robbie's arm is presenting granulomas.

15. What is the primary difference between sprains and strains?

    a. Sprains can be managed at home, while strains require surgery
    b. Sprains refer to injuries of muscles and tendons, while strains refer to injuries of ligaments
    c. Sprains refer to injuries of ligaments, while strains refer to injuries of muscles and tendons
    d. There is no difference; the two terms can be used interchangeably

16. Which of the following scales is used to characterize ocular burns?

    a. Roper-Hall scale
    b. Likert scale
    c. Visual acuity scale
    d. Likemann's scale

17. What is one way to reduce the intensity of phantom limb syndrome?

    a. Cognitive-behavioral therapy focused on positive acceptance of the situation and a prosthesis
    b. Updating the prosthesis each time a technological advance is made
    c. Prescription antipsychotics
    d. Unfortunately, the intensity of phantom limb syndrome cannot be reduced

18. In deep lacerations or lacerations that are older than a day, what is an important note to remember in treatment?

    a. Amputation of the area may be necessary.
    b. The deepest layer of skin affected should be treated first, and superficial layers of skin should be repaired in order after each deeper layer fully heals.
    c. The entire wound should be closed immediately.
    d. A physical therapist should provide the initial assessment to ensure that treatment aligns with the rehabilitation program.

19. Osteoporosis is associated with which type of fracture?

    a. Open
    b. Closed
    c. Simple
    d. Pathological

20. If left untreated, which of the following viruses will lead to blindness within six months?

    a. Human Immunodeficiency Virus
    b. H1N1 influenza
    c. Cytomegalovirus
    d. Meningococcus

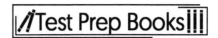

21. What is one evidence-based reason that some microbial bacteria have become resistant to antibiotics?
   a. Patients who are prescribed antibiotics fail to finish the dosage
   b. Climate change
   c. The presence of genetically modified organisms in the food system
   d. Overly sterile hospital environments

Answer Explanations

1. B: Abscesses are common complications of invasive dental procedures such as root canals. Halitosis and impacted wisdom teeth are dental conditions, but are not a risk during root canal recovery. Plantar abscesses occur in the feet and have nothing to do with root canals.

2. A: Epistaxis refers to nose bleeding, which is normally a relatively minor condition unless the patient was in a traumatic injury involving the face. It can commonly occur in dry conditions. Since Jake is visiting a very dry, elevated climate from a humid sea-level climate, experiencing a nosebleed is common. Pinching the bridge of his nose and tilting his head is the best immediate action to take, as this can stop bleeding. He likely will not need emergency services. Leftover antibiotics should never be taken for any reason, and nosebleeds are not related to type 1 diabetes.

3. A: Open angle glaucoma is characterized by slow fluid buildup in the eye, which then causes pressure in the eye to increase. Angle closure glaucoma is characterized by less gradual fluid buildup. Retinal detachment is more likely to result in floaters and vision loss. Hypertension near the eye normally results from clotting or plaque buildup in the blood vessels.

4. C: A history of hypertension increases the chances that plaque or clots will block, or occlude, the retinal artery. The other options listed are not related to this condition.

5. A: Acute compartment syndrome, characterized by swelling and pain from fluid buildup in a section of muscle and fascia, is common after crushing injuries. Shock would not cause the calf to swell or cause the patient to hallucinate an injury. Deep vein thrombosis normally occurs from inactivity and poor circulation, not from injury. The sciatic nerve is not located in the calf and injuries to it do not cause localized swelling.

6. C: These are the characteristics of cauda equina syndrome, which refers to major nerve damage to a group of nerve endings that control the bowels, bladder, and legs. The other symptoms listed do not relate to this syndrome.

7. D: Stepping on nails is the most common cause of puncture wounds, and the sole of the foot is the most commonly affected area of puncture wounds.

8. A: High-pressure injection guns can inject at pressures up to 12,000 psi; as a result, they can cause extremely widespread damage to muscles, bones, and nerves.

9. B: Pressure ulcers can develop in bony spots when a person remains immobile for a long period of time, causing irritation and pain to areas that make contact with a bed or wheelchair. While Marina does appear to be experiencing emotional distress, it is unlikely to physically present in her tailbone. Pain from her femur bones would not occur near her tailbone. A broken tailbone would have been noticed during treatment of her injuries, as opposed to an injury that came on suddenly.

10. D: Blast injuries are common in combat war zones, where military personnel are most likely to be.

11. B: When the retina becomes detached, it results in excessive floaters, vision loss, and tunnel vision. It will continue to cause symptoms until the retina is re-attached. However, this is a routine surgery which normally has a positive prognosis. The other conditions listed do not usually require immediate surgery, except in a few rare cases.

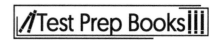

12. B: Ocular ulceration is common in patients with rheumatoid arthritis due to the autoimmune response that occurs in these patients. While Elizabeth may experience the other conditions listed, they are not likely to be related to her rheumatoid arthritis.

13. C: Chronic compartment syndrome is most likely to affect healthy, active individuals under the age of forty who play repetitive sports. Ray fits every risk factor.

14. D: Granulomas are inflamed or infected tissues that look like thick bumps under the surface of the skin. They develop around microscopic foreign bodies. Patients who are in emergency situations tend to have higher rates of experiencing foreign body complications, as these can get overlooked when emergency teams are focused on life-sustaining measures instead. The presence of bumps on Robbie's arm are not indicative of the other options.

15. C: Strains occur when muscle fibers and tendons are overloaded and become unstable. Sprains are injuries to ligaments; a common sprain occurs at the ankle. Both mild strains and sprains respond to at-home treatment. The other options do not apply.

16. A: The Roper-Hall scale is divided into four categories, with Grade 1 burns having positive prognoses and Grade 4 burns being irreparable cases. The other scales listed do not apply to ocular health or are fictional.

17. A: Phantom limb syndrome is most likely to diminish if the patient mentally feels comfortable with the prosthesis and accepts it as an artificial limb, therefore allowing the brain to perceive that area of body as missing. This changes the brain's neural processing for the area over time.

18. B: In order to prevent infection and needing to reopen the wound, the deepest layer of the wound should be repaired and allowed to heal fully before treating the next layers of skin. The superficial layers of skin should be kept sterile and covered during recovery. The other options listed are not relevant to the process.

19. D: Osteoporosis is associated with pathologic fractures, in which bone shatters under levels of force that would otherwise be considered normal. The other types of fractures listed can occur in people with any kind of bone health.

20. C: Cytomegalovirus is a viral infection of the retina that primarily affects immunocompromised patients. If left untreated, patients will go blind in six months. Immunocompromised patients are at high risk of this due to the fact that administering treatment can be rejected by or difficult for their bodies. The other options listed do not result in blindness within six months, or are not a virus.

21. A: There is a documented tendency for patients who are prescribed antibiotics to stop taking the dosage once their symptoms subside. This is problematic because stopping a prescription antibiotic before the dose is completed does not kill all of the harmful bacteria. The bacteria that remain evolve to become resistant to the antibiotic, and the medicine is no longer effective. Other reasons for resistance include over-prescription for medical cases that do not necessarily require antibiotics.

Environment and Toxicology Emergencies and Communicable Diseases

Environment

An environmental hazard is defined as a material or event that may negatively affect an individual's health or wellbeing. Some environmental hazards that emergency department nurses may face include fires, electrocutions, radiation or chemical burns, and chemical exposures such as poisoning (accidental and intentional).

Burns

A burn injury occurs when layers of the skin are destroyed by extreme heat, an electrical current, or exposure to harmful radiation or corrosive chemicals. Burns are classified by size and extent of tissue damage. The severity of tissue damage directly correlates with the amount of time the area is exposed to the harmful agent and the agent's intensity. How quickly a burn heals is contingent upon how expeditiously treatment is rendered.

<u>Types of Burns</u>
- First-degree (superficial thickness) burns affect only the top layer of the skin, cause localized redness and pain, and typically heal within three to six days.

- Second-degree (superficial partial thickness) burns are deeper (e.g., a sunburn) and consist of skin bubbling, a weepy surface, and eventual peeling away of damaged skin; these usually heal between ten days and three weeks with no scarring.

- Second-degree (deep partial thickness) burns are deeper still, affecting more than one skin layer and resulting in scarring and possible skin grafting. This type of burn may heal anywhere from three to six weeks, but this depends on treatment and patient compliance with medical recommendations.

- Third-degree (full thickness) burns result when injury and destruction of deeper layers of skin is so severe that the wound will not heal by itself. Eschar (dead tissue) will form over the damaged area and must peel or be scrubbed off for the burn to begin the healing process. Nerve damage and decreased blood supply cause reduced or absent sensation. Depending on the patient's preexisting comorbidities, healing may take weeks to months.

- Fourth-degree (deep full thickness) burns are the deepest burns and extend through all skin layers to muscles, tendons, and bone; there is no pain because nerve endings have been irrevocably damaged.

Complications resulting from a burn injury largely depend on the burn location. Burns of the upper body (head, neck, and chest) are associated with pulmonary issues. Burns involving the extremities require immediate therapy to prevent immobility caused by contractures (shortening and hardening of muscles and tendons, leading to extremity inflexibility and disfigurement), which may occur further into the healing process. Any burn in the perineal area is at an increased risk to develop infection from urine and feces.

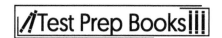

Nursing considerations when caring for a patient with any type of burn injury must focus on the following phases: emergent, acute, and resuscitative/rehabilitative. In the emergent phase, hypovolemic shock is a concern, as well as impaired cognition or altered mental status as a result of severe pain. Thorough patient assessment and rapid response are essential in this phase to prevent potential complications. The nurse must assess adequacy of air exchange, monitor fluid loss, administer pain medication, and thoroughly cleanse and dress the wound.

During the acute phase of the burn, wounds form eschar (partial-thickness burn), and re-epithelialization, or wound healing, presents as the beginning of pinkish scar tissue. In this phase, wound infection is very likely, and prophylactic antibiotic treatment should be initiated. The main interventions during this phase consist of rigorous wound care, pain management, infection prevention, and psychosocial care.

While in the rehabilitative phase, a patient may experience more mature repair of the injury with the formation of new, short scar tissue and healing itching. The nurse should encourage the patient and caregiver to actively participate in the plan of care and treatment goals; this is imperative in the facilitation of the healing process. Topical ointments and lotions should be used and applied to affected areas to promote healing and keep skin moisturized, as well as to reduce itching. The patient is encouraged to remain compliant in continuing physical and occupational therapies.

Education revolves around explanation of the burn process, phases of healing, and expected outcomes related to burn management. Infection control (i.e., handwashing, keeping the affected area clean and dry, and performing necessary dressing changes) must be discussed with the patient and caregiver upon discharge from the facility. The patient should be able to recognize signs and symptoms of infection so that treatment may begin immediately. Nurses should be able to refer to the appropriate mental/emotional health providers in the community, and referrals to family and support groups will assist in long-term emotional management, manage self-esteem issues, and setting reasonable expectations.

Chemical Exposure

Chemical exposure refers to contact with or exposure to a chemical substance by touching, inhaling, or consuming it. Poisoning, which is one type of chemical exposure, is defined as the ingestion of, inhalation of, or skin contact with a substance that impairs health or kills a living organism.

There are treatments available only for certain types of poisons, and the possibility of an individual recovering from an accidental or intentional ingestion or inhalation of a harmful, poisonous agent is fundamentally determined by the amount of the agent absorbed by the body and how swiftly treatment to reverse the toxic effects of the poison is initiated. Some poisons can be detrimental to the lungs if inhaled and injurious to the esophagus and stomach lining if swallowed. Central nervous system (CNS) impairment can occur from alcohol poisoning or overdosing on prescription pain medications or antidepressants.

Young children are at an increased risk of accidental poisoning, as they are naturally inquisitive and curious about the world around them. To help prevent poisoning in children, all lower and upper cabinets in the home, especially in the kitchen and bathrooms, should be locked and bottles should be childproofed. The visual attractiveness of some cleaning products today makes it such that they are particularly alluring for children. For this reason, such products (e.g., Tide Pods, Fabuloso) should be kept out of reach of very young children. The elderly are also at a heightened probability of poisoning due to diminished eyesight and impaired memory. Under these circumstances, all medications should be locked away from the elderly person and only administered by a medical professional or a family member who has been educated about the dosage, route, reason for the medication, common side effects, and drug interactions and contraindications.

Some agents that are used for everyday gardening and farming, like pesticides, can be harmful to the eyes and skin if an individual does not take the proper protective precautions. There are three levels of pesticide poisoning: mild, moderate, and severe.

Signs and symptoms of mild pesticide poisoning include, but are not limited to, mucous membrane, throat, and skin irritation; headache; dizziness; thirst; nausea; diarrhea; sweating; weakness or fatigue; and changes in mood. Moderate pesticide poisoning symptoms include excessive salivation, vomiting, abdominal cramps, difficulty swallowing or breathing, diaphoresis, trembling, inability to control muscular movements, and mental confusion. Severe pesticide poisoning signs include inability to breathe, chemical burns on the skin, loss of reflexes, unconsciousness, and death. In this type of poisoning, the CNS is severely affected.

When caring for a patient who has ingested, inhaled, or been exposed to any harmful or poisonous substance, a nurse must know what was absorbed, how it was absorbed, and how much was absorbed. Knowing this information will allow a nurse to determine the best course of medical treatment. Basic therapies for the management of acute poisoning and exposure include washing the affected area (skin, eyes) with soap and water and inducing vomiting, but these are only applicable and effective with certain types of contaminants. If a corrosive cleaning agent (e.g., bleach, sodium hydroxide) is swallowed, vomiting is not the best way to rid the system of it. Anything caustic that is ingested burns the throat, esophagus, and small intestine as it makes its descent downward into the stomach, so it stands to reason that if that same product is forcibly removed from the digestive system through vomiting, it will also burn coming back up.

Gastric lavage is usually indicated when the patient has ingested a possibly life-threatening amount of a harmful substance and presents to the emergency department within one hour of intake. It involves flushing the stomach with saline in an attempt to remove the poison. Activated charcoal is sometimes given and has been proven to reduce the amount of poison absorbed if administered within one hour of ingestion.

Electrical Injuries

An electrical injury (electrocution) is defined as an instance in which an electrical current passes through a living organism. This type of injury occurs when electrical equipment is not stored properly, maintained in good working order, or grounded. Before operating any electrical equipment, an individual should inspect all electrical cords and outlets for uncovered, fraying, or damaged wires. One should never operate any unfamiliar electrical equipment or any electrical equipment near water or a water source.

There are different types of electrical burns: direct contact, electrical arcs, flame, and flash. With a direct contact burn, the current will pass straight through the body and cause damage to both the surface of the skin and deeper tissues. Electrical arc burns result when current sparks are formed between objects and cause deep thermal burns when they come into contact with the skin. A flame burn occurs when clothing ignites and burns the skin. A flash burn is the result of heat from a nearby electrical arc causing a thermal burn but not entering the body. Electrical injuries can result in temporary or prolonged

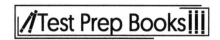

unconsciousness, cardiac or respiratory arrest, renal failure, permanent brain damage, and, in some instances, death.

A patient presenting to the emergency department after an electrical injury may be unconscious, have suffered some sort of arrest, and/or have severe burns. A nurse must perform a thorough assessment to determine the type of burn and full extent of the injuries. Lab studies to perform include, but are not limited to, complete blood count (CBC), electrolyte panel, creatinine, and arterial blood gases (ABGs). Imaging studies to be considered include head computed tomography (CT) (especially if the patient was thrown from the electrical source), chest radiography, and cervical/spine imaging. An ECG will usually be done on any adult who has suffered an electrical injury, especially if that patient suffered a loss of consciousness, chest pain, arrhythmia, or myocardial infarction (heart attack).

Immediate nursing care will focus on maintaining a patent airway, monitoring circulation and establishing intravenous (IV) access, cervical spine immobilization, wound care, and, in extreme electrical burn instances, surgical consultation. If the electrical burn is very severe, the patient may be transferred to a burn and trauma center for more specialized treatment and therapy.

Complications that may arise after an electrical injury mainly depend on whether the injury was low voltage (less than 1000 volts) or high voltage (1000 volts or greater). With a low-voltage injury, recovery centers around the occurrence and interval of unconsciousness. The longer the patient was unconscious, the worse the prognosis. Any patient unconscious for 24 hours or greater has a slim chance of a full recovery. With low-voltage injuries, disfigurement can be minimized, but scarring is almost a certainty. In the event of a high-voltage injury, a patient can survive with massive burns, but potential amputation remains a concern, and traumatic injury significantly increases the rate of mortality.

Envenomation Emergencies

Envenomation is defined as the injection of a venomous substance by a bite or sting. Spider, snake, shark, and alligator bites, as well as bee, wasp, and stingray stings can all carry life-threatening consequences, especially if an individual has an allergy to a particular bite or sting. In the case of spider bites, almost all are venomous, but most are not harmful. Any bite from a brown recluse, black widow, or tarantula can be lethal to a human. A bite from a black widow or tarantula may seem similar in appearance as a small, erythematous papule; however, a bite from the brown recluse may present as a skin laceration or even a necrotic wound.

Some snake bites are poisonous and can therefore cause a severe systemic reaction in the victim. One who suffers a snake bite should instantly be transported to a safer area and rest to reduce venom flow throughout the circulatory system. The affected extremity is immobilized below heart level. Swelling may occur, so constrictive clothing and jewelry must be removed.

Shark bites, while not all that common, are still dangerous. Sharks have heightened senses of sight and smell, which make their prey easy to locate. All shark bites, no matter how small, require urgent medical attention. Although not venomous, shark bites can cause severe infection due to their oral bacteria. Immediately after a bite, the affected area must be thoroughly rinsed with water and compressed with a bandage to stop bleeding.

Most alligators are afraid of humans, but this does not mean they will not bite a human. Many alligator bites occur in or around water, and although they hunt best while immersed in water, they have been known to lunge at prey who are on land and in close proximity to them. Severe infection can occur from an alligator bite, and interim care until the individual reaches the hospital includes stopping bleeding, cleaning, and disinfecting the wound as much as possible.

A bee or wasp sting often presents as a raised, pruritic area of skin. An individual with an allergy to bee or wasp stings may suffer an anaphylactic reaction (hives, pruritus, swelling of lips and tongue, and narrowing of the airway), so immediate administration of epinephrine (EpiPen®) is necessary to maintain airway patency and prevent further complications.

A stingray leaves behind pieces of itself (spinal fragments) after it attacks; therefore, the wound must be irrigated to remove as many of these as possible before starting medical treatment. The best venue to do this is in the water where the attack occurred, which is usually seawater. To relieve pain, the affected area may be soaked in hot water and then cleansed and bandaged. Emergency department attention is still required after a stingray injury to continue care, remove remaining stingray barbs and spine, perform x-rays, and administer necessary medications (antibiotics and possibly tetanus vaccine).

Nursing care for a patient suffering from an envenomation emergency is highly contingent upon the type of injury sustained. Initial interventions with most injuries consist of pain management, thorough wound irrigation and cleansing, stopping bleeding/administering blood or blood products, and preventing infection through the dispensation of antibiotics. Tetanus vaccine administration may be necessary for tarantula bites and stingray injuries, and for some snake bites, giving antivenom is required. Complications such as swelling, neurotoxicity (toxic effect on nerve tissue), life-threatening blood loss, and death may occur if medical treatment is not delivered right away. Once the patient is discharged from the hospital, the focus of rehabilitative therapy is continual pain management, thorough wound cleansing, and monitoring the injury for signs and symptoms of infection.

Food Poisoning

Food poisoning is commonly caused by bacteria or other toxins in food, which may result in severe gastrointestinal (GI) upset such as vomiting and diarrhea. Two of the most common bacteria that trigger food poisoning are *Salmonella* and *Escherichia coli* (*E. coli*). These bacteria are often found in undercooked foods like eggs, chicken, and pork; raw fruit and vegetables; and sometimes, in unclean or untreated drinking water.

Signs and symptoms of *Salmonella* poisoning include vomiting, diarrhea, abdominal cramping, fever, chills, and bloody stool. These symptoms may last for about a week, but it may take longer for the GI system to fully recover. *Salmonella* resides in the small intestines of humans and animals, but most infections occur when consumed food has been contaminated by fecal matter. This is most often because not everyone washes their hands after using the restroom, and then they prepare food for others. Infection can also occur if one touches something tainted with *Salmonella* and then puts that hand in his or her mouth. Frequent international travel, particularly to underdeveloped third-world countries, and being an owner of a bird or reptile also places an individual at increased risk for *Salmonella* infection. Additionally, to those who are immunocompromised because of illness (e.g., acquired immunodeficiency syndrome, or AIDS) or taking antirejection medications after an organ transplant, *Salmonella* infection will be a threat.

The development of complications resulting from *Salmonella* poisoning are largely relevant to the age group infected (infants, young children, elderly adults), immunocompromised individuals, and pregnant women. Dehydration remains the most common problem, as diarrhea may be persistent. Dry lips and mucous membranes, sunken eyes, and decreased urine output are all signs of severe dehydration.

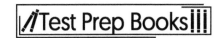

Bacteremia (bacteria in the bloodstream) is an issue if *Salmonella* is not treated quickly and enters the bloodstream. The circulatory system transports the bacteria throughout the body, causing infection and inflammation in the brain, heart, and bones or bone marrow.

Medical intervention revolves around reversal of dehydration due to constant vomiting and diarrhea. Intravenous fluids will often be administered, as well as antibiotics. A CBC is ordered to determine the level of infection by way of the white blood cell count. Most people don't seek medical treatment, because symptoms clear the system in three to four days. Because the immune systems of infants and young children are not fully developed, if untreated, GI issues continuing longer than two to three days can contribute to the development of more serious complications (sepsis, severe dehydration).

Escherichia coli lives in the digestive tracts of humans and animals. Most strains are harmless, while others cause GI upset and some urinary tract infections, which can lead to renal failure if untreated and, subsequently, death. Contact with the feces of humans or animals intensifies the possibility of contracting *E. coli*. Again, this contact will most likely come from consumption of fecal-contaminated food or water. Human and animal feces infected with *E. coli* may also be present in some lakes and rivers and drinking water that has not been properly treated.

Escherichia coli can also get into some meats during processing, and any food coming in contact with these meats will also be tainted. Unpasteurized milk and dairy products, as well as raw fruits and vegetables, can also be a source of *E. coli*, as dairy products may have been in contact with bacteria from the cow's udders, and fruits and vegetables may have animal feces on them. It is imperative that all meat (especially unprocessed meat, like wild game) is cooked to at least 160 degrees Fahrenheit (71 degrees Celsius) to rid it of all bacteria; milk and dairy products must be "pasteurized," and raw fruits and vegetables need to be thoroughly washed.

The main signs and symptoms of *E. coli* infection are nausea, vomiting, abdominal cramps, and bloody diarrhea. These symptoms usually start a few days after infection, although some adults never experience any symptoms. If left untreated after symptoms appear, the infection may worsen to cause a fever, generalized weakness, and oliguria (decreased urine output). Medical testing and treatment will usually include testing a stool sample for the bacteria, and again, dehydration is a concern. For persistent vomiting/diarrhea, IV fluids will be given, as well as antibiotics. In the case of bloody diarrhea, it's best not to use over-the-counter (OTC) antidiarrheal medication, as this will cause the *E. coli* infection to remain in the patient's system, therefore increasing absorption of the bacteria.

Parasite and Fungal infestations

A parasite is an organism that attaches itself to a host organism to obtain nutrients essential for the parasitic organism's growth. A common parasite is **Giardia** (a.k.a giardiasis), which commonly affects children. It seems to prevail and thrive in highly crowded environments, such as classrooms and daycare centers, but may also be found in unclean areas of the world, some bodies of water, and untreated drinking water. It can be transmitted through food and human-to-human contact via fecal matter.

Signs and symptoms of giardiasis include vomiting, diarrhea, bloating, and abdominal cramps. In children, there may also be a failure to thrive, and some people may even develop lactose intolerance. Much like *E. coli*, some people never suffer any symptoms, but this doesn't mean that the parasite cannot still be spread to another person. Medical testing and treatment are similar to that of *E. coli*, and common antibiotic treatment includes metronidazole (Flagyl®), tinidazole (Tidamax®), and nitazoxanide

(Alinia®). In pregnant women with mild symptoms, obstetricians may delay treatment until after the first trimester, as the recommended medications carry the potential of harmful effects to the fetus.

Another common parasitic infection is scabies, which is caused by an infestation of **Sarcoptes scabiei**. Similar to giardiasis, scabies is generally found in extremely populated areas as a result of close contact. A mite will burrow into the skin of the host, lay eggs, and expire, and the larvae will mature and complete their life cycle. The most common symptom of scabies is a pruritic, papular rash, and medical treatment consists of topical application of a scabicide called permethrin (Elimite®), which will eliminate the mite infestation. Education to caregivers about scabies and the use of Elimite® includes frequent handwashing and washing of clothing and bed linens daily in hot water.

Fungal infections are those that commonly cause a fungal inflammation of the skin, nails, and sometimes, internal organs. Ringworm is one such infection that is characterized by a circular or ring-like appearance on the skin. Although this is the main characteristic, it is not always present. Ringworm is most common in children, but it can happen to anyone at any age. It is commonly spread via person-to-person contact or if one comes in contact with infected flakes of skin or objects that an infected person has touched. Individuals who already have skin problems (eczema, psoriasis) seem to be at an increased risk for contracting ringworm.

Symptoms of ringworm include a ring-like-shaped patch of skin on the body or a blister, if severe. It may show up in clusters of ring-like shapes or only one and may be prominent in the scalp, feet, and groin areas. Itching, scaly areas of skin, crusting, and patchy hair loss may occur. It is fairly simple to diagnose, and treatment usually consists of a topical antibiotic cream or ointment to be applied to the affected areas several times a day.

Radiation Exposure

Exposure to radiation occurs naturally with exposure to the sun; however, too much exposure to the sun's ultraviolet rays can cause severe sunburns and skin cancer. Man-made radiation, such as that used in x-rays and treatment for cancer, is generally less harmful, as it is administered in small controlled doses. Radiation that originates from a nuclear weapon or nuclear power plant is serious and can have detrimental effects (e.g., cancer, genetic mutations), as a large dose of radiation at once almost has the same effects as smaller doses of radiation over a prolonged period of time.

Anyone employed at a nuclear power plant or who frequently handles materials that emit radiation should make sure all potentially radioactive materials handled are labeled properly, wear the appropriate personal protective equipment (PPE) to reduce the risk of exposure, limit the time spent near the radioactive source, and whenever possible, increase the distance from the source.

Radiation sickness may occur after an individual has been exposed to a large amount of radiation over a short period of time. Signs and symptoms include nausea and hair loss, and in extreme cases, reduced internal organ performance and death. The severity of these symptoms directly correlates to the amount of time exposed to the radiation. Immediate radiation sickness will most likely predispose the individual to an exponentially greater risk of leukemia or some other form of cancer later in life.

To determine the absorbed dose of radiation, a nurse or other medical professional must perform a thorough assessment and ask the patient or caregiver appropriate questions pertaining to the source of and distance from the radiation, the type of radiation, and when the signs and symptoms of radiation sickness began. The answers to these inquiries will assist the medical professional in establishing the most appropriate course of treatment.

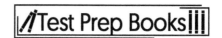

Submersion Injury

Submersion is defined as the condition of being placed under the surface of a fluid medium. A near-drowning experience is one that results in the survival of a living organism for at least 24 hours after submersion under water or other liquid. Hypoxemia and asphyxiation are main concerns, as these result in widespread cell and organ damage. Brain cells sustain permanent impairment after four to six minutes of submersion, and cardiac arrest is another complication that is considered a direct consequence of hypoxemia. Aspiration pneumonia, although rare, is nevertheless an outcome when the submersion occurs in stagnant and warm fresh water. Uncommon bacteria that reside in these types of waters may cause the pneumonia as well as other categories of infections in the lungs, sinuses, and CNS. Hypothermia is another issue to consider if submersion was prolonged and occurred in water that was below freezing temperatures.

Infants and very young children are at increased susceptibility to near-drownings and actual drownings, as their muscle strength is still developing and they often cannot hold themselves or their heads up and out of water. Babies have been known to drown in an inch or less of water; this usually occurs in the bathtub when a caregiver has left the room for just a matter of seconds.

The prognosis after a near-drowning is primarily based on the length of time an individual was submerged, the age of the individual, the degree of contamination in the fluid medium, the temperature of the medium, the symptoms displayed after the submersion, and any underlying comorbidities. Other factors include the timing of the resuscitative efforts and the physical and mental response of the victim to those efforts. The outcome may be hopeful if the submersion was five minutes or less and the person shows positive neurological responsiveness, reactive pupils, and normal cardiac rhythm. An individual, especially a child, who has been submerged for 10 minutes or more and does not respond to cardiopulmonary resuscitation (CPR) within a half hour after submersion has an extremely unfortunate prognosis, consisting of either severe neurological damage, death, or both.

A patient presenting to the emergency department who is symptomatic after a submersion injury will demonstrate altered vital signs (decreased core body temperature, tachycardia, or bradycardia), altered level of consciousness, anxiety, wheezing, and coughing. Medical interventions for an individual who has suffered a submersion injury focus on immediate adequate ventilation, as the primary target organ of submersion is the lungs (endotracheal intubation and mechanical ventilation may be necessary), circulatory support, temperature management, and close and continual assessment of neurological condition while awaiting a bed in the intensive care unit (ICU). If the individual does not exhibit unprompted, purposeful extremity mobility and normal brain stem function 24 hours after the incident, it is highly likely he or she has sustained serious neurological sequelae. Tests including ABGs, CBC, electrolyte levels, and renal function will be done to determine the level of multisystem organ involvement, as well as chest x-rays, CT, and ECG for a patient who has a significant cardiac history.

Outpatient care is determined by the characteristics and level of residual functional neurological impairment. Rehabilitative attention for one who has suffered severe neurological injury after submersion will revolve around frequent physical, occupational, and speech therapies. Neurosurgical and orthopedic consultation will most likely be necessary for those patients suffering significant head or neck damage. After initial recuperation, an individual may experience non-pulmonary issues, such as osteomyelitis and brain abscesses. Surgical consultation may be required for such conditions, as they sometimes don't respond to antibiotic or antimicrobial therapy alone. Medication therapy that is effective after recovery may include an inhaled beta-agonist bronchodilator, such as albuterol, which relaxes smooth muscles in the bronchi of the lungs.

Temperature-Related Emergencies

Heat Illnesses

A heat emergency, also known as heat illness, is a health catastrophe caused by prolonged exposure to a hot climate and sunlight. Being locked in a vehicle without adequate air ventilation for an extended period of time will also cause such a crisis. This happens because the body's temperature control system is overloaded. Heat emergencies usually have three stages: heat cramps, heat exhaustion, and heatstroke. Heat cramps (caused by excessive salt loss) usually occur after being physically active in the heat but can also happen if an individual has *not* been active. Muscle pain and tightness are the main symptoms and this condition generally befalls small children, the elderly, and those who are overweight, have consumed alcohol, or are ill or taking certain medications. Signs of heat exhaustion (caused by serious dehydration) include dizziness, mild confusion, headache, extreme thirst, irritability, diaphoresis, nausea or vomiting, and fainting. Someone experiencing heatstroke may exhibit all the signs of heat exhaustion, in addition to dangerously increased core body temperature (104 degrees Fahrenheit or greater), irrational behavior, hallucinations, seizures, and loss of consciousness.

Immediate intervention in all stages of heat emergency involves relocating the individual to a cooler area (out of the sun), applying ice packs or cool cloths to the body, massaging the cramping muscles, loosening constrictive clothing, and offering water if the person is conscious. Heatstroke requires urgent medical attention, as brain swelling may occur if the individual is not treated immediately. Other complications include shock and bluish lips and fingernails.

Once in the emergency department, the heatstroke patient will need to be treated for shock and severe dehydration. High concentrations of oxygen are a necessity, as is placing the patient in a cool pool or ice bath. When doing so, the nurse or other health care professional must ensure that the patient, in his or her weakened condition, does not drown. Vital signs, especially body temperature, must be frequently monitored.

Hypothermia, or an abnormally low core body temperature, occurs when the body is exposed to cold temperatures for an extended period of time, therefore making it almost impossible to produce heat as quickly as it is lost. Hypothermia occurs most often at very cold temperatures but can also happen in cool temperatures if an individual becomes chilled after being in the rain or submerged in cold water. It also can occur after significant sweating. Warning signs of hypothermia include shivering, incoherent thoughts and speech, confusion, and drowsiness. This becomes a medical emergency when the person's core body temperature is 95 degrees Fahrenheit or below.

If immediate medical attention is not possible, one must begin warming the individual as follows:

- Relocate the individual to a warm room or shelter.

- Remove any wet clothing.

- Warm the center (core) of the body initially: the chest, neck, abdomen, and groin using an electric warming device (blanket) or skin-to-skin contact under loose and dry layers of blankets or sheets.

- Warm, nonalcoholic beverages can help, but the individual must be conscious to drink them.

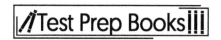

- Once the core temperature has increased, the individual should be wrapped in a warm, dry blanket.

- Seek medical care as soon as possible.

If an individual becomes unconscious during hypothermia, CPR should always be initiated, even if the person appears to be deceased. CPR should continue through the warming process of the victim.

Frostbite

Frostbite occurs as the result of prolonged exposure to freezing or below-freezing temperatures. It causes a loss of sensation and color in affected body areas and most frequently involves the nose, ears, cheeks, chin, fingers, and toes. The frostbitten area is normally numb.

Symptoms of frostbite generally occur in stages: first degree, second degree, third degree, and fourth degree. During the first-degree stage, the affected area consists of a white plaque surrounded by hyperemia and swelling. At the second-degree stage, the area involves a large, fluid-filled eruption with partial-thickness skin death. The third-degree stage consists of the development of small hemorrhagic blisters, followed by eschar formation that includes the hypodermis and requires debridement. In the fourth-degree stage, there is no longer any blistering or edema. Full-thickness necrosis, with extensive, visible tissue loss is present, which may result in gangrene. Amputation at this stage is usually required.

Interventions for frostbite are similar to those for hypothermia; the exception is that the affected area must be handled gently and immobilized, and rubbing or excessive touching of the area should be avoided to prevent further tissue damage. The rewarming process will be painful and most likely require the administration of analgesics. Tetanus prophylaxis is necessary, as well as topical and systemic antibiotic treatment.

Vector-Borne Illnesses

A vector-borne illness is termed as a bacterial or viral disease that is transmitted by mosquitoes, ticks, fleas, and some mammals. Examples of these include rabies, Lyme disease, and Rocky Mountain spotted fever.

Rabies

Rabies is a viral illness most often transmitted from one mammal to another through saliva after a bite from a rabid animal, typically a wild raccoon, fox, or bat. Non-bite exposures, while uncommon, still may occur if scratches, abrasions, open wounds, or mucous membranes are contaminated with the saliva of a rabid animal. The virus then travels from the affected area to the brain via the nerves. Early symptoms of rabies infection are similar to those of the flu and include generalized signs such as fever, headache, and overall malaise. During disease progression, the more specific symptoms consist of insomnia, anxiety, confusion, slight or partial paralysis, hallucinations, hypersalivation, and difficulty swallowing.

Medical attention is urgent because once the individual begins to show signs of infection, survival is rare. Diagnosis of the rabies virus involves performing several necessary tests, as no one test is adequate. Saliva, spinal, and serum samples are collected for testing, and biopsies of skin follicles at the nape of the neck are implemented.

For most bite wounds, thorough washing with water or diluted povidone-iodine solution is helpful in decreasing the incidence of bacterial infection. For anyone who has not been previously vaccinated against rabies, post-exposure care should always involve administration of the passive rabies antibody as well as the vaccine. This prophylactic treatment, if given immediately, will prevent the development of rabies, and therefore eliminate the risk of transmitting rabies to another human.

Lyme Disease

Lyme disease is a spirochetal infection caused by the Borrelia burgdorferi bacteria. It is spread to humans through the bite of an infected tick. Characteristics of infection are similar to those of rabies; the exception is a distinct skin rash known as erythema migrans (EM). This ring-shaped rash does not occur in all victims of Lyme disease, as many people don't even develop a rash. If EM does develop, it usually occurs at the site of the tick bite (but not always) within three to thirty days after exposure. Loss of muscle tone in the face may also happen, manifesting itself as Bell's palsy. Symptoms will usually resolve over a period of weeks or months, even if left untreated; however, nontreatment is risky because the infection can disseminate to the heart, joints, and CNS. Carditis (inflammation of the heart) is a potential complication, along with arthritic pain and edema of the large joints.

Diagnosis of Lyme disease is contingent upon clinical manifestations, with particular attention paid to the EM lesion. A two-step lab test is recommended to confirm diagnosis. The first step is enzyme immunoassay (EIA), which will be positive for individuals exposed to Lyme disease. If the EIA is positive or inconclusive, a Western blot test will be done, which will confirm the presence of the disease in the system. In individuals with neurologic involvement, cerebrospinal fluid (CSF) should also be examined.

Nursing interventions for the patient with a definitive diagnosis of or suspected exposer to Lyme disease will consist of the administration of oral antibiotics for active skin lesions and amoxicillin or other antibiotics to prevent progression of the disease.

Rocky Mountain Spotted Fever

Rocky Mountain spotted fever is a bacterial infection caused by a tick from a mammal, most often a wild rodent or dog. The causative agent is **Rickettsia rickettsii**. Early signs and symptoms of infection include fever, malaise, severe headache, and vomiting, but these may not present themselves for an incubation period of two to fourteen days. A few days after the initial signs appear, the infection manifests as a maculopapular or petechial rash around the wrists and ankles and may spread to the palms of the hands and soles of the feet. Like Lyme disease, this rash is distinctive and specific to this infection, and again, some individuals don't develop a rash, which makes diagnosis more difficult.

Rocky Mountain spotted fever destroys the lining of small blood vessels, which results in leakage or increased clot formation. These complications may cause encephalitis, carditis, pneumonitis, renal failure, and possible amputation of fingers and toes due to decreased blood supply from the damaged small vessels. If left untreated, it has a death rate of nearly 75 percent.

Diagnosis involves lab tests that check a blood sample, rash specimen, or the tick itself to determine the organism that caused the infection. Before the conclusive lab results are available, treatment is begun, as early antibiotic therapy is important in the initial stages to prevent progression and life-threatening complications; treatment as early as five days after suspected exposure is recommended to avoid such problems. Doxycycline is the most effectual antibiotic therapy in the treatment of Rocky Mountain spotted fever, but it's contraindicated in pregnancy, so the physician may prescribe chloramphenicol instead.

As with all tick, mosquito, and flea bites, prevention is key. When working or vacationing outdoors, especially in heavily wooded areas, wearing long-sleeved shirts and long pants and using insect or tick repellent will assist in the prevention of bites and subsequent vector-borne illnesses.

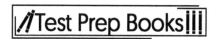

Toxicology

Toxicology is defined as the study of hazardous chemical substances and drugs and the way in which a human or other living organism reacts to them.

Acids and Alkalis

An acid is a chemical substance that deactivates alkalis, liquefies certain metals, and is typically a caustic or sour-tasting material. Acidic products include most household cleansers, such as toilet cleaners and bleach, and battery acid and chemicals added to gasoline. Acids can cause injury, which is dependent on the type and strength of acid and the length of time the skin was exposed to it. Acid exposure generally stays within the affected area and very rarely involves deeper tissues. It is imperative to contact the Poison Control Center initially after a chemical burn, as not all acidic burns are treated in the same manner. The rule of thumb is to immediately rinse the area with cool water, but this is not always effective with all chemicals, as some acid burns react negatively with water. Examples of these include the following:

- Carbolic acid, or phenol: Rinse affected area first with rubbing alcohol (it does not mix with water).

- Sulfuric acid: Flush with a mild soapy solution if burn doesn't appear to be serious; water will make the injury feel hot.

- Hydrofluoric acid: Initially flush area with a baking soda (bicarbonate of soda) solution, and then flush with a large amount of water. NEVER flush the eye with baking soda solution in the event of a hydrofluoric acid burn.

- Some metal compounds that are treated with mineral oil.

An alkali is a material that tastes bitter and forms a salt when combined with an acid. Similar to acids, alkalis are found in many household cleaning agents such as CLR (Calcium, Lime, and Rust), oven and drain cleaners, certain dishwasher powders, and some fertilizers. As with acid exposure, the extent of injury is contingent upon the type and strength of the agent and the length of time the affected area was subjected to it. Some alkali burns, like acid, react negatively with water. These include the following:

- Dry powders: These need to be brushed away first, as adding liquid will create a compound that burns. After the powder is brushed away, the area should be flushed with water.

- Metal compounds treated with mineral oil.

Chemical burns to the eye are comparable to skin burns with regard to the degree of damage and the most appropriate way to initially treat them. Contact lenses must be removed before flushing the eye, but if this is not possible, one may flush with the lenses in. As previously mentioned, the Poison Control Center will know the best way to care for an acid or alkali injury to the eye, so they should be consulted immediately. Sticky compounds, such as glue, can result in complications for the eye because attempted removal of the compound may produce more damage. Many water-based glues can be flushed out of the eye with water, but superglue requires immediate medical attention, and an ophthalmologist may need to be seen.

A patient presenting to the emergency department with an acid or alkali burn to the skin or eye will require a thorough assessment to determine the severity of injury sustained and if further complications can be avoided. A very severe chemical burn to the skin will be closely evaluated and may need to be dressed, and antibiotics will be administered. A critical chemical burn to the eye will most likely necessitate the care of an ophthalmologist once initial treatment is rendered and the patient is stable.

Carbon Monoxide

Carbon monoxide (CO) is a colorless, odorless, and tasteless gas and, for this reason, has been dubbed as the "silent killer." It has a binding capacity that is two hundred times greater than that of oxygen (O_2). During CO poisoning, O_2 molecules are moved, and CO binds to hemoglobin to form carboxyhemoglobin. Tissue hypoxia will then occur because of the decreased O_2-carrying ability of hemoglobin.

CO is created by everyday household appliances, and if an area is not properly ventilated, the concentration of CO released by these machines builds up in the air. Customary sources of CO are vehicle exhaust (especially from large vehicles like sports utility vehicles and eighteen-wheelers), smoke from fires, engine fumes, and nonelectric heaters. Other sources include (but are not limited to) gasoline-operated water heaters, charcoal grills, cigarette smoke, spray paints, paint removers, solvents, and degreasers. The best protection against CO poisoning is to install a CO alarm in the home as an initial line of defense. Adequate ventilation around gas ovens, ranges, and clothes dryers will also prevent inhalation of CO fumes.

Clinical manifestations of CO poisoning are contingent upon the percentage of CO in the blood and directly correlate with the amount absorbed by the body. Mild poisoning (11 to 20 percent) will cause symptoms such as headache, flushing, decreased visual acuity and cerebral function, and slight breathlessness. Moderate poisoning (21 to 40 percent) presents with headache, nausea and vomiting, drowsiness, vertigo, confusion and stupor, decreased blood pressure, and an increase or irregularity in heart rate. Severe poisoning (41 to 60 percent) involves coma and death, and fatal poisoning (61 to 80 percent) is just that—fatal. Once CO poisoning is suspected or symptoms are exhibited, one should immediately seek medical attention. Prognosis is difficult to predict, as CO will have different effects on those with underlying medical conditions. Even with appropriate treatment, long-term brain damage can occur, resulting in such issues as memory loss and difficulty thinking or focusing.

Diagnosis requires a specific blood test to be performed, as the signs and symptoms of CO poisoning are unspecific and mimic the indicators of other illnesses. Treatment for CO poisoning begins with high concentrations of O_2, normally via a face mask attached to an O_2 reserve bag. CO levels in the blood may be evaluated on a consistent basis until they appear low enough to discharge the patient from emergency care.

Cyanide

Cyanide is a very poisonous chemical substance that exists in gaseous, liquid, and solid forms. Cyanide toxicity is usually considered to be an uncommon form of poisoning, but exposure to it often occurs in patients presenting to the emergency department who have suffered smoke inhalation from a residential or industrial fire. Many investigated homicides are due to long-term poisoning from consumed cyanide-containing food and drink. Additionally, it occurs naturally in foods such as cassava root and apricot seeds, so continual consumption of these foods will also lead to cyanide poisoning.

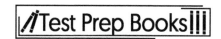

Cyanide toxicity can result from absorption through the ocular, nasal, and oral passageways (inhalation), consumption (ingestion), and absorption through the skin. Once absorbed, cyanide enters the circulatory system and is transported throughout the body to all tissues and organs. Clinical signs and symptoms vary and are highly reliant upon the dose and route of exposure. Manifestations may range from minor upper airway irritation to collapse, coma, and death within minutes. For near-fatal cases, immediate and aggressive supportive care and antidote administration can be lifesaving.

Prognosis is positive for patients who only display minor symptoms and therefore do not require antidote therapy, and reasonably good for those who are moderately affected but have received urgent medical care. Suicidal poisonings will usually carry a negative outcome because the amount of cyanide ingested or absorbed is large. Individuals who survive cyanide poisoning are at an increased risk for developing CNS dysfunction, such as anoxic encephalopathy. Acute and deferred neurologic symptoms such as Parkinson-like syndrome and other neuropsychiatric sequelae have also been chronicled.

Drug Interactions

A drug interaction occurs when two or more different drugs taken together produce a chemical or physiological outcome. An interaction does not necessarily have to involve only medications and can also comprise interactions of drugs with foods, drinks, and even certain health disorders. Drug interactions can hinder the effects of some drugs, cause unexpected adverse effects, or even increase the mechanism of action of a particular drug.

Drug interactions fall into three categories: drug-drug, drug-food/beverage, and drug-medical condition.

- Drug-drug interactions occur when two or more medicines react with one another. This may result in an unanticipated side effect.

- Drug-food/beverage interactions are the result of a particular drug reacting with a certain food or beverage.

- Drug-medical condition reactions may happen when a preexisting health issue renders specific drugs as potentially detrimental.

OTC medication labels contain useful information about medication ingredients (active and inactive), indications for usage, warnings, directions on how to administer, and possible drug interactions. It is important for an individual to read and understand this information, and consulting a physician to learn more about potential drug interactions is always a sensible action to take.

As the development and self-administration of dietary supplements has taken root over the last couple of decades, one should be mindful that these, too, can have potentially negative adverse effects when combined with certain medications. Federal law defines dietary supplements as products taken orally that contain a "dietary ingredient." Such ingredients include vitamins, minerals, amino acids, and herbs. Some dietary supplements, as well as certain herbs, are considered "alternative therapies" and should still be regarded as an agent that may potentially cause an interaction with a medication.

The following are some examples of supplements that react with particular medications:

- St. John's wort: An herb that is known to reduce the strength of medications in the bloodstream.

- Vitamin E: Can be life-threatening if taken with certain anticoagulants, as it can increase anticlotting activity and may result in an increased risk of bleeding.

- Ginseng: An herb that may enhance the bleeding effect of heparin, Coumadin, aspirin, and nonsteroidal anti-inflammatory drugs (NSAIDS), such as ibuprofen (Advil) and naproxen (Aleve); additionally, combining ginseng with drugs like Nardil® and Parnate® (monoamine oxidase inhibitors, or MAOIs) can cause headaches, insomnia, and hyperactivity.

It is imperative that the emergency department nurse or other health care professional performs a comprehensive assessment on the patient presenting with unexpected adverse effects as a result of a drug interaction. A thorough history and physical consisting of existing medical conditions, prescribed medications, OTC medications, dietary supplements, and prior incidence of drug interactions must be completed. Laboratory tests, particularly prothrombin time (PT) and partial thromboplastin time (PTT), will most likely be drawn to determine blood clotting time in those individuals who have ingested ginseng and vitamin E with other anticoagulants. With severe cases of drug interactions, a neurological evaluation will also be completed to establish the extent of damage, if any, that has occurred as a result of the interaction.

Overdoses and Ingestions

The definition of an overdose, in simplest terms, is a dangerously high amount of something that is generally considered too much. Drug overdoses may be through accidental overuse or intentional misuse. Illicit drugs, which are used to achieve or maintain a euphoric state, may be used hazardously when the body's metabolism cannot detoxify the substance rapidly enough to avoid unplanned side effects.

Accidental overdoses normally occur either with very young children or elderly adults. Young children, as discussed previously, are curious and at a developmental stage when everything goes into their mouths. The elderly are usually coping with failing vision and memory impairment, so they may misread the directions on a bottle or retake something they've already taken. Adolescents and adults are most likely to overdose on one or more substances, either illicit or prescribed, for the purpose of intentionally harming themselves.

Drug overdose symptoms vary with the type of drug taken, but typically they reflect a heightened level of the therapeutic effects seen with prescribed use. In an overdose, the anticipated side effects are more distinct, and other effects that would not normally occur with recommended usage will appear. Vital signs will be erratic (pulse, respirations), mental state will most likely be altered (confusion, intense sleepiness, stupor), angina (chest pain) is possible if overdose caused heart or lung damage, and GI symptoms, such as nausea and vomiting, may be apparent.

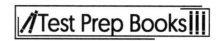

Some commonly-abused drugs include (but are not limited to) the following:

- Barbiturates: Sedatives like Nembutal® and Seconal®, which are usually prescribed to manage anxiety, panic attacks, and insomnia

- Benzodiazepines: Sedatives such as Valium® and Xanax®, used to manage anxiety and panic attacks

- Sleep medications: Ambien®, Lunesta®, Sonata®

- Opioids: Pain management drugs such as codeine, morphine, Oxycontin®, Percocet®, and Percodan®

- Opioids plus acetaminophen for pain management: Vicodin®, Lortab®, Lorcet®

- Amphetamines: Stimulants like Adderall® and Dexedrine®; also known as *speed*

- Dextromethorphan (DXM): Common ingredient in OTC medications normally used for cough and other cold symptoms; effective when administered in the correct dosage, but too much causes a euphoric state and hallucinations.

- Pseudoephedrine: Common ingredient in OTC decongestants; it is also a main component of methamphetamine ("meth") and, for this reason, is stored behind the pharmacist's counter

Illicit drug (marijuana, cocaine, heroin) use is at an all-time high, and abuse of one or more of these can lead to detrimental, if not fatal, effects. The youth of America seem especially vulnerable to the risk of overdose of illegal substances, as they are still physically and psychologically developing. Marijuana continues to be the most commonplace prohibited drug used by young people, while cocaine and heroin overdose-related events seem to be chiefly among adults in their mid-to-late thirties.

Substance Abuse

Substance abuse is defined, most simply, as extreme use of a drug. Abuse occurs for many reasons, such as mental health instability, inability to cope with everyday life stressors, the loss of a loved one, or enjoyment of the euphoric state that the overindulgence in a substance causes. Abused substances create some type of intoxication that alters decision-making, awareness, attentiveness, or physical impulses.

Substance abuse results in tolerance, withdrawal, and compulsive drug-taking behavior. Tolerance occurs when increased amounts of the substance are needed to achieve the desired effects. Withdrawal manifests as physiological and substance-specific cognitive symptoms (e.g., cold sweats, shivering, nausea, vomiting, paranoia, hallucinations). Withdrawal does not only happen when an individual stops abusing the substance, but also occurs when he or she attempts to reduce the amount taken in an effort to stop using altogether.

Some of the most commonly abused substances include the following:

Tobacco
People abuse tobacco either in cigarette, cigar, pipe, or snuff form. People report many reasons for tobacco use, including a calming effect, suppression of appetite, and relief of depression. The primary addictive component in tobacco is nicotine, and tobacco smoke also contains about seven hundred

carcinogens (cancer-causing agents) that may result in lung and throat cancers, as well as heart disease, emphysema, peptic ulcer disease, and stroke. Withdrawal indicators include insomnia, irritability, overwhelming nicotine craving, anxiety, and depression.

Alcohol

Some individuals need a drink to "smooth out the edges," as it is a CNS depressant, which tends to calm and soothe individuals and lower inhibitions. However, it also slurs speech and impairs muscle control, coordination, and reflex time. Alcohol abuse can cause cirrhosis of the liver; liver, esophagus, and stomach cancers; heart enlargement; chronic inflammation of the pancreas; vitamin deficiencies; certain anemias; and brain damage. Physical dependence is a biological need for alcohol to avoid physical withdrawal symptoms, which include anxiety, erratic pulse rate, tremors, seizures, and hallucinations. In its most serious form, withdrawal combined with malnourishment can lead to a potentially fatal condition known as **delirium tremens** (DTs), which is a psychotic disorder that involves tremors, disorientation, and hallucinations.

Other Prescriptions

Prescription medications, such as anti-anxiety, sleep, and pain medications.

Marijuana

Marijuana is considered the most frequently abused illicit drug in the United States. General effects of marijuana use include pleasure, relaxation, and weakened dexterity and memory. The active addictive ingredient in marijuana is tetrahydrocannabinol (THC). It is normally smoked (but can be eaten), and its smoke has more carcinogens than that of tobacco. The individual withdrawing from marijuana will experience increased irritability and anxiety.

Cocaine

Cocaine is a stimulant that is also known as *coke, snow,* or *rock*. It can be smoked, injected, snorted, or swallowed. Reported effects include pleasure, enhanced alertness, and increased energy. Both temporary and prolonged use have been known to contribute to damage to the brain, heart, lungs, and kidneys. Withdrawal symptoms include severe depression and reduced energy.

Heroin

Also known as *smack* and *horse,* heroin use continues to increase. Effects of heroin abuse include pleasure, slower respirations, and drowsiness. Overdose and/or overuse of heroin can cause respiratory depression, resulting in death. Use of heroin as an injectable substance can lead to other complications such as heart valve damage, tetanus, botulism, hepatitis B, or human immunodeficiency virus (HIV)/AIDS infection from sharing dirty needles. Withdrawal is usually intense and will demonstrate as vomiting, abdominal cramps, diarrhea, confusion, body aches, and diaphoresis.

Methamphetamines

Also known as *meth, crank,* and *crystal,* methamphetamine use also continues to increase, especially in the West and Midwest regions of the United States. A methamphetamine is categorized as a stimulant that produces such effects as pleasure, increased alertness, and decreased appetite. Similar to cocaine, it can be snorted, smoked, or injected and eaten as well. Like cocaine, it shares many of the same detrimental effects, such as myocardial infarction, hypertension, and stroke. Other prolonged usage effects include paranoia, hallucinations, damage to and loss of dentition, and heart damage. Withdrawal symptoms involve depression, abdominal cramps, and increased appetite.

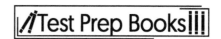

Nursing interventions for the individual addicted to tobacco, alcohol, and other drugs centers around the prevention of relapse, and treatment depends on the individual and the substance that is abused. Behavioral treatment assists with recognition of abuse triggers, habits, and drug cravings, as well as providing the tactics to help one cope with these issues. A physician may prescribe nicotine patches for the tobacco abuser and methadone or Suboxone to manage withdrawal symptoms and certain drug yearnings.

Withdrawal Syndrome

Withdrawal syndrome, also known as discontinuation syndrome, commonly manifests as anxiety, irritability, insomnia, and decreased attention span. It is defined as the occurrence of a substance-specific condition that follows the termination of, or decline in, the consumption of a psychoactive element that the individual habitually abused.

Signs and symptoms of withdrawal syndrome, as well as management and treatment, are predicated upon the type of substance that was discontinued. The emergency department nurse must collect a comprehensive history and physical to determine the type of drug, amount and duration used, time of last ingestion, reason for the current cessation, alternative therapies used to manage withdrawal symptoms, and baseline vital signs. He or she must also remove unnecessary items from the environment, provide a quiet and calm atmosphere with minimal stimuli, maintain patient orientation (to person, place, and time), ensure patient safety by implementing seizure precautions, initiate security devices if necessary and as prescribed (verbal or written order by physician) to prevent the individual from harming himself/herself and others, and administer medications, as advised, to lessen withdrawal symptoms.

Alcohol

Patients presenting with mild alcohol withdrawal may be treated on an outpatient basis, provided that no comorbidities require the individual to be admitted as an inpatient. Moderate or severe alcohol withdrawal, along with the presence of DTs, requires hospitalization and possible ICU admission. This is because the mortality rate from severe alcohol withdrawal with DTs has been as extreme as 20 percent if left untreated. Sedatives are the chief medications for treatment of alcohol withdrawal syndrome because they are cross-tolerant drugs that modulate GABA (Gamma-Aminobutyric Acid) function. GABA receptors are the major inhibitory neurotransmitter receptors in the brain. These drugs commonly consist of benzodiazepines and barbiturates.

Sedative-Hypnotics

Withdrawal syndrome from sedative-hypnotics is treated using an extended release substitution medication (either a benzodiazepine or phenobarbital) in a maintenance dosage for a few days, followed by a steadily decreasing dose over the next two to three weeks.

Stimulants

Withdrawal syndrome (also known as **washout syndrome**) from stimulants is treated only with observation and does not require any specific medications.

Communicable Diseases

A communicable disease is defined as an infectious disease easily transmitted from person to person by direct contact with an infected individual or an infected individual's bodily fluids/discharges (sputum, semen, blood, or mucus).

Difficile

Clostridium difficile (*C. diff*) is a bacterium known for causing infectious diarrhea and a more serious condition called *C. diff* colitis. The symptoms of infection can range from minor (frequent watery diarrhea, abdominal pain and tenderness) to lethal (as many as fifteen watery stools/day, severe abdominal pain, anorexia, fever, weight loss, and blood or pus in stool).

If an individual suspects that he or she may be infected, that person may want to consult a physician before self-administering an antidiarrheal medication, as stopping the diarrhea will almost certainly make the *C. diff* infection worse, thus leading to other complications.

In the health care setting, *C. diff* is spread mainly by hand-to-hand contact. Healthy people can occasionally fall prey to *C. diff* infection; however, individuals at greatest risk for contracting *C. diff* are mainly those who are hospitalized or in long-term care (LTC) facilities. Patients who are under a multiple-antibiotic regimen also have an increased chance to be infected, as the wide range of broad-spectrum antibiotics administered will eradicate the "good" intestinal bacteria that can prevent overgrowth of *C. diff*. Other risk factors include (but are not limited to) GI tract surgery, certain diseases of the colon such as inflammatory bowel disease and colorectal cancer, use of chemotherapy drugs, previous infection with *C. diff*, age sixty-five years or older, and kidney disease.

Nursing considerations when caring for a patient presenting to the emergency department for *C. diff* will focus on immediate hydration and pain management. Stabilization of vital signs is required if the patient presents with fever and hematochezia (bright red blood in stool). A CBC as well as a basic metabolic panel (BASEMET or BMP) or comprehensive metabolic panel (COMPMET or CMP) will be collected to determine any metabolic disturbances as a result of frequent diarrhea, and a stool sample may be necessary. A physician will typically prescribe a ten- to fourteen-day course of antibiotic therapy consisting of one of the following: metronidazole (Flagyl®), fidaxomicin (Dificid®), or vancomycin (Vancocin®). An improvement of symptoms will usually occur about 72 hours after starting antibiotics, but diarrhea may still reappear briefly. In addition to prescribed medications, probiotics may also be considered as an alternative treatment. Upon discharge from the health care facility, the patient will need to remember to continue drinking a lot of water to prevent dehydration from recurrent diarrhea (if and when it persists).

Prevention of the illness focuses on excellent hygiene; frequent handwashing after coming into contact with an infected individual, using chlorine bleach-based cleaning agents for home use, and washing soiled clothing with detergent and bleach are a few of the ways to reduce or eliminate the possibility of a *C. diff* infection.

Childhood Diseases

Rubeola (measles), mumps, pertussis (whooping cough), chicken pox (varicella), and diphtheria are all common, contagious viruses that usually strike during childhood.

Measles

Measles (rubeola) is caused by the infectious agent paramyxovirus. It is transmitted via airborne particles and direct contact with infectious droplets, and it also crosses the placental barrier to the fetus. The highest concentration of the measles virus resides in the respiratory tract secretions, blood, or urine of an infected individual. It has an incubation period of ten to twenty days but is considered communicable between four days before the rash appears to five days after. Signs and symptoms of

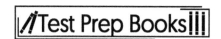

measles virus are fever, malaise, coryza (head cold with a runny nose), cough, conjunctivitis, and a red, erythematous, maculopapular rash. These eruptions normally start on the face and spread downward to the feet and will gradually turn a brownish color. The individual may also display "Koplik's spots," which are small red spots with a bluish-white center and red base, commonly located in the mouth.

Nursing interventions associated with the care of the individual with measles involve the rigorous adherence to airborne droplet and contact precautions if the child is hospitalized, using a cool mist vaporizer for cough and coryza, and administering antipyretics for fever along with vitamin A supplementation, as prescribed.

Mumps

Mumps is another infection caused by paramyxovirus. It is transmitted the same way as measles, with the highest concentration of the virus existing in an infected individual's saliva or urine. The incubation period of the mumps is fourteen to twenty-one days and is communicable immediately before and after the beginning of parotid gland swelling. The patient presenting with mumps will have a fever, headache and malaise, anorexia, jaw or ear pain aggravated by chewing, followed by parotid gland swelling, and orchitis (inflammation of one or both testicles), as well as aseptic meningitis.

When caring for the individual with mumps, the nurse or other health care provider must: Initiate droplet and contact precautions; encourage bedrest until gland edema decreases, as well as a soft or liquid diet to prevent chewing; apply hot or cold compresses as prescribed to the neck area; provide warmth and local support with well-fitting undergarments to relieve pain and discomfort associated with orchitis; and monitor for signs of meningitis.

Pertussis

Pertussis, otherwise referred to as "whooping cough," is caused by the infectious agent *Bordatella pertussis*. It is spread through direct contact or droplets from an infected person and incidental contact with recently tainted items of clothing and bedclothes; the main source of the bacterium is discharge from the respiratory tract of an infected individual. Incubation can be anywhere from five to twenty-one days but is generally ten days. The communicable period is greatest during the time when discharge from respiratory secretions ensues. Physical indicators of pertussis include symptoms of respiratory infection followed by increased severity of cough, with a loud "whooping" respiration, possible cyanosis, respiratory distress, restlessness, irritability, and anorexia.

Implementation of care focuses on compliance with strict airborne and droplet precautions during the catarrhal stage (when respiratory secretion discharge is present), especially if the individual is hospitalized. Administration of antimicrobial therapy as prescribed, reduction of cough-causing environmental factors (dust, smoke, sudden alterations in temperature), and encouragement of adequate hydration and nutrition. Monitoring of vital signs, cardiopulmonary status, and pulse oximetry are other interventions involved.

Chicken Pox

Chicken pox (varicella) is a result of the highly contagious varicella-zoster virus. It is transferred via direct contact, droplet (airborne), and contaminated items. The concentration is greatest in the respiratory tract secretions and skin lesions of the infected individual. Incubation is anywhere from thirteen to seventeen days and is transmissible from one to two days before the onset of the rash to six days after the first vesicles appear and when skin lesion crusts have formed. Signs and symptoms of infection include slight fever, malaise, and anorexia, followed by a macular skin outbreak that first develops on the trunk and scalp and then moves to the face and extremities. The rash may also appear in the mouth and genital and rectal areas. Lesions become eruptions, begin to dry out, and create a crust.

Nursing care involves initiation of severe contact and droplet provisions if the person is hospitalized. At home, the individual must be isolated from others until the vesicles have dried. The antiviral agent acyclovir (Zovirax®) may be used to treat chicken pox in vulnerable immunocompromised individuals to lessen the number of lesions, shorten fever time, and decrease itching, lethargy, and anorexia. The use of VCZ immune globulin (VariZIG®) or IV immune globulin (IVIG) is suggested for immunocompromised children who have no previous history of varicella and are most susceptible to contracting the virus and have complications as a result.

Diphtheria

Diphtheria is caused by the contagious *Corynebacterium diphtheriae* and is virulent during direct contact with the infected person, carrier, or contaminated articles. Its source is the discharge from the mucous membrane of the nose and nasopharynx, skin, and other lesions of the infected. The incubation period is between two and five days, with the transferrable period being variable and dependent on the absence of virulent bacilli (three cultures of discharge from the nose, nasopharynx, skin, and other lesions must be negative), usually two to four weeks.

The person presenting with diphtheria infection will experience a low-grade fever; malaise; sore throat; foul-smelling, mucopurulent nasal discharge; lymphadenitis (inflammation of lymph gland); and neck edema.

Care consists of isolation of the hospitalized individual, administration of antibiotics and diphtheria antitoxin as prescribed (after a skin or conjunctival test to rule out sensitivity to horse serum), and tracheostomy care if a tracheotomy is required.

Herpes Zoster

Herpes zoster, also referred to as shingles, normally attacks individuals with a history of chicken pox infection. It usually occurs in adulthood and is a result of the reactivation of the varicella-zoster virus. The possibility of infection is especially likely in persons who are immunocompromised. Flare-ups occur in a segmental distribution pattern on the skin area along the infected nerve (the once-dormant virus is located in the dorsal nerve root ganglia of the sensory cranial and spinal nerves) and will appear after several days of irritation in the area. It is contagious to those who have never had chicken pox and have not been vaccinated against the virus.

The patient with shingles will present with unilaterally clustered skin lesions along peripheral sensory nerves on the trunk, thorax, or face. The person will generally be suffering fever, malaise, burning and pain in the affected area(s), paresthesia (numbness and tingling), and pruritus. Diagnosis is determined by visual evaluation, Tzanck smear, and a viral culture that is specific to the identification of the causative agent.

When caring for the individual with shingles, the health care professional must isolate the patient (standard and contact precautions) because exudate from the lesions contains the virus. Vital signs, the skin, and the eyes will be monitored for infection. In some cases, skin necrosis may occur. Neurovascular status and seventh cranial nerve function must also be assessed, as Bell's palsy is a potential complication. Another possibility is post-herpetic neuralgia (severe pain), which can remain after the lesions heal. The environment must remain cool, as warmth and touch aggravate the pain. Loose and

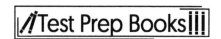

lightweight cotton clothing is encouraged to prevent irritation, and prevention of scratching or rubbing the affected area is key. Patient education revolves around the use of astringent compresses to relieve irritation and promote crust formation and healing, keeping the affected areas clean and dry to prevent infection, and following the prescribed medication regimen (topical treatments, antiviral meds).

Mononucleosis

Mononucleosis is a common infection caused by the Epstein-Barr virus. It is transferrable via direct intimate contact; its most customary source is oral secretions, but it can also be spread through the secretions from the nasal cavity and oropharynx, and sometimes tears. Incubation may be anywhere from four to six weeks, and the communicable period is unknown. It is most often assessed in teenagers and young adults, particularly those who are sexually active. It is important to remember that those who have been exposed to mononucleosis will always carry the virus, even after infection indicators have resolved. Signs and symptoms usually manifest as a high fever, severe sore throat, swollen lymph nodes/tonsils, nausea, abdominal pain, weakness, and fatigue. Hepatosplenomegaly (enlargement of the liver and spleen) may occur, and the patient may also present with a distinct macular rash that is most prominent over the trunk.

Nursing care will involve a complete head-to-toe assessment, comprehensive history and physical, and a CBC. Normally, self-care is sufficient to manage the signs and symptoms of infection, but splenic rupture due to splenomegaly is a possible problem, so the patient should be prohibited from heavy lifting and engaging in any contact sports. Plenty of rest, sore throat lozenges, and Tylenol® or Advil® are encouraged to assist with resolution of residual symptoms.

Multidrug-Resistant Organisms

Multidrug-resistant organisms (MDROs) are defined as bacteria that have become impervious to certain antibiotics and can therefore no longer be used to kill the bacteria. MDROs commonly develop when antibiotics are self-administered longer than necessary or when they are not needed at all but still taken.

Staphylococcus aureus (*S. aureus*) is a bacterium that is generally located on the skin or in the nasal passages of healthy people. When present without symptoms, it is known as colonization, and when symptoms are present, it is an infection. Methicillin-resistant *Staphylococcus aureus* (MRSA) is a strain of *S. aureus* that is resistant to methicillin and most often occurs in individuals who have been hospitalized for an extended period of time or frequently visit a health care facility (hospital acquired) for treatment of an illness (e.g., dialysis).

Infection can also ensue as community-associated MRSA, which occurs in healthy individuals who have not recently been hospitalized or treated for an illness in a facility. People at risk for this type of MRSA consist of athletes, prisoners, daycare attendees, military recruits, IV drug abusers, and those who live in crowded settings, have poor hygiene practices, and are immunocompromised. Community-associated MRSA is communicated through human-to-human contact, contact with MRSA-contaminated items, or infection of a preexisting abrasion or wound that has not been dressed.

MRSA enters the bloodstream via this kind of abrasion and can cause sepsis, cellulitis, endocarditis (inflammation of the inner lining of the heart), osteomyelitis, septic arthritis, toxic shock syndrome, organ failure, and death. Prevention of infection focuses on strict handwashing, practicing good personal hygiene, avoiding sharing personal items (toothbrushes, mouth guards, clothing, bedclothes), and thoroughly cleansing an abrasion or wound.

The individual infected with MRSA will present with a fever and the appearance of an erythematous, edematous skin area, which is warm to the touch, painful, and draining pus. A more severe infection will manifest as the previously described rash, chest pain, cough, fatigue, chills, fever, malaise, headache, muscle aches, and shortness of breath.

Interventions to be implemented upon initiating care for the individual infected with MRSA consist of a detailed assessment of skin lesions; anticipation of drainage of an infected skin site and culturing of secretions; preparation of blood, sputum, and urine culture; administration of antibiotics; and in-depth education of the patient and caregivers with regard to causes and modes of transmission, signs and symptoms, and the importance of adherence to recommended treatment measures.

Vancomycin-resistant enterococci (VRE) are enterococci that have developed a resistance to many antibiotics, particularly vancomycin. Enterococci live in the intestines and on the skin and normally do not cause any issues until they become unaffected by certain antibiotic therapies. Common sites of infection include the intestines, the urinary tract, and wounds. VRE, similar to many other bacteria, can be spread by casual contact or contact with contaminated objects. Akin to MRSA, VRE are most commonly communicated from a health care worker to those who are hospitalized or in a nursing home. Additionally, those who are immunocompromised, have long-term illnesses, have had a major surgery, or have been treated with multiple antibiotics have a greater chance of becoming infected. Understandably, VRE seem to prevail most heavily in individuals who have used vancomycin often.

Healthy people are at little to no risk for infection by VRE, and even if one has been exposed to VRE or the bacteria are present in his or her system, subsequent illness from infection is rare. Hindrance of VRE infection is maintained through the use of a strict handwashing regimen; using alcohol-based hand sanitizers; keeping skin abrasions clean, dry, and covered with a bandage; and avoiding other people's wounds. Refraining from sharing personal items such as towels and razors can prevent infection with VRE, as well as keeping one's living environment clean by disinfecting all frequently used surfaces (doorknobs, light switches, kitchen counter tops, refrigerator handles, cabinet knobs and drawer handles, faucet handles, and bathroom counter tops). When prescribed antibiotics, one should take them as recommended and be mindful that, while antibiotics can help treat a bacterial infection, they do not cure viral infections.

Signs and symptoms of a VRE infection depend largely on where the infection is located. If VRE are present in a wound, the affected area will be erythematous and painful to the touch. One who is suffering a urinary tract infection caused by VRE will exhibit flank pain and burning and pain upon urination. Some people have general symptoms such as fever, diarrhea, and generalized weakness.

Diagnosis of VRE starts with a blood, wound culture, urine, or stool sample to determine the cause of the illness. Severe VRE infections are treated with caution, and the hospitalized individual is isolated to prevent the spread of infection to others. Health care providers entering the room of the infected should don a disposable gown and gloves and remove them before exiting the room. VRE infections, by nature, are difficult to manage due to the antibiotic resistance of the strain. Antibiotic treatment may consist of oral agents as well as IV, and blood, urine, and stool samples will be sent to the lab for testing after initiation of antibiotic therapy to determine if VRE bacteria are still present in the body.

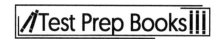

Tuberculosis (TB)

Tuberculosis (TB) is a highly communicable disease caused by the infectious bacteria *Mycobacterium tuberculosis*. *M. tuberculosis* is an acid-fast rod that secretes niacin; when the bacteria reach a vulnerable site, they multiply quickly. Because it is an aerobic bacterium, meaning it grows in the presence of oxygen, it principally affects the upper lobes of the lungs where the O_2 concentration is the greatest. It can also affect the brain, intestines, peritoneum, kidneys, joints, and liver. It is transmitted via the airborne route, with the primary source of the bacterium being saliva and lung secretions. TB has a dangerous onset, and many individuals are not aware of infection until it is well advanced. TB infection progresses as follows:

- Infected droplets enter the lungs, and the bacteria form a tubercle lesion.

- The body's defense systems capture the tubercle, leaving a blemish.

- If capture does not occur, the bacteria may enter the lymph system and travel to the lymph nodes, causing an inflammatory response called granulomatous inflammation.

- Initial lesions form and may become dormant, but can be revived and become a secondary infection when re-exposure to the bacterium occurs.

- Once active, TB is known to cause necrosis and cavitation (formation of a hole) in the lesions, which leads to rupture, the spread of necrotic tissue, and destruction to various areas of the body.

Rapid identification of those in close contact with the infected individual is important so that they may be tested and receive necessary treatment, and once identified, they will be assessed with a tuberculin skin test and chest x-rays to determine if they have been infected with TB. The risk of transmission of the infection is significantly decreased once the infected individual has been taking TB medication for two to three weeks.

TB infection generally manifests as fatigue, lethargy, anorexia, weight loss, low-grade fever, chills, night sweats, incessant cough with the production of mucoid and mucopurulent sputum (sometimes blood streaked), chest tightness, and a dull, aching chest pain. In the advanced stages of the illness, dullness with percussion over affected parenchymal areas, bronchial breath sounds, rhonchi, and crackles will be present. Partial obstruction of a bronchus caused by endobronchial disease or compression by edematous lymph nodes may create localized wheezing and dyspnea.

The main goals of treatment involve preventing transmission, managing symptoms, and inhibiting progression of the disease. Diagnosis consists of many factors, including collection of an all-inclusive patient history, which will detail the following:

- History of TB exposure

- Country of origin and travel to regions in which the incidence of TB is increased

- Recent history of flu, pneumonia, febrile illness, or foul-smelling sputum production

- Previous tests performed to determine the presence of *M. tuberculosis* in the body and the results of those tests

- Recent bacilli Calmette-Guerin vaccine, a vaccine that contains attenuated (dead) tubercle bacilli and is usually administered to those who reside in foreign countries or are traveling to foreign countries to create increased resistance to TB

Diagnostic efforts will also revolve around results of a physical examination of the chest, auscultation of breath sounds, and inquiring about chest tightness or a dull, achy chest pain. A chest x-ray is not considered a definitive diagnostic tool, but the presence of multinodular infiltrates with deposits of calcium phosphate in the upper lung lobes is suggestive of TB. If the disease is active, it will appear on a chest x-ray as lung inflammation, and it will form a TB-specific necrosis, in which diseased tissue devolves into a firm, dry mass (caseation), also apparent on an x-ray.

Additionally, the attending physician will most likely order a specific blood analysis test to determine the presence of TB in the body (QuantiFERON-TB Gold). This test is quite sensitive and rapid, and results can be available in as little as 24 hours. Sputum cultures positive for *M. tuberculosis* are considered confirmatory of the diagnosis, and after the administration of medications has begun, sputum samples are obtained again to establish the effectiveness of therapy. A positive TB skin test does not mean that active TB is present, but it is indicative of previous exposure or the presence of inactive disease. Once it is positive, it will remain so throughout an individual's lifetime.

Once diagnosis has confirmed infection, the patient with active TB infection is admitted and placed under airborne isolation precautions in a negative-pressure room (to maintain this, the room door must be tightly closed). The room should have at least six exchanges of fresh air per hour and be ventilated to the outside, if possible. The patient's nurse wears a particulate respirator (special individually fitted mask) and a gown when the probability of clothing contamination exists. Thorough handwashing is required before and after caring for the patient, as well as after leaving his or her room. The patient should be required to wear a surgical mask if he or she needs to leave the room for a test or procedure. Respiratory isolation is discontinued after the patient is no longer considered contagious.

The medications used for active TB infection consist of first-line and second-line drugs. First-line medications include isoniazid, rifampin, ethambutol, pyrazinamide, rifabutin, and rifapentine. These medications provide the most effective anti-TB activity. Second-line agents (amikacin, ciprofloxacin, and kanamycin) are used in conjunction with first-line agents but are more toxic to the body's systems. Active TB is treated with a combination of medications to which it is vulnerable, and this approach is instituted because of resistant strains of the organism.

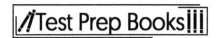

Education upon discharge consists of the following:

- Providing the patient and caregivers with information about TB and allaying concerns about the contagious aspect of the illness

- Encouraging the patient to follow the medication regimen exactly as prescribed

- Advising the patient that the medication regimen is continued over a six- to twelve-month period, depending on the situation

- Informing the patient of the side effects/adverse effects of the medications and ways to minimize them to maintain compliance

- Instructing the patient to resume activities gradually, as he or she is still in the recovery period

- Instructing the patient to cover his or her mouth and nose when coughing/sneezing and to place used tissues into plastic bags for disposal

- Informing the patient that a sputum culture is necessary every two to four weeks once medication therapy is initiated, and once the results of three consecutive cultures (about three months of treatment) are negative, he or she is no longer considered infectious

- Advising the patient to avoid excessive exposure to silicone or dust because these materials can cause further lung damage

- Informing the patient of the importance of compliance with treatment, follow-up care, and collection of sputum cultures as prescribed

Practice Questions

1. A 64-year-old Caucasian male enters the emergency department with a burn to his left forearm. You notice that the top layer of skin is discolored and darkened and has started to peel off. He is also complaining of "not being able to feel my arm." You know, based on the initial physical assessment and his complaints, that he is suffering from which of the following?
    a. A second-degree burn
    b. A third-degree burn
    c. A first-degree burn
    d. A fourth-degree burn

2. During the emergent phase of a burn injury, which of the following might a nurse expect to see?
    a. Decreased blood pressure
    b. Increased urine output
    c. Decreased heart rate
    d. Pink skin

3. A 22-year-old female presents with severe burns covering the neck, chest, and abdomen. Which of the following statements is correct and applicable to this patient?
    a. Burns in that area are associated with hepatic issues and the nurse should expect to see jaundice.
    b. Burns in that area are associated with ocular issues and the nurse should expect to see corneal abrasion.
    c. Burns in that area are associated with pulmonary issues and the nurse should expect to see difficulty breathing.
    d. Burns in that area are associated with vascular compromise issues and the nurse should expect to see compartment syndrome.

4. A frantic woman calls the emergency department and tells you that she caught her two-year-old son drinking bleach from under the kitchen sink. What should you tell her to do *first*?
    a. "Try to make him throw up."
    b. "Call the Poison Control Center."
    c. "See if he will drink some water."
    d. "Bring him to the ER."

5. A 12-year-old male comes into the ER with vomiting and bloody diarrhea. From the patient history that his father is able to give, yesterday the boy drank some milk from the cow on their farm. Based on this information, you know that he is most likely infected with which of the following?
    a. *Escherichia coli*
    b. *Salmonella*
    c. *Clostridium botulinum*
    d. *Giardia lamblia*

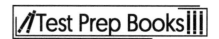

6. A 26-year-old woman wanders into the emergency department shivering and babbling incoherently. You know that it has been raining outside, it's cold, and the woman's clothing is soaked through. You recognize this as hypothermia, and after you escort her to a warm room and remove her wet clothing, what is the next thing you should do?

    a. Give her something warm to drink.

    b. Wrap a warm, dry blanket around her.

    c. Assess her vital signs.

    d. Warm her chest, neck, abdomen, and groin with an electric blanket or some other warming device.

7. A 40-year-old male presents to the ED with large blisters covering all the toes of his right foot. He tells you that he is homeless, has no shoes, and has had prolonged exposure to outside's freezing temperatures, especially at night. You ascertain from this information that he is suffering from which of the following?

    a. Second-degree frostbite

    b. Fourth-degree frostbite

    c. First-degree frostbite

    d. Third-degree frostbite

8. A man approaches you in the emergency room with complaints of malaise, insomnia, and difficulty swallowing. You notice that while he's speaking, he is drooling and keeps wiping his mouth. He says he was hunting yesterday and was bitten on his ankle by a fox. Based on his symptoms, you deduce that he is most likely infected with which of the following?

    a. Zika virus

    b. Rabies

    c. Rocky Mountain spotted fever

    d. Lyme disease

9. A 17-year-old girl is admitted to the ER with a moderate burn to her left hand. She tells you that she was cleaning the toilet with a chemical toilet-bowl cleaner and accidentally spilled some on her hand. She shows you the bottle, and you notice that one of the active ingredients is sulfuric acid. She said that she called Poison Control as soon as the spill happened. You know that they told her to initially do which of the following?

    a. "Rinse it with water first."

    b. "Treat the affected area with rubbing alcohol first."

    c. "Flush the area with a mild soapy solution first."

    d. "Just continue to evaluate the affected area for pain, redness, or blistering."

10. A 53-year-old woman presents to the ED complaining of generalized weakness, dizziness, and difficulty breathing. You collect a patient history, and she discloses that she frequently consumes apricot seeds as a snack and has done so for the past 15 years pretty regularly. You suspect, based on this information, that she has fallen victim to which of the following?

    a. Carbon monoxide poisoning

    b. Food poisoning

    c. Alcohol poisoning

    d. Cyanide poisoning

11. A mother brings her 15-year-old son into the emergency room with a fever, headache, and swelling around his neck. She tells you that she remembers catching her son deeply kissing his girlfriend about two weeks ago. After completing a detailed patient history and head-to-toe assessment, you ascertain that he may be suffering from the mumps. After speaking with the attending ED physician, you notice that he orders airborne/droplet precautions. What else should the physician order?

    a. Resumption of normal activity once stabilized

    b. Regular diet

    c. Soft or liquid diet

    d. Four-point restraints, in case patient becomes delirious and combative

12. Why is it MOST important to educate the patient recovering from mononucleosis about refraining from heavy lifting?

    a. The patient needs to rest as much as possible to facilitate healing.

    b. Heavy lifting may exacerbate residual symptoms.

    c. Straining from heavy lifting may trigger a vasovagal response.

    d. Splenic rupture due to hepatosplenomegaly is a concern.

13. *Mycobacterium tuberculosis* is an aerobic bacterium. What does this mean?

    a. It can sustain itself without the presence of oxygen.

    b. It grows in the presence of oxygen.

    c. It cannot detoxify oxygen.

    d. It does not use dissolved oxygen for its metabolic reactions.

14. While collecting a history and physical of a patient who may be infected with tuberculosis (TB), the nurse would ask all EXCEPT for which of the following?

    a. "Have you ever been exposed to tuberculosis?"

    b. "Have you traveled outside the country to places where TB is prevalent?"

    c. "Have you noticed that your appetite has increased lately?"

    d. "Have you recently had the flu, pneumonia, or foul-smelling saliva?"

15. You are discharging a patient who was hospitalized for TB infection. During the education of the patient, you inform the patient that he or she will no longer be considered infectious after how many negative sputum cultures?

    a. Three

    b. Four

    c. Two

    d. Six

Answer Explanations

1. B: Third-degree burns are characterized by darkened, dead tissue (eschar) that must be peeled or scrubbed off for the healing process to begin. There is also reduced or absent sensations due to nerve damage and decreased blood supply. A second-degree burn is deep, but loss of sensation in the affected area doesn't occur. A first-degree burn affects only the top layer of skin, and a fourth-degree burn extends through all skin layers, and there is no pain due to the destruction of nerve endings.

2. A: In the emergent phase, hypovolemic shock is a potential issue due to excessive fluid and/or blood loss, which will cause a drop in blood pressure. Increased urine output is unlikely unless the patient is in fluid overload. With a drop in blood pressure, heart rate will increase due to increased myocardial contractility, and vasoconstriction will occur. A person in hypovolemic shock will have pale, clammy skin due to decreased fluid or blood volume in the body.

3. C: Burns of the head, neck, and chest are associated with pulmonary issues. No hepatic insufficiency would be displayed with a burn of this type, but it may if a deep burn is sustained in the abdominal area. Corneal abrasions are most common when a direct burn to the face and eyes has occurred. Circumferential burns of the extremities can create a tourniquet-like effect and lead to vascular compromise.

4. B: The Poison Control Center is most appropriate, as different substances require different interventions. Induced vomiting of a caustic substance will cause more damage to the esophagus and throat. Water can dilute the bleach but would not be the initial thing to do. Bringing the child to the ER is not appropriate unless Poison Control recommends doing so.

5. A: Some of the main sources of *E. coli* are undercooked ground beef and unpasteurized milk or dairy products. *Salmonella* infection usually occurs when food has been tainted with fecal matter (fecal-oral route). *Clostridium botulinum* mainly comes from improperly canned foods, smoked or salted fish, and other foods kept too long at warm temperatures. The primary sources of *Giardia lamblia* are raw produce and contaminated, untreated water. It can also be spread by an infected food handler.

6. D: After the patient has been relocated to a warmer room and wet clothes have been removed, his or her core should immediately be warmed with a warming device. Giving something warm to drink is helpful, but should occur only after the core temperature has begun to stabilize. Vital signs at this point wouldn't be assessed; temperature needs to have an opportunity to become stable. Wrapping a warm, dry blanket around the patient should happen after a significant amount of time is spent increasing core body temperature; the patient should initially be warmed from the inside out, not the other way around.

7. A: Second-degree frostbite presents as large, fluid-filled blisters with partial-thickness skin necrosis. Fourth-degree frostbite has no blistering or edema, and there is full-thickness necrosis. The signs of first-degree frostbite are a whitish plaque area surrounded by hyperemia and edema. Third-degree frostbite consists of small hemorrhagic blisters, followed by eschar formation.

8. B: Rabies infection presents as generalized poor feeling, difficulty sleeping and swallowing, and hypersalivation. Most people infected with the Zika virus will only have mild symptoms, if any. Rocky Mountain spotted fever originates from a tick from a mammal and usually presents as headache, vomiting, and a petechial (spotty) rash around the wrists and ankles, and the signs and symptoms could take as long as 14 days to appear. Lyme disease has similar characteristics to rabies, but normally results from the bite of an infected tick, rarely a wild animal.

9. C: Because the agent contains sulfuric acid, Poison Control would advise the patient to rinse the affected area with a mild, soapy solution, as straight water will make the injury feel hot and may possibly do more damage. Rubbing alcohol is effective in treating a hydrofluoric acid burn, not sulfuric acid. Interval assessment of the affected area, without treatment, will most likely cause further damage, as a burn of this sort must be cared for immediately.

10. D: Cyanide occurs naturally in apricot seeds, and the patient has consumed them quite frequently for over a decade. Carbon monoxide poisoning can manifest itself in many different ways, depending on how much is absorbed by the body. Food poisoning signs and symptoms usually consist of nausea, vomiting, and diarrhea, but not necessarily weakness and difficulty breathing. Alcohol poisoning will usually manifest as decreased respirations (less than eight breaths per minute), vomiting, blue-tinged or pale skin, and unconsciousness.

11. C: A soft or liquid diet is recommended to reduce jaw or ear pain that is caused by edematous parotid glands. Even if the patient is stable, he or she is encouraged to rest until gland edema subsides. A regular diet is not appropriate here, as chewing exacerbates jaw and neck pain. There is no indication for four-point restraints, as a mumps infection does not generally cause agitation, delirium, or combative behavior.

12. D: Hepatosplenomegaly is a potential issue among those infected with mononucleosis, so splenic rupture is a definite possibility, and one should refrain from heavy lifting or contact sports. Rest is encouraged after mononucleosis infection, but it is not the most important reason for refraining from heavy lifting. Residual symptoms are common, but they usually consist of a slightly sore throat and weakness; heavy lifting isn't considered a factor. A vasovagal response is possible but is normally triggered by prolonged standing and straining while moving bowels and not necessarily lifting heavy objects.

13. B: Aerobic bacteria grow in the presence of oxygen, while anaerobic bacteria can grow without available oxygen. Aerobic bacteria can actually detoxify oxygen through the use of certain enzymes to convert superoxide (an oxygen derivative, which is toxic to all organisms) to oxygen and hydrogen peroxide. Aerobic bacteria need oxygen for metabolic reactions, while anaerobic bacteria do not.

14. C: One of the symptoms in TB infection is anorexia, or decreased appetite. The individual will also most likely exhibit a significant drop in weight. A comprehensive health history will inquire about past exposure to TB; recent travel to countries where TB is increased; and history of influenza, pneumonia, or foul-smelling sputum.

15. A: The patient recovering from tuberculosis is considered noninfectious after about three months of treatment, or when the results of three consecutive sputum cultures are negative. Four- and six-month cultures are not generally done, and two cultures are too few to determine whether the patient is still contagious.

Professional Issues

Nurse

Critical Incident Stress Management

The Critical Incident Stress Management (CISM) model is a framework that nursing staff can use to manage stress that results from working with emergency cases, which can often be horrific in nature, long, complex, and taxing on the nursing staff's physical, emotional, and mental health. Beyond providing routine medical care, nurses are also often tasked with comforting the patient and the patient's family, whose lives have been altered. The CISM model includes a progressive series of stress management tools to help alleviate the acute stress that nursing staff may feel during emergency cases, and to provide tools for maintaining their health and wellness moving forward.

Pre-Crisis Stage Intervention is the first stage of the model. It is an educational activity that occurs before patients are seen, and allows the nursing staff time to physically relax and mentally prepare for the challenges of a traumatic case. Additionally, nursing staff may learn coping mechanisms that they can hopefully revisit should they feel overwhelmed during or after the case. This can include tools like short meditations, breathing techniques that soothe the central nervous system, and maintaining emotional boundaries from their work. Acute Crisis Stage Intervention is the next stage of the model, which occurs right after the case arrives into the department and the situation has been assessed. This can be a short period—under twenty minutes—that allows nursing staff to come together, communicate any personal or professional concerns related to the case, and work as a team to determine next steps for treatment.

If possible, some time may be set after this meeting to allow the team to process any mental, emotional, or physical discomfort they may be experiencing. At the end of the day, it is recommended that the team come together again for approximately an hour to discuss the nursing staff's emotions from the day and to provide tools for any prolonged emotional duress they may be experiencing. This session is referred to as defusing. However, group meetings that take place a few days later, or between a single nurse and a staff leader, can also provide therapeutic benefit. These meetings should allow nursing staff that were part of traumatic cases to openly express their concerns, discuss the emotions they feel from working on such cases, and to receive support from their colleagues and leaders. Finally, these events can also extend to the families of the nursing staff. Families may benefit from receiving tools that help them support the nurse, and to help the family unit cope with the demands of a physically and emotionally demanding career.

Finally, Post-Crisis Stage Intervention refers to situations where some weeks have passed but staff members still feel affected by a certain incident. In this stage, professional psychological services may be useful.

Ethical Dilemmas

Healthcare providers routinely face situations with patients where they must analyze various moral and ethical considerations. In the emergency department, where quick judgment and action is necessary to care and where patients are often not fully sound in body or mind, ethical dilemmas can arise without much time to process resolutions.

The Emergency Nurses Association adheres to an established Code of Ethics, which states moral and ethical guidelines that nurses should incorporate into their practice. Above all else, nurses have the responsibility to do no harm while advocating for, promoting good health outcomes for, minimizing injury to, and protecting the overall health and function of their patients. It is important to consider the patient holistically when applying these values, such as considering what the patient may view as a good quality of life, what family values the patient holds, other family members that may be affected (such as a spouse or children), legal considerations, and logistical considerations (such as how much time and medical resources are available). When patients are unable to make decisions autonomously, or even to indicate consent to treatment (as can be common in emergency cases), nurses should act from these responsibilities to make wise and compassionate decisions on the patients' behalf.

Dilemmas that can arise for nursing staff include situations where the patient may have cultural or personal beliefs that prevent lifesaving treatment. For example, a female emergency patient may not want to be treated by any male staff, or a patient that needs a blood transfusion may not accept this procedure due to religious beliefs. In cases where the patient is able to directly communicate their wishes, the nurse may need to defer to the patient's wishes in order to preserve the patient's autonomy. This may mean providing alternative means of care (such as finding available female medical providers to assist with the female patient that does not wanted to be treated by male staff). It may mean withholding treatment that the patient refuses.

If the patient's life is in question and rapid medical action is necessary to save the patient's life, nursing staff may need to intervene even if it is against the patient's wishes. Ethical considerations like these will vary by case and patient, and will depend on the severity of the case, the medical and personal history of the patient, and the judgment of the nurse in question. In all cases, it is ideal if the nurse and patient are able to communicate openly with each other about the case and potential medical options, and hope that the resolution is able to be for the greatest good.

Evidence-Based Practice

Evidence-based practice (EBP) is a research-driven and facts-based methodology that allows healthcare providers to make scientifically supported, reliable, and validated decisions in delivering care. EBP takes into account rigorously tested, peer-reviewed, and published research relating to the case, the knowledge and experience of the healthcare provider, and clinical guidelines established by reputable governing bodies. This framework allows healthcare providers to reach case resolutions that result in positive patient outcomes in the most efficient manner, therefore allowing the organization to provide the best care using the least resources.

There are seven steps to successfully utilizing EBP as a methodology in the nursing field. First, the work culture should be one of a "spirit of inquiry." This culture allows staff to ask questions to promote continuous improvement and positive process change to workflow, clinical routines, and non-clinical duties.

Second, the PICOT framework should be utilized when searching for an effective intervention, or working with a specific interest, in a case. The PICOT framework encourages nurses to develop a specific, measurable, goal-oriented research question that accounts for the patient population and demographics (P) involved in the case, the proposed intervention or issue of interest (I), a relevant comparison (C) group in which a defined outcomes (O) has been positive, and the amount of time (T) needed to implement the intervention or address the issue.

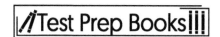

Once this question has been developed, staff can move onto the third step, which is to research. In this step, staff will explore reputable sources of literature (such as peer-reviewed scholarly journals, interviews with subject matter experts, or widely accepted textbooks) to find studies and narratives with evidence that supports a resolution for their question.

Once all research has been compiled, it must be thoroughly analyzed. This is the fourth step. This step ensures that the staff is using unbiased research with stringent methodology, statistically significant outcomes, reliable and valid research designs, and that all information collected is actually applicable to their patient. (For example, if a certain treatment worked with statistical significance in a longitudinal study of pediatric patients with a large sample size, and all other influencing variables were controlled, this treatment may not necessarily work in a middle-aged adult. Therefore, though the research collected is scientifically backed and evidence-based for a pediatric population, it does not support EBP for an older population.)

The fifth step is to integrate the evidence to create a treatment or intervention plan for the patient.

The sixth step is to monitor the implementation of the treatment or intervention and evaluate whether it was associated with positive health outcomes in the patient.

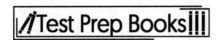

Finally, practitioners have a moral obligation to share the results with colleagues at the organization and across the field, so that it may be best utilized (or not) for other patients.

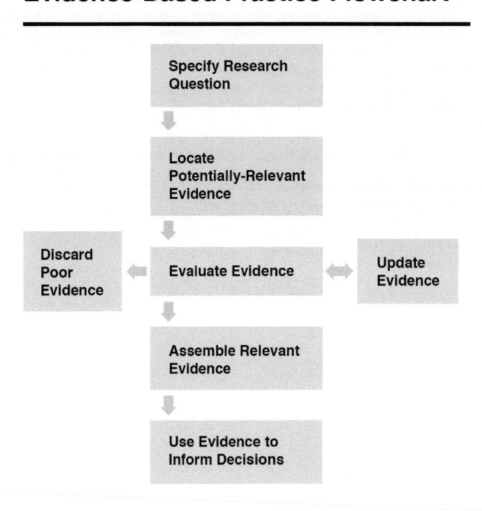

Lifelong Learning

Since the medical and healthcare fields are always rapidly changing due to technological advances, new research, organizational and governmental regulations, and through continuous process improvements in healthcare delivery, nurses can expect to continue their education throughout the course of their careers. Consequently, the ability to learn new topics will be a necessary skill in order to remain a competent practitioner. Lifelong learning and continuing education are associated with improved patient outcomes, job satisfaction, personal validation and achievement, and obtaining skills that were not taught or available at the time that the nurse was enrolled in a formal education program. The most crucial association with lifelong learning activities is the improvement in quality of care. Incompetent or unaware nursing staff means a great deal of risk for the patient. By constantly striving to improve their knowledge and practical skills, nurses decrease the chance that they will be held liable for negligence or

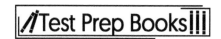

malpractice, and they are taking tangible actions to adhere to the ethical tenets of the healthcare profession.

While avenues to continue professional development in the nursing field may be formal (such as obtaining extra relevant degrees or certifications, publishing research, or enrolling in trainings offered by the nurse's workplace), many opportunities require intrinsic motivation, such as taking personal initiative to keep abreast of current relevant literature, consulting with mentors, or experiencing different responsibilities within the field. However, even with these varied opportunities and with the multitude of personal and professional benefits that engaging in lifelong learning activities bring, there are still some barriers for nurses. These include obstacles like disinterest, lack of time on the job or outside of the job to participate in activities, an inability to balance work and life needs with job demands, and lack of financial resources (to pay for educational activities and/or to take the time off to participate in them). In this regard, it is helpful for leadership and subordinate employees to work together to overcome these barriers.

Nurses who are in positions of leadership can help push for organizational support for development activities, and promote a culture of top-down change and support. In the events that development activities are free or hosted by the nurse's workplace, it is imperative that the nurse realizes this is a valuable opportunity and take the time to attend and fully engage in the experience. This shows that such activities are in demand and valued, and is likely to make affordable and accessible professional development activities part of the workplace culture.

Research

Nursing research is a crucial component of EBP, high quality healthcare delivery, and positive patient outcomes. Effective nursing research creates and compiles bodies of knowledge relating to all clinical and non-clinical aspects of nursing. Nurses who play a role in nursing research are typically advanced-level, senior practitioners who have the necessary experience to contribute further to existing bodies of nursing knowledge through personal expertise, the ability to run or be involved in conducting research trials, and in accurately collecting and analyzing data.

Nurse researchers typically have advanced educational degrees, such as a Master's or doctorate degree, and may work in specialized fields as a nurse practitioner. However, as entry-level nurses spend more time and gain more exposure to different aspects of the field, they should keep in mind that a nurse researcher is a highly skilled and rewarding career path that is critical to the development and advancement of the nursing field. High quality nursing research shapes the scope of clinical education for entry-level and experienced nurses; influences healthcare policy at the local, state, and federal levels; and enhances standard operating procedures within a healthcare organization. Together, these allow for organizations to deliver the highest level of care to patients who need them at the lowest costs.

Nurses who choose to pursue research as a career can expect to become involved in different aspects of research design and the research process. Nurse researchers will need to pass training modules that review the legalities and ethics of working with human populations in research, which is a different avenue than treating patients for disease or injury. Nurse researchers can expect to learn how to write research proposals, which serves as a large component of applying for funding, in addition to becoming familiar with seeking out viable funding sources. Depending on the end goal of the study, nurse researchers may learn how to design objective study trials, collect data through laboratory work or through sample surveys, conduct and interpret statistical data analysis, and write conclusive discussions about their findings. Upon completion, nurse researchers can expect to be involved in the publication process, where a formal manuscript detailing the design and findings of the research study are submitted to scholarly journals. Journals often require extensive revisions and editing, so nurses should be prepared to follow up with their manuscripts.

Most research projects include collaboration with doctorate-level researchers from other disciplines who share a vested interest in the topic or have skills to contribute to the project. For example, health research teams often include a biostatistician whose primary contribution is to compile, analyze, and interpret collected data. Entry-level nurses, interns, or students may choose to assist with simpler, but necessary, tasks such as survey administration or data entry. Recruiting individuals to help with these sorts of tasks can provide a great support to the research team.

The National League for Nursing (NLN) is an organization in the United States that promotes research activities through networking, support, guidelines, and funding. The NLN publishes research priorities every four years. Current priorities include further investigating evidence-based practices, promoting research exposure to student learners in order to set the foundation for health promotion and disease prevention, and evaluating best practices relating to end-of-life and other life transitional care for both patients and their families. The NLN's website, www.nln.org, is an excellent resource for current nurses to find continuing education opportunities and explore research tools to support and enhance their career paths.

Patient

Discharge Planning

Nurses are commonly tasked with discharge planning—the set of procedures that guide patient experiences once they have received written clearance by a physician to leave the medical facility. This transition is a critical one for the patient, who may be physiologically able to leave the inpatient setting, but may still require physical and psychological follow-up care in the home. Additionally, some patients may transition to another department, a rehabilitation facility, a hospice home, or somewhere else that is not their primary residence. The patient may also require medical appointments at regular intervals to monitor recovery. Finally, caregivers of the patient may also need counseling on this transition.

Effective discharge planning covers several different areas with the primary goals of ensuring a stress-free transition for the patient and decreasing the chance that the patient will need to be readmitted for any issues related to their current medical case. Discharge planning should begin with noting the health status of the patient, ideally by an interdisciplinary group of healthcare providers. This analysis should be discussed in detail with the patient and any relevant caregivers, with ample opportunity for both the patient and the caregiver(s) to discuss any questions or concerns. Assuming all questions and concerns have been discussed satisfactorily, logistical planning for the transition can begin. This may include determining how and where the patient will be physically moved, what equipment or medical staff may be needed in the next place that the patient will be residing, instructions for caregivers, and instructions for the patients. If extra support or professional support is needed after discharge, the nurse should provide referral information or arrange the referral for the patient. Finally, any follow-up appointments should be scheduled and reminder cards provided.

Poor discharge planning that is conducted without reviewing these options or done in a rushed manner can result in poor patient satisfaction, poor patient health outcomes, re-admittance, and/or costly medical errors. Having strict and standardized operating procedures for discharge planning in which all

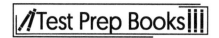

medical staff are cross-trained can help the overall process be comprehensive and beneficial for both the patient and the organization.

End of Life Issues

End of life issues can be complicated from both a logistical and an emotional perspective. For many patients, end of life issues may not have been discussed or resolved with family members; a nurse or other medical staff member may have to step in the role of facilitating this sensitive subject. Even when the situation has been planned for, it can come unexpectedly for both the patient and family members. Most end of life situations will require managing the physical and emotional pain of the patient and family members, helping the patient transition in a dignified manner, and dealing with legal paperwork. Many healthcare providers report not feeling emotionally equipped to handle these aspects, do not feel they have time on the job to adequately do so, or feel there is no financial compensation to provide these services. Being aware that job duties may require these uncomfortable tasks can be the first step in being able to provide some level of effective end of life support for the patient and family. Understanding common end of life issues can also help.

Organ donation and tissue donation refer to the process of removing healthy, functional organs or tissues from the patient's body after death and transplanting them to another patient in need. This may be a topic that the patient has already considered; for example, many people make this decision when applying for a driver's license and have it notated on their card. Common organs that can be donated include the heart, lungs, liver, and kidneys. Common tissues that can be donated include heart, skin, components of the eyeball, and bone.

Advanced directives are legal documents that note how a patient would like to receive or guide medical treatments in the case of terminal cases, cases where the patient is in a vegetative state, or in other end of life contexts. Having this document prepared in advance is extremely helpful for healthcare providers and the patient's family, as the patient's personal decisions are known and can be accounted for. However, many people do not take the time to develop these. Advance directives may only be utilized when a physician has declared the patient to be in an end of life state. Other rules may vary by state, so it is useful to be informed of the particular guidelines set forth by the state in which providers are practicing. In emergency cases, support staff do not usually have the legal rights to follow instructions written in an advanced directive until a physician confirms that the patient will not recover. Therefore, support staff must continue to provide comprehensive, life-sustaining care unless otherwise instructed.

More healthcare organizations are beginning to allow family members to be present during end of life procedures, including intense procedures that can be harrowing to watch. New research shows this can be beneficial for family members as they cope in the long-term. While remaining present with the patient is often the wish of family members, they may be unaware of the emotional upheaval they may feel when watching a loved one go through resuscitative procedures. Nursing staff should be equipped to be able to continue working even with the presence of distraught family members, and be able to provide compassionate and honest support if needed.

Withholding and withdrawing treatments are a component of palliative care. They are most commonly seen in tragic, traumatic events or in hospice care. These procedures occur when a patient is believed to be terminal, and interventions that were previously being utilized to sustain the patient are gradually ceased in order to let the patient pass comfortably. Withholding and withdrawing treatments are often requested by patients who are aware of their situation and are ready to move on, but may also be done at the request of family members or medical proxy if the patient is in a vegetative state.

Forensic Evidence Collection

The emergency department often sees patients who are victims of criminal activities that are still under investigation. Therefore, nursing staff play a role in collecting and submitting appropriate evidence to the necessary authorities. While forensic nursing is a specialty skill, all nurses should have some knowledge of how to identify and distribute important forensic evidence. Overlooking forensic evidence on a victim could affect the outcome of a prosecution.

Collecting forensic evidence often begins in the emergency department. If possible, nurses should obtain informed consent from the patient and explain to them what kind of evidence they will be searching for and collecting, and to whom the evidence will be submitted. If a nurse is able to establish good rapport with the patient, the patient may feel ready to share sensitive information about the case that the nurse can document, such as details relating to the reason for the visit or to the alleged assailant. It is also important to document if the patient seems uncomfortable to share information or will not do so.

The most common forensic evidence tool is photography. With consent, nurses may choose to photograph physical abuse, damaged accessories, injuries, or other images that appear out of the ordinary. Notes submitted with the photograph should confirm details like date, time, physical area, and bodily structures involved. Nurses should be mindful to preserve the patient's dignity during this process.

Next, nurses may be able to collect different biological and organic agents from the patient, such as tissue and fluid samples, hair or debris (especially if it does not seem to be an article that belongs to the patient), and pieces of clothing that appear to be torn or stained. Non-biological pieces of evidence, such as bullets, may also be collected. The medical organization should have sterile tweezers with which to handle these items, and sterile bags in which to place these pieces of evidence.

Finally, nurses who work with victims of criminal activities should be able and willing to testify in court, and discuss any forensic evidence that was collected.

Pain Management and Procedural Sedation

Pain is the most commonly seen symptom in the emergency department, as most emergency situations cases cause patients to have a high level of pain. However, since cases in the emergency department often vary widely in scope and every patient will have a different personal threshold for pain tolerance, best practices are difficult to develop when it comes to pain management. It is often done on a case by case basis. However, when a patient's pain is not managed in a way that seems appropriate to that individual, it can cause patient and family dissatisfaction in the healthcare organization. As a result, medical staff must try to provide effective and safe pain management options that can make the patient comfortable at the present time, but that also do not cause harm over time. In some cases, like a sprained muscle, ice therapy and time can provide adequate pain management. More serious cases, defined as pain that does not subside after an objectively reasonable period of time for the injury, may require topical, intramuscular, or oral pain medication. These can include stronger doses of common over-the-counter pain medications, or prescription pain medications.

Prescription pain medications, especially opioids and muscle relaxers, are known for causing debilitating addiction, so when prescribing them to a patient, the lowest dose and dosing frequency necessary should be utilized. Additionally, patients should be closely monitored for their reactions to their pain

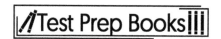

medications. Finally, some individuals who are addicted to prescription pain killers and muscle relaxers may feign injuries in order to receive another prescription. Therefore, all patients' medical histories should be thoroughly evaluated to note their history of pain medication usage. Patients should also be assessed for showing any signs of drug abuse history and withdrawal symptoms (such as damaged teeth, shaking, and agitation).

Procedural sedation allows patients to remain somewhat alert during medical procedures that may be uncomfortable but not unbearably painful, such as resetting bones. Unlike general anesthesia, where patients are completely sedated and do not feel any sensations, procedural sedation allows patients to be somewhat conscious and aware of bodily functions. It can be utilized with or without pain-relieving medications. Practitioner awareness is crucial when administering procedural sedation, especially when pain relief is also utilized. Recently, overuse and improper use of common procedural sedation agents, such as propofol, and common pain relief medications that are often used in conjunction, such as fentanyl, have caused high profile deaths.

Patient Safety

Patient safety is a fundamental component of healthcare delivery. Preventing errors that could endanger patient safety is a quality issue and one that all medical personnel should take seriously. Errors that compromise patient safety include lack of attention that leads to infections, injury, medication dosing errors, and failing to account for medical history (such as administering a medication to which the patient is allergic).

In the emergency department, patient safety can become compromised due to the fast-paced nature of the job, the available staffing at a particular facility, and the demographics of the patients who come to that particular department. Since emergency situations usually warrant immediate life-sustaining treatment, smaller aspects may become overlooked. For example, an emergency patient may be more susceptible to medical staff overlooking small foreign bodies as they work to keep the patient's vital signs stable. However, these can cause serious infections at a later time that ultimately compromises the patient's safety again.

Additionally, emergency departments are notorious for becoming overcrowded, especially in times of catastrophe or when the population served lacks access to primary health care so they utilize the emergency department for general medical needs. Medical staff may be limited in number, sleep deprived, or unable to take regular breaks due to staffing needs. All of these issues can affect human alertness and performance on the job. The patients themselves may require extra resources outside of the scope of care that the emergency department can provide. For example, some patients who visit the emergency department may not have the means to pay, may not adhere to discharge protocol, or may have language barriers that prevent effective treatment from taking place.

Finally, some smaller or rural departments may not have adequate security measures in place, such as personnel and cameras that keep the physical location safe, or secure data management systems that work to protect patient privacy.

Not all of these issues can be mitigated by nursing staff at the micro-level. However, nurses can work to set systems in place that address how to best cope with common issues such as overcrowding and security. For example, nurses can develop an internal system with how to best treat large groups of patients, such as shared appointments with patients' consent. Nurses can also practice safe recordkeeping measures, such as ensuring patient data is not left where others can view them.

Patient Satisfaction

Patient satisfaction is a highly valued benchmark of healthcare quality. Data relating to patient satisfaction can be collected internally by a healthcare organization or through external institutions that focus on healthcare quality. In the business of healthcare, patient satisfaction often serves as the "demand" in a supply and demand economy. Higher patient satisfaction scores are associated with better patient health outcomes, and consequently associated with happier patients, patients who are more likely to return to and recommend a particular healthcare organization, higher quality of medical staff that the healthcare organization retains, increased level of outside funding that the healthcare organization receives, and fewer medical malpractice suits. Patients report higher satisfaction when they receive care that they find to be tailored to their needs, care that is safe yet efficient, and care that is accessible. In this regard, healthcare delivery requires a nuanced level of customer service; however, rather than delivering a tangible manufactured product, medical staff deliver a product that affects the patient's ability to live well and their long-term physical, mental, and emotional state.

All medical staff are able to provide exceptional patient service by being welcoming and concerned about the patient, allowing space for the patient to voice their concerns and fears, treating the patient like a person rather than a medical case, respecting the patient and showing concern for the patient's family, and being reliable and punctual in their interactions with the patient. Many burdensome aspects of care that could be looked at negatively, such as patient wait times, can be alleviated by simple communication that explains the reasoning behind the issue. Communication and transparency are simple tools that often serve as the key players in managing patient expectations. Medical staff can also maintain communication with the patient after discharge, such as through an online patient portal, to ensure adequate care continues through the patient's full recovery and make the patient feel valued.

Transfer and Stabilization

Patients in the emergency department are susceptible to experiencing a number of transfers. The initial transfer is often from the scene of the patient's emergency to the emergency department. From there, the patient may need to be transferred to another part of the healthcare facility, or to an entirely new healthcare facility. This is dependent on the patient's needs and the resources available at the facility. For example, a patient who is initially brought to a trauma center may be moved to standard facility as he or she progresses in recovery, but before a full discharge is a viable option. Or, a patient that requires urgent care may be brought to a hospital that is understaffed and needs to be moved to a facility with available beds. A risk and benefit analysis of moving a patient should be carefully considered before making the decision, as transferring a patient is never a low-risk process. It is associated with negative outcomes for most patients with a high risk of additional injury or death for patients who are already in critical condition.

In each transfer, the patient will need to be carefully monitored for any changes in vital signs. The intention is to keep the patient stable throughout the course of the transfer; however, medical staff should be ready to re-stabilize the patient if needed. Before transfer, medical staff should make themselves aware of what the patient is at risk of experiencing during transfer, since each patient's risk will be different based on medical history and health status. Medical staff should know what actions they will take for any negative events that could potentially occur for the patient at hand.

Stabilization of the patient requires monitoring five important aspects: the patient's airway, the patient's breathing, the patient's circulation, the presence of any disabilities or dehydration, and the exposure of any visibly suspect changes (such as suddenly flushed or clammy skin). This is referred to as

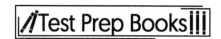

the ABCDE approach and is a commonly used tool for stabilizing patients, set forth by the World Health Organization.

Transitions of Care

Transitioning care refers to any context where the patient's care level and/or specific caregiver changes. This could be a case as simple as a nursing shift change, where the nurse attending to a particular patient changes, or as complex as moving the patient from a healthcare facility to their place of residence but requiring that the patient needs in-home medical staff and equipment. Any time there is a change in care level, there is an opportunity for the quality of care to decline. This can be due to a lack of communication between healthcare providers, a lack of communication between healthcare providers and the patient, a lack of education provided to the patient about their care, a paperwork mix-up, or some other type of unintentional error. Therefore, standardizing transition procedures and documentation can be a critical and valuable component to quality patient care.

Initial patient boarding is an important moment of data collection. Whether it is the patient's first admission into the healthcare system or a transition into a new system, documenting as much information about the patient's personal history, medical history, the condition that brought the patient into the facility, any documentation of advanced directives or medical proxies, and initial health assessments can be valuable as the patient's time in care progresses. Ideally, a standardized electronic medical record that can be continuously accessed and updated by all healthcare providers who play a role in the patient's care can prevent complications that arise from lack of communication. Otherwise, comprehensive intake forms at each transition can help minimize the chance of the patient receiving inadequate or improper care.

A standardized shift handoff procedure can provide a seamless transition between two different medical staff members who may be providing care for the same patient. It can provide detailed and crucial information about the patient and the case; equally importantly, it can as serve as a tool that indicates official responsibility has moved from one provider to another. This provides a clear mechanism for providing accountability on who is overseeing specific tasks between staff members.

Internal handoffs occur within the same healthcare facility, including, but not limited to, shift handoffs and inter-department handoffs (i.e., a physical therapist is working with a patient in the orthopedic surgery ward). All established healthcare facilities will have their own internal handoff protocols. This can include procedures such as formal handoff training for new staff, continuing training for established staff, verbal handoff protocols, written handoff forms, and stringent repercussions for staff members who fail to meet handoff standards.

External handoffs occur within two separate healthcare entities or during a transition of care. Unless the two systems involved have similar procedures, external handoffs can be compromising situations for the patients, and prone to errors.

Errors in handoffs can occur when procedures are not standardized—that is, they do not occur in the exact same manner and convey the exact same information each time a handoff occurs. Developing formal, written standard operating procedures can eliminate various human errors from occurring. Standardizing a process may look like (but is not limited to) a written checklist, a process flowchart, a meaningful acronym, or an audit tool for staff members to follow. Additionally, errors in handoffs can occur when established standard operating procedures are ignored, written poorly, or are too broad for the scope of the procedure. Errors in handoffs can also occur if medical staff are rushed, are unsure of the team members they are working with, or receive incorrect information anywhere along the duration of a patient's stay.

Cultural Considerations

Patients will come from all backgrounds and cultures, and medical providers should be aware of the different cultural needs that may present themselves in the emergency department. Culture can encompass anything from a person's geographical location, race, ethnicity, age, socioeconomic status, and religious beliefs that influence the behaviors, traditions, and rituals that he or she chooses to engage in each day. It is important to note that cultural considerations will present themselves daily. Some patients may be unable to speak English and will need interpretive services. Some patients may request that only same-sex providers treat them. Some patients may need to keep culturally valuable adornments in place that could interfere with treatment (i.e., a metal symbol on a patient that needs magnetic resonance imaging, a procedure where metal poses an extreme danger). Respecting and attending to different cultural needs will provide the patient with a better healthcare experience, lead to increased patient satisfaction, and impact overall health outcomes (as patients will be more likely to seek out care if they feel comfortable doing so).

Medical providers can show that they consider cultural differences by kindly and compassionately asking patients to share cultural viewpoints, to share aspects of the medical system and services that make them comfortable or uncomfortable, and to continuously create rapport that allows the patient to feel comfortable in voicing their concerns. Medical providers should be mindful of any preconceived notions that they hold of certain cultures, and if possible, actively work to dispel these. Medical providers should also be mindful to not make presumptions, even if those presumptions come from an intention to be empathetic. For example, a patient who looks to be of Asian descent may have been born and raised in the United States and not identify well with any part of Asian culture. Finally, many healthcare organizations offer internal trainings that cover cultural considerations and cultural diversity. For staff that feel their knowledge and experience is limited in this aspect, these trainings can provide an avenue for personal and professional growth.

Having a diverse emergency department staff can be extremely beneficial when servicing a patient demographic that encompasses many cultures. Having a medical provider who is able to relate directly with a patient's culture can make the patient feel more comfortable and open. Additionally, a diverse emergency department staff can overcome common obstacles such as language barriers or lack of patient education. In this regard, healthcare organizations and nursing leadership should work to actively recruit a diverse workforce.

System

Delegation of tasks to assistive personnel

Nursing staff take on many responsibilities that can be delegated to other clinical and non-clinical colleagues. However, learning how to effectively and safely delegate tasks, while still making patients feel cared for, is a skill that can take time to develop. It requires knowing not only what the needs of the patient are, but also the strengths and weaknesses of assistive personnel and how to best communicate professional needs with them. It also requires personal development in becoming comfortable with outsourcing responsibilities, as the nurse who delegates still remains accountable for the patient.

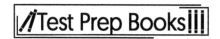

Assistive personnel may be supervised by nurses, but clinical assistive staff can provide basic medical assistance such as monitoring patients' vital signs, assisting with caretaking duties, monitoring any abnormalities or changes in the patient, maintaining a sterile and safe environment, and any other request made directly by nursing staff. Non-clinical assistive personnel, such as front desk staff, can assist with patient communication (such as wait times), managing paperwork and ensuring it is complete, and performing any other administrative task that may support the nursing staff's cases.

When nursing staff choose to delegate tasks, they may feel worried about risking their own accountability or work ethic. However, relating with assistive personnel, understanding their strengths and weaknesses, understanding their interests, and remaining transparent about the needs that are present in the department can ensure that delegated tasks are a good fit for the person who is taking the responsibility. In this regard, nursing staff take on a leadership and managerial role that requires developing their problem-solving, time management, and interpersonal skills. Some effective tools for delegation can include standardized checklists that cover the procedure that is being delegated, formal and informal meetings about assistive personnel's comfort levels and interests in performing certain tasks, and matching professional needs with individual qualifications. When delegation is effective, it can help the entire department work in a more efficient manner. Additionally, both nursing staff and assistive personnel are more likely to feel like part of a cohesive team and less likely to feel overworked or undervalued.

Disaster Management

A disaster emergency refers to any event that may bring a large influx of patients into the medical setting, such as a natural disaster or a mass casualty situation. They tend to be events marked by horror, calamity, and chaos, and nursing staff play a vital role in managing the complex mental, emotional, and physical demands of a community.

All healthcare organizations will have internal standards and resources in place for responding to a disaster. These may be tailored to the geographical area; for example, a coastal healthcare facility may have specific guidelines for hurricane events, while a Midwestern facility have specific guidelines for tornado events. Additionally, guidelines may be amended as new potential threats arise. For example, if an infectious disease outbreak is occurring in a certain area within the country, all healthcare facilities may implement standards to follow for that specific disease. Staying current on emerging threads, knowing the facility's capacity for treatment during a time of crisis, and planning for vulnerable populations (such as young children and the elderly) is a crucial component of disaster preparation. It allows medical staff to anticipate potential risks and the logistics of responding to them.

If a disaster does occur, nursing staff should utilize the tools prepared to navigate the event. This may require setting up work stations outside of the usual spaces, managing crowds, triaging incoming patients, working with assistive personnel, keeping patients calm, and determining the flow of treatment. It will be imperative for staff to cooperate in teams, follow a chain of command, and remain in constant communication with one another. Actual response to the disaster may encompass procedures like triaging existing patients, providing care as needed, and referring more serious cases to the appropriate medical staff member.

Recovery begins as the disastrous event ends, and can last for a long time. It accounts for providing a safe space for patients to heal, promoting a sense of calm in the community, providing basic needs to patients (such as food and shelter), and evacuating stable patients as needed. As patients' initial injuries heal, managing infections becomes vital. Patients may return with post-traumatic stress, depression, fear, anxiety, or suicidal tendencies. Through all this, nursing staff must also learn to support themselves and their colleagues so that they may healthfully tend to the needs of the rest of the community.

Federal Regulations

The healthcare industry must adhere to a number of federal regulations that intend to protect patient's rights, privacy, and safety.

The Emergency Medical Treatment and Labor Act (EMTALA) was passed in 1986. This act set forth regulations that allowed all individuals seen in an emergency department to receive emergency treatment regardless of insurance status or financial status. The primary impetus for this act was in response to hospitals turning patients away who did not have the ability to pay. Healthcare facilities do not receive any government assistance to subsidize patients that cannot pay, and this has influenced overall healthcare costs. Healthcare facilities do have some control over determining what constitutes as an emergency need, and can refuse treatment if they deem the patient as not requiring emergency care.

The Health Insurance Portability and Accountability Act (HIPAA) was passed in 1996. This act set forth regulations that required healthcare facilities and providers to protect patient's private information (such as demographics, health history, prescriptions, etc.) that could identify them. Additionally, this act has undergone revisions to account for technological advances to health information systems in order to keep both written and electronic individual health information protected. HIPAA requires organizations to have security measures in place, such as data encryption, limited access to patient files, and ongoing training requirements for staff to stay familiar with safeguarding techniques. HIPAA also included provisions that amended other laws pertaining to healthcare coverage continuation in the event of job loss, voluntary resignation, or retirement.

The Patient Protection and Affordable Care Act was passed in 2010. Key components of this act included expanding Medicaid eligibility requirements, increasing healthcare facility quality standards, and reforming individual insurance markets by requiring that all individuals are given the same opportunity to purchase health insurance. This act increased the number of people that were able to purchase health insurance, therefore potentially bringing more people into the healthcare system. It also required stringent electronic record implementation and security, which required many healthcare facilities to overhaul their internal systems. This legislation is considered to be one of the most monumental reforms to the healthcare industry in the last fifty years.

Patient Consent for Treatment

Ideally, patients should always provide written consent for treatment. This should also include discussion between the healthcare provider and the patient about what treatment will entail, what the end goal is of treatment, the risks and benefits of the treatment, and the opportunity for the patient to voice any questions and concerns. Patient consent decreases liability for the healthcare provider and increases patient reports of empowerment. Patients also have the right to revoke previously given consent at any time.

However, problems with patient consent do exist. In many healthcare facilities, the consent process can be a rushed one; often, patients receive a large packet of paperwork in which the consent form is included. Many patients sign without reading, or do not understand what they are signing but complete the form out of fear, pressure, or to appear informed when they actually do not feel that way. Often, verbal exchange about the form or treatment does not occur. Legally, healthcare providers do not have

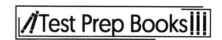

to provide an explanation of information that is accepted as common knowledge. However, medical topics are often not part of the average person's body of knowledge, and this gap can be complicated to bridge without thorough communication. Healthcare providers can attempt to resolve these problems by taking the time to discuss the consent form with the patient, simplifying consent forms, and providing additional media (such as literature or video links) to patients, especially in the event of more complex procedures.

In the emergency department, informed consent can be tricky as patients may arrive in an unconscious state or may require immediate treatment without the time to discuss the procedure. Most healthcare providers who work in the emergency room utilize the concept of implied consent, assuming that an unconscious or critical patient would voluntarily consent to life-sustaining treatment.

Performance Improvement

Performance improvement is a mechanism to continuously review and improve processes in a system to ensure that work is completed in the most cost-effective manner while producing the best possible outcomes. Healthcare facilities are constantly hoping to drive down cost and increase reimbursements while delivering the highest quality of healthcare, and utilize analytical methods to achieve this. These analyses and implementations may be done by top administrative employees at the organization and be executed across the healthcare system, or within a particular department. Leadership support is always crucial for positive change to occur and sustain itself.

All processes should be regularly monitored for opportunities to improve. Common opportunities include areas of reported patient dissatisfaction; federal, state, or internal benchmarks that are not being met; areas of financial loss; and common complaints among staff. While multiple opportunities for improvement may exist, focusing on one at a time usually produces the greatest outcome. When choosing a process to improve, it is important to select a process that can actually be changed by the members involved (i.e., medical staff often do not have control over external funding sources). Processes where minimal resources are required for change, but that can produce positive end results, are also preferable to costlier improvements. Once the process has been selected, a group of stakeholders that are regularly involved in the process should map out each step of the process while noting areas of wasted resource or process variation. From here, stakeholders can develop a change to test.

The PDCA cycle provides a framework for implementing process improvements. Plan, the first step, involves planning the change. This will include accounting for all workflow changes, the staff members involved, and logistics of implementation. It should also include baseline data relating to the problem. Do, the second step, involves implementing the change. During this step, data collection is crucial. For example, if a department believes that implementing mobile work stations will decrease nurses' wait time between patients, the department should keep a detailed record of the time spent with and between each patient. Check, the third step, involves checking data relating to the change with the baseline data and determining if the change improved the process. Act, the final step, involves making the change permanent and monitoring it for sustainability.

Risk Management

In a healthcare facility, human lives are the focus of services provided and risks are inherently present in the work. These risks include lawsuits, malpractice claims, financial loss, and harm (whether intentional or unintentional) to the patients. Effectively managing risk in order to reduce the probability of a negative outcome encompasses a number of theoretical and analytical steps.

Identifying potential causes of risk can come both from theoretical brainstorming, as well as reviewing concrete evidence. Key stakeholders can examine existing processes and hypothesize how they may present risk. Additionally, reviewing documented instances where risks came to fruition can bring attention to what the healthcare facility and providers should avoid. Documented instances can be those that occurred at another facility, which can serve as a learning lesson for the industry, or they can be instances that occurred internally, such as a filed patient lawsuit or complaint. Regular risk assessments, similar in nature to an audit, can pinpoint areas of risk. These should be system-wide and conducted at regular intervals, with extra assessments conducted any time a new system is implemented or a new healthcare regulation comes into effect.

Once potential causes of risk have been identified, stakeholders should objectively identify which have the possibility to cause the most overall harm, whether it is to the organization, to medical staff, or to patients. These should then be listed in order of urgency, and individual solutions should be discussed. The PDCA cycle of process and quality improvement can be a useful tool when determining an effective yet streamlined solution, as it encompasses many of the qualities that a risk-mitigating solution will need.

Finally, a system should be in place that allows all medical staff to voice areas of risk that they see on the job. As the front line in many of the processes that take place in a healthcare facility, medical staff are able to provide valuable insight regarding risk. Medical staff should feel comfortable reporting causes of risk in the workplace, and a standardized procedure for reporting risks should be in place. In the event that a negative outcome due to preventable or unavoidable risk does occur, it is important that all staff members know how to best respond to the event in order to mitigate its effects on the organization's reputation, business operations, staff members, and patients.

Symptom Surveillance

An emergency department nurse may be one of the first people who recognizes that a disease outbreak is occurring in a community. Noticing and detecting symptoms that occur repeatedly can indicate an outbreak, and early detection can prevent widespread transmission. Nursing staff often have the most contact with patients that present symptoms of an infectious disease, so developing basic skills in epidemiology—the study of health disease patterns—can be a tremendous public health benefit. Having an established surveillance system in place within the healthcare facility can make epidemiological reporting easier for nursing staff.

Most community-oriented epidemiological projects are conducted by county and state health departments. When an outbreak occurs, epidemiologists attempt to track the first person diagnosed with the disease and map out that person's activities and interactions in hopes of limiting the disease's spread. This often results in collaborative work with the healthcare facility in which the patient was initially seen.

Additionally, most states require that incidences of certain potentially catastrophic infectious diseases seen in healthcare facilities are reported within a certain timeframe so that action may be taken. Standardized reporting forms that account for well-known symptom clusters are a helpful tool for nurses to survey patients and submit these findings.

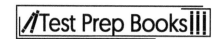

However, many healthcare providers are unsure of these details, which can serve as an obstacle to rapid, thorough reporting. Healthcare providers also report feeling like they may be violating patient privacy by disclosing these details to state or county health departments. In this regard, training medical staff on the nature of public health epidemiology and how accurate, detailed reporting can be a service to the patient population may be a valuable endeavor.

In addition, a number of healthcare systems are implementing infectious disease surveillance programs in which nursing staff are encouraged to take leadership roles. Truly effective disease surveillance will require collaboration between government health programs and healthcare facilities.

Triage

Triage refers to prioritizing patients based on urgency of care, and is a common component of the emergency department and disaster contexts. Often, one or a team of nurses will be in charge of only triaging patients. Incoming patients may be marked by colors which indicate the level of their needs, which are assessed using the ABCDE protocol mentioned in the Transfer and Stabilization section. Green tags indicate the patient has relatively minor injuries. Yellow tags indicate that the patient does require serious care but may be able to wait until critical patients, marked with red tags, are treated. Patients with red tags need immediate intervention. Patients who are marked with black tags are deceased or expectant—individuals expected not to survive. The triage process occurs at regular intervals, and patients may change priorities as their health status changes.

Triage may be simple, where incoming patients are quickly and physically sorted into *stable*, *in need of observation*, or *in need of immediate treatment* groups. Personal information, initial assessment of the patient's health needs, and overall risks are documented. All incoming living patients are likely to receive some form of treatment. Advanced triage takes place during catastrophic events where many victims and fatalities are likely. In these situations, the medical burden can become overwhelming. Medical staff may notice that some incoming patients, while living, have injuries that cannot be easily treated or where treatment will prolong the time until impending death. In these cases, medical staff may make judgments to forego offering interventions to these patients in order to better utilize available manpower, medical resources, and time.

In this context, healthcare providers may also discharge patients earlier than normal in order to accommodate more patients. Often, advanced triage selections have to be made within a minute or less of seeing the patient, and care may be given in any physical space that is available. Overall, this experience can be a moral and ethical dilemma for many healthcare providers. Once an event requiring advanced triage has passed, it is important for medical staff to assess their own health needs and mental state, as well.

Practice Questions

1. Susan is the head nurse in an emergency department. Each morning, she asks her entire staff to convene in the break room for fifteen minutes. During this time, she gives everyone the opportunity to share any concerns for the day. She also goes around the room and asks everyone to briefly share, in one sentence, the biggest event occurring in their personal lives. She closes this session with a minute-long group meditation. Each morning, she also provides a card that has a relaxation exercise to each of her staff members to try during the day. In which stage of the CISM model is Susan engaging her staff?
   a. Pre-Crisis
   b. Acute
   c. Post
   d. Recovery

2. During triage, which color band signifies patients who do not need immediate treatment, but need to be closely monitored?
   a. Green
   b. Yellow
   c. Red
   d. Black

3. Which of the following contexts would likely require advanced triage processes?
   a. A pediatric clinic early in the morning
   b. A makeshift clinic set up to assist victims of a major avalanche
   c. A free flu shot clinic
   d. An emergency department clinic that is fully staffed, has empty beds, and a slow morning

4. When healthcare providers see patients who are unconscious or not of a sound state of mind, what principle is utilized in order to provide treatment?
   a. Assumption
   b. Risky consent
   c. Informed consent
   d. Implied consent

5. A small group of clinical nurses is choosing to improve an existing process relating to patient discharge. They have identified that patients have a high re-admittance rate during the summer months. After mapping the current process, they note that patients leave the printout of discharge instructions that they are provided in their hospital room approximately 65% of the time. The nurses set up a meeting to review potential solutions. In which part of the PDCA cycle is this performance improvement plan?
   a. Plan
   b. Do
   c. Check
   d. Act

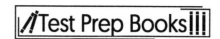

6. An OB/GYN clinic requires patients to fill out their name, address, phone number, and insurance type on a clipboard upon check-in. The clipboard stays at the front reception until the front desk staff are able to remove the sign-in sheets and check the patients in electronically. What is a legal issue in this procedure?

   a. All patients should check themselves in electronically, rather than using pen and paper, according to the Affordable Care Act of 2010.

   b. OB/GYN patients are more likely to have small children with them, so requiring them to fill out paperwork in the office could be a liability.

   c. Patient privacy is compromised during the time that the clipboard remains on the front desk.

   d. Some patients may not be able to write, so this is a violation of the American Disabilities Act.

7. Which set of laws comprised the biggest healthcare reform in the last fifty years?

   a. The Patient Protection and Affordable Care Act

   b. The Privacy Act

   c. The HiTech PHI Act

   d. The Emergency Medical Treatment and Labor Act

8. Which field of public health can nursing staff support by establishing symptom surveillance systems?

   a. Health policy

   b. Nutrition services

   c. Epidemiology

   d. Health promotion

9. What is the final step of a health research project?

   a. Analyzing and interpreting data

   b. Receiving funds to pay incentives to study participants

   c. Publication of a manuscript detailing the study in scholarly literature

   d. Destroying personal information of participants in the data collection system

10. At what time during a patient's stay are medical errors most likely to be made?

    a. During bloodwork

    b. During labor for pregnant patients

    c. When extra tests are ordered

    d. During any transition of care

11. Which set of laws was enacted in order to prevent healthcare facilities from turning away patients that needed life-sustaining care, regardless of ability to pay?

    a. The Patient Protection and Affordable Care Act of 2010

    b. The American Health Care Act of 2017

    c. The Emergency Medical Treatment and Labor Act of 1986

    d. The Medicare Introduction Act of 1965

12. Which of the following is an example of a healthcare provider showing cultural consideration to a patient?

a. A healthcare provider does not allow a patient's same-sex spouse to visit in the recovery room due to the healthcare provider's religious beliefs.

b. A healthcare provider allows a patient of the Islamic faith to keep her headscarf on during a physical exam.

c. A healthcare provider tells a person who identifies as Asian on his intake form that she does not like Chinese food.

d. A healthcare provider tells an older patient that unless he or she enrolls in the online patient portal, the provider will not provide treatment.

13. Gemma is a nurse at a small clinic who is feeling overwhelmed with too many things to do. She walks by the front desk and notices the waiting room has no patients, and that the front desk staff are chatting and looking at pictures from a recent wedding. How can Gemma delegate some of her responsibilities in this situation?

a. She can ask a front desk staff member to perform bloodwork for the patient who is waiting in a back room.

b. She can ask a front desk staff member to get her a snack.

c. She can provide a list of patients who are about to be discharged to a front desk staff member and ask the member to print out discharge paperwork.

d. She can ask one of the front desk staff members to write a new job posting advertising for a new nurse and post it on a job board

14. Knowing the geographical risks to a healthcare facility and resources available to the community is a component of which aspect of nursing?

a. Disaster management

b. Epidemiology

c. Community service

d. Continuing education

15. With what variables are high patient satisfaction scores associated?

a. Rural locations

b. Female patients between the ages of fifteen and thirty who are in relatively good health

c. Better patient outcomes and higher patient retention

d. Lower patient weight over time

16. Elias has been a registered nurse since he received his Bachelor of Science in Nursing in 2005. He loves his job and has decided he would like to return to school to receive his Master's degree. What is this an example of?

a. A promotion

b. Continuing education

c. Specializing

d. Work-life balance

Answer Explanations

1. A: The Pre-Crisis stage of the CISM model provides tools for nursing staff to relax, mentally prepare any traumatic incidences, and voice any concerns they have for the day. The other stages listed address actions during and after traumatic incidences.

2. B: Yellow bands signify patients that need to be observed. Green bands signify patients with minor issues. Red bands signify critical patients that need immediate care. Black bands signify deceased patients.

3. B: Advanced triage processes are normally used in catastrophic events, such as an avalanche. The other options listed probably would not require fast-paced triage processes of any kind.

4. D: When patients are physically or psychologically unable to provide verbal or written consent to treatment, healthcare providers rely on implied consent, acting on the belief that the patient would like the best treatment to benefit his or her life.

5. A: The nurses are in the planning stage. When they develop a change to implement, they'll be in the Do stage. Once the change has been implemented, they'll check the results and compare it to their baseline re-admittance and printout retention rates. Finally, they'll act to sustain any positive changes.

6. C: Patient information that is left on the clipboard is visible to other patients who are using the clipboard to check in. This is a direct violation of HIPAA laws, which has a privacy clause stating that identifiable patient information should remain private and safeguarded. The other options do not apply.

7. A: Passed under President Barack Obama's term, the Patient Protection and Affordable Care Act of 2010 reformed individual health insurance markets and expanded Medicaid coverage. Overall, it cut uninsured patient numbers by approximately half. It is the largest healthcare reform since Medicaid and Medicare programs were developed in the 1960s.

8. C: Epidemiology is the study of health symptom clusters and patterns of disease outbreak in a community. Since nursing staff are often the first people to notice repetitive symptoms in a community, their services can be a great benefit to public health workers.

9. C: When research studies are complete, they should be officially disseminated to colleagues in the field through academic and scholarly publications. This gives credence to the study and allows it to influence both future research and current fieldwork. Receiving funds and interpreting data are earlier stages of a research project. Participant data does not necessarily need to be destroyed as long as it remains safeguarded and the participants give their permission for their data to remain with study materials.

10. D: Transition of care requires many changes that almost always lead to a slight or major decline in quality of care. This can be mediated with strict standard operating procedures for transition and high levels of communication between caregivers.

11. C: The Emergency Medical Treatment and Labor Act of 1986 (EMTALA) was a direct response to healthcare facilities turning away patients that were unable to pay for treatment, even in life or death situations. However, facilities are not reimbursed for losses by this law, and this has had an effect on overall healthcare costs.

12. B: In this case, the healthcare provider considered religious and cultural beliefs of the patient to make her feel comfortable during the exam. Effective cultural considerations improve patient satisfaction scores. In the other options listed, the healthcare providers act inconsiderately, insultingly, and make assumptions about the patient's culture.

13. C: While all are examples of handing over responsibilities of Gemma's, Choice *C* is the only feasible, legal option. The front desk staff cannot legally perform clinical roles such as drawing blood. They also are not Gemma's personal assistants, and cannot complete tasks for her personal needs. They can help her with administrative tasks relating to the patients, however, and are skilled in doing so. When delegating tasks, it is important to make sure those tasks can be performed competently and safely by assistive personnel.

14. A: These are direct components of preparing for a local or nearby disaster, which sets the foundation for disaster management.

15. C: In addition to these two factors, patient satisfaction is also associated with more resources for the organization and retention of high-quality staff. The other options do not apply.

16. B: Elias is choosing to further his education, which is a component of lifelong learning. While this may lead to promotion, specializing in a particular field of nursing, or work-life balance, pursuing an advanced degree is directly related to maintaining competence in his field. Nurses should expect to continue their education throughout the course of their careers, as technology, regulations, and other external factors influence the shape of the industry.

Index

Dear CEN Test Taker,

We would like to start by thanking you for purchasing this study guide for your CEN exam. We hope that we exceeded your expectations.

Our goal in creating this study guide was to cover all of the topics that you will see on the test. We also strove to make our practice questions as similar as possible to what you will encounter on test day. With that being said, if you found something that you feel was not up to your standards, please send us an email and let us know.

We have study guides in a wide variety of fields. If you're interested in one, try searching for it on Amazon or send us an email.

Thanks Again and Happy Testing!
Product Development Team
info@studyguideteam.com

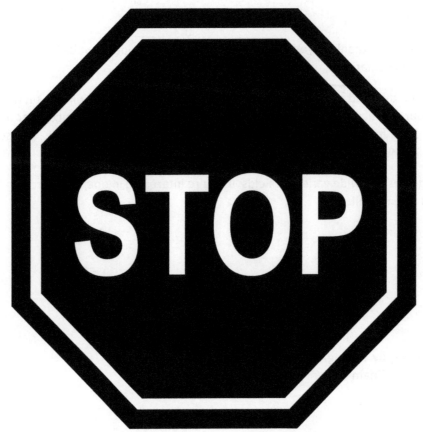

FREE Test Taking Tips DVD Offer

To help us better serve you, we have developed a Test Taking Tips DVD that we would like to give you for FREE. **This DVD covers world-class test taking tips that you can use to be even more successful when you are taking your test.**

All that we ask is that you email us your feedback about your study guide. Please let us know what you thought about it – whether that is good, bad or indifferent.

To get your **FREE Test Taking Tips DVD**, email freedvd@studyguideteam.com with "FREE DVD" in the subject line and the following information in the body of the email:

    a. The title of your study guide.

    b. Your product rating on a scale of 1-5, with 5 being the highest rating.

    c. Your feedback about the study guide. What did you think of it?

    d. Your full name and shipping address to send your free DVD.

If you have any questions or concerns, please don't hesitate to contact us at freedvd@studyguideteam.com.

Thanks again!

CPSIA information can be obtained
at www.ICGtesting.com
Printed in the USA
BVHW012235270422
635376BV00024B/1137

9 781628 459050